BAD CHOICES

BAD CHOICES

A Look Inside Planned Parenthood

Douglas R. Scott

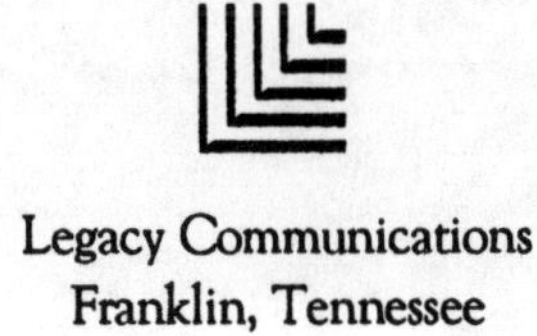

Legacy Communications
Franklin, Tennessee

Published July 1992. First Edition.
Printed in the United States of America.
97 96 95 94 93 92 8 7 6 5 4 3 2 1

Legacy Communications
P. O. Box 680365
Franklin, Tennessee 37068

Library of Congress Cataloging-in-Publication Data

Scott, Douglas R.
Bad choices : a look inside Planned Parenthood / Douglas R. Scott.
— 1st ed.
p. cm.
Includes bibliographical references and index.
ISBN 1-880692-02-3
1. Planned Parenthood Federation of American. 2. Birth control-
-Religious aspects—Christianity. 3. Pro-life movement—United
States. I. Title.
HQ766.5.U5S43 1992 92-19401
363.9'6—dc20 CIP

Dedicated to
the "Patriarch of the Pro-Life Movement,"
Joseph R. Stanton, M.D.,

and to those in the fields of medicine,
law, and education who support the right to life
in the face of strident opposition within their professions

ABOUT THIS BOOK

Bad Choices: A Look Inside Planned Parenthood details the activities of the world's primary advocate of legal abortion. While this book may be useful to pro-life activists, its format is designed for a general audience. *Bad Choices: A Look Inside Planned Parenthood* should be made available to pro-life volunteers, supporters of legal abortion, Planned Parenthood workers, and those who are undecided about Planned Parenthood.

Some of the material in *Bad Choices: A Look Inside Planned Parenthood* is not suitable for children. After much prayer and deliberation it was decided that direct quotations from Planned Parenthood literature should be included herein, even though the text of these materials is often explicit and offensive. Planned Parenthood is making this material available to children without parental knowledge or consent. The material included in this book is designed to provoke godly action by parents to put an end to this intolerable crime against North America's youth.

Every effort has been made to assure the accuracy of the information in *Bad Choices: A Look Inside Planned Parenthood.* Quotations have been checked and rechecked to be sure they are used in context and to assure the accuracy of their reprinting.

[I]f a lie is told often enough
people begin to believe it
and lies can kill.

Gloria Allred

CONTENTS

FOREWORD

There was a time, not long ago, when politics was about political issues—not things like the balancing of interests between labor and management, or between farmers and manufacturers, the adjudication of civil rights, the interplay of nations, and the maintenance of peace and freedom. These questions were and are serious and often have provoked bitter conflict. But political debate in the past was conducted within an over arching framework which took for granted certain cultural premises.

It would once have been inconceivable for anyone to assert that the Constitution contains a right to kill unborn children, or that government programs should have been set up to give contraceptives and instruction in how to use them to adolescents, or that the state should concern itself with how many children married couples have. These things were outside the political discussion because they had to do with the cultural norms on which civil society was based. They were, in the strictest sense, private matters.

It is ironic that questions such as these have recently been dragged into the political arena in the name of privacy. It is disquieting that the very premises which provide a framework for society have themselves become the subject of political controversy.

This amounts, in fact, to a cultural revolution. No society can exist without certain unspoken premises, taken for granted by virtually everyone, which provide some common ground within which differences can be aired. For the past generation these premises have been under attack. Cultural radicals of various kinds have been steadily working to unravel the cultural norms that hold our society together. The central issues in American politics today deal not with the traditional balancing of political interests, but with the battle over these cultural affirmations that give society its very identity.

This cultural revolution is broader than the sexual revolution, but the sexual revolution is a major component in the assault on traditional standards. It calls into question matters that have been taken for granted not only in North America, but in every successful society in history—matters such as the unique dignity of marriage and the family, the sanctity of human life, and the norms of responsible sexual behavior.

The sexual revolution, in turn, is broader than the agenda of Planned Parenthood or any other single organization. But revolutions of any kind do not just happen. They are made by people who implement ideas through organizations. The ideas which Planned Parenthood has been advancing for the past generation strike at the heart of some basic institutions of our society—the family, education, and even the definition of who is and who is not a member of the human community.

Without a group such as Planned Parenthood, it would be difficult to imagine the sexual revolution getting very far and without the sexual revolution, the broader cultural revolution could not have touched the most basic aspects of life. Planned Parenthood, therefore, has played and continues to play a key role in the unraveling of the American community. *Bad Choices: A Look Inside Planned Parenthood* offers a clear and readable summary of how that has happened.

PAUL M. WEYRICH
President, Free Congress Foundation

PREFACE

For the past two decades, Americans have witnessed what historians will someday call the era of the Questioning of Standards. Standards in the areas of monetary policy, human life, and human sexuality have been questioned.

The political left has been deeply involved in promoting abortion. This interest did not develop by accident. The religion of the political left is secular humanism, which denies the existence of God and the standards which God gave us through His Word to mankind, the Bible. When a political movement denies God and the rules He gave to man for direction, we should not be surprised that such a movement will seek to destroy human life by protecting abortion and, in the case of teenagers, seek to substitute its judgment for the proper role of parents in teaching human sexuality.

The high moral ground for the pro-life movement is described in excellent detail by Douglas R. Scott. *Bad Choices: A Look Inside Planned Parenthood* details not only what Planned Parenthood has been doing with tax money, supporting and performing abortions, but explains how concerned citizens can shift community resources to activities which promote and sustain life.

Douglas R. Scott is to be congratulated on producing a needed exposé on what Planned Parenthood has been doing in North America and worldwide.

WILLIAM E. DANNEMEYER
United States House of Representatives
California, 1979–1993

PREFACE

ACKNOWLEDGMENTS

My thanks first go to my parents for instilling personal values at an early age. Also, many friends have participated in the preparation of this book by showing their support. I wish to thank Walter "Red" and Patricia Bainbridge, Matthew Endrizzi, John Murphy, Jay Nenninger, Andrew Taylor, Jim Giese and family, Joan Poulin, and my friends at Iowans for LIFE.

Thanks, too, to all of those who have waited many months for this book to be completed.

The following persons supplied information for inclusion in this book: Patricia P. Bainbridge, Michael P. Bobic, Gloria Carr, Sharon Clow, Marjorie Dannenfelser, Ken Freeman, Jim Giese, Cathy Hetzler, Eric Kennerk, Jeanne Pitkus, Ann Polka, Jim Backlin, James Wanke, Michael Pauley, and Professionals for Life. Thanks to all others who supplied information as well.

A special thanks to Patricia P. Bainbridge for volunteering countless hours using her excellent research expertise. If it needs to be found, she can do so. Thanks to Walter "Red" Bainbridge, the former national champion and Olympic ice skater, for his technical and other assistance.

INTRODUCTION

You may be one of the millions of Americans who believe Planned Parenthood is a credible and caring "family planning" organization. You have been told that Planned Parenthood offers needed education to youngsters which, in turn, leads to a reduction in the high rate of teen pregnancies and sexually transmitted diseases.

You may be aware of the variety of services offered by Planned Parenthood in your community, such as tests for sexually transmitted diseases and pregnancy, birth control, counseling, and educational programs. Planned Parenthood speakers go into schools to talk about sexual matters. Its teen drama groups are kept busy. Most people hear of the services offered by Planned Parenthood and say, "Now there's a worthy charity." Planned Parenthood sounds like the kind of organization every community needs.

Bad Choices: A Look Inside Planned Parenthood will shatter your preconceived beliefs. As you read the evidence, judge for yourself the truth about Planned Parenthood, as stated in its own publications.

Bad Choices: A Look Inside Planned Parenthood examines the life of Planned Parenthood's founder, Margaret Sanger. Who was this woman? What did she believe? Does Planned Parenthood still hold to her philosophy?

Information is presented on what Planned Parenthood is teaching young people in schools. Planned Parenthood leaders make it clear that they believe young people should not be taught abstinence as a sexual lifestyle. Rather, they believe teens should be taught to accept all forms of sexual expression.

You will discover how distrust between parent and child is promoted. While parents are urged to communicate with their children, Planned Parenthood tells children they may not want to communicate with their parents.

Learn about Planned Parenthood's abortion connection. As the primary advocate and beneficiary of abortions, Planned Parenthood has spent millions of dollars to keep abortion legal. Yet, the public is not fully aware of the trauma experienced by women who have visited Planned Parenthood clinics. Such tragic testimonies are detailed.

The power and influence of Planned Parenthood is examined. The media is generally known to be supportive of Planned Parenthood. Could there be a connection between these two groups? Planned Parenthood has a vast financial empire which, through direct-mail appeals, foundation support, and government grants, enables it to enjoy an annual multi-million dollar budget. Through its involvement at all levels of government, from local school boards to international politics, Planned Parenthood has influenced public policy.

Planned Parenthood has hundreds of affiliates and facilities throughout North America and you will discover how they are connected, both organizationally and philosophically. Local leaders occasionally attempt to escape the wrath of those who point out the irresponsibility of Planned Parenthood's programs by denying that their chapter does such things. ("Maybe that Planned Parenthood group does such things but we don't.") Yet indisputable evidence shows the international network of chapters are closely knit together by a philosophy, strategy, and agenda that links them to an overall game plan.

The aggressive reaction of Planned Parenthood leaders toward their critics is examined. While they have viciously and personally attacked those who vocally oppose the Planned Parenthood philosophy, the organization has not been invulnerable to thoughtful counterattacks. *Bad Choices: A Look Inside Planned Parenthood* details how citizens have successfully challenged Planned Parenthood in their communities.

Bad Choices: A Look Inside Planned Parenthood examines what you can do about Planned Parenthood and its agenda, which is aggressively promoted at the local level. Planned Parenthood programs are all around us. It is important that every citizen learn how these programs, often paid for with tax dollars, impact our lives, the lives of our neighbors, and especially the lives of our children.

After reading this book, you undoubtedly will feel a sense of urgency to counter Planned Parenthood's lethal ethic, which is destroying lives.

1

FOUNDATION FOR SOCIAL CHANGE

Margaret Higgins Sanger Slee could be described as one of the world's most unique women. While many people view Margaret Sanger as one of the greatest women ever born, others see her as one of the most evil. She has been compared to Martin Luther King, Jr., and Adolf Hitler. As one Sanger biographer put it, "people either worshipped Margaret Sanger or couldn't bear her."[1]

Margaret Sanger is known throughout the world as founder of the international birth control movement and what is now called Planned Parenthood. It was this movement which led to the use of the phrase "birth control."[2]

PARENTS

Michael Higgins proposed to his girlfriend when he was 19 years old. Anne Purcell was "a rather nondescript girl from a strict Catholic family. Her parents objected to the union because Michael was a freethinker, but he was so handsome and persuasive he whittled down their objections, and the marriage soon took place."[3] After marriage, Anne Higgins stopped attending mass.

Michael Higgins settled in Corning, New York, where he became politically active. As an outspoken and "freethinking Socialist" living in a Catholic community, he was not the most popular man in town.[4] Higgins would invite infamous men to Corning, such as agnostic Robert Ingersoll, who is known for having advocated birth control as a way "to limit the number of unwanted children in charitable and public institutions."[5] In order to bring social reformer Henry George to Corning, Higgins, during a financially lean period when the family was surviving on the small incomes of the three oldest children, "took what was left of the household money and spent it all at once to subsidize" the trip.[6]

Higgins was labeled a heretic and his offspring were branded "children of the Devil, atheists and heretics."[7] His political and anti-Christian activities made it difficult to secure work in Corning. A stonecutter, Higgins was often forced to leave town to find work. Anne Higgins became proficient at caring for her family on the meager income provided by her husband.

While Anne Higgins was a Catholic, Michael Higgins was often scorned by leaders of the church. This was exacerbated when he joined the Knights of Labor, a group dedicated to ending "the stream of unskilled immigrants from Catholic countries."[8] Anne Higgins, on the other hand, was a "[g]entle, patient, forbearing" woman[9] who "had a selfless courage . . ."[10]

EARLY YEARS

Margaret Higgins was born in Corning on September 14, 1879, though she claimed to have been born in 1883. The sixth born, Higgins had seven brothers and three sisters. With the exception of one brother who died at the age of four following a brief illness, she reported that her siblings had been strong and healthy.[11]

Margaret Higgins experienced great scorn because of her father's activism. In fact, when she was "about six years old and was standing in line to get one of the free Christmas gifts that were being handed out to the youngsters. . . . the priest caught sight of her . . . [and] said sharply, 'Get out of line, you child of the devil.'"[12] Higgins did, however, have a significant advantage over others who were similarly ostracized. As a beautiful and graceful young woman, she was seldom without male admirers.

Anne Higgins died of tuberculosis when Margaret Higgins was 20 years old. The death left a lasting impression on the family, particularly on Michael Higgins who changed from a loving father to "an irritable tyrant."[13] Michael Higgins became highly critical of his children. Due to the change in her father's demeanor, Margaret Higgins' relationship with her father became seriously strained. Although she had never been close to her mother, Margaret Higgins became angry with her father and blamed him for her mother's death:

> Dammit [sic], you killed my mother. She was only forty-nine when she died. But those eighteen pregnancies didn't hurt you a bit. You—you'll live forever![14]

Margaret Higgins was interested in an acting career, but she later became interested in studying to be a doctor. Events in her life made that impossible. Higgins planned to become a registered nurse but she only worked as a nurse probationer and, though she had been accepted, never entered nursing school.

FIRST MARRIAGE

William Sanger and Margaret Higgins met at a party. An architect, William Sanger picked up Higgins one day in 1902 and took her off to be married. Margaret Sanger expressed both outrage and joy at what Sanger had done.

William Sanger was another "freethinker." He and Margaret Sanger attended meetings with labor and socialist leaders. Margaret Sanger wrote several series of articles for *The Call,* a socialist newspaper. The articles were solicited after she began speaking at socialist meetings. Sanger's first series of articles were titled "What Every Mother Should Know." The follow-up series was titled "What Every Girl Should Know." They addressed matters relating to sexuality.

The Sangers had three children. Their first child, Stuart Sanger, was born in 1903. Grant Sanger was born in 1908 and was the closest to his mother. It was not expected that this would be the case as Margaret Sanger had favored Peggy Sanger, her third child, who was born in 1911. Peggy Sanger died of pneumonia at the age of four while her mother was in Europe. Referring to her daughter's death many years later, Margaret Sanger wrote, "The joy in the fullness of life went out of it then and has never quite returned."[15]

Margaret Sanger once claimed to have had a respect for birth:

> To see a baby born is one of the greatest experiences that a human being can have. Birth to me has always been more awe-inspiring than death. As often as I have witnessed the miracle, held the perfect creature with its tiny hands and tiny feet, each time I have felt as though I were entering a cathedral with prayer in my heart.[16]

BIRTH OF A CRUSADE

Several Margaret Sanger biographers, as well as her autobiography, refer to alleged incidents involving Sadie Sachs. According to the story, Sachs attempted to abort herself. Sanger reportedly went to the Sachs' home, at the pleading of Sadie Sachs' husband. Sachs recovered, but Sanger was called to the house months later for the same reason. Sachs died soon after Sanger arrived. It was this event, according to Sanger and several biographers, that turned Sanger from a revolutionary into a crusader. She "was resolved, no matter what it cost, to do something to give women control over their own bodies."[17]

Did the Sachs events really take place as described? Historian David M. Kennedy, reflecting on this alleged event, writes, "Margaret Sanger's reliance on the Sadie Sachs episode to account for the beginnings of her career resembled a common autobiographical ploy of reformers."[18]

Sanger believed that women should have as many children as they wanted, so long as they could be cared for and they did not damage the health of the mother. Later in life, Sanger began to view the rapidly increasing world population as a problem requiring "voluntary family limitation for all." Her immediate goal, however, was to give every woman the "right to decide" how many children she would bear.[19] Sanger became interested in the work of John Stuart Mill who "regarded the production of large families in the same light as drunkenness . . ."[20]

Sanger saw herself as "The woman's rights activist of the twentieth century. Her criticism of the limited vision of other feminists was often shrill."[21] As a result, Sanger had a difficult time getting along with the feminists of her day:

> Feminists were trying to free women from economic and social slavery. Margaret wanted to free women from biological slavery. An alliance between the feminists and the birth control movement seemed logical, but Margaret's ideas were far too advanced. . . .
>
> Unable to obtain more than a token support from feminists, Margaret turned to the Socialists and trade unionists. She had already decided that a magazine would serve as a good rallying point for the new movement. She had made plans to publish *The Woman Rebel* . . .[22]

Sanger served as "editor, manager, circulation department, [and] bookkeeper" for the *Woman Rebel*.[23] She was solely responsible for all aspects of the magazine.

The first issue, published in March 1914, discusses Sanger's effort to make woman "the absolute mistress of her own body" and to give her "the absolute right to dispose or withhold herself, to procreate or to suppress the germ of life." She urged women to stop bearing children they were not "physically, mentally or financially prepared to take care of."[24] The masthead of the *Woman Rebel* was "NO GODS NO MASTERS."

Margaret Sanger's movement ran headlong against the Comstock Law of the day. Named for its sponsor, Anthony Comstock, the law forbade the distribution of birth control and birth control literature by mail. It was also illegal for women to seek birth control information, though Sanger charged that wealthy women were able to obtain it. Material relating to birth control was labeled "lewd and lascivious" under the 1873 law.[25] Sanger had several confrontations with the Postal Service which was charged with enforcing the Comstock Law with regard to materials sent through the mail.

It was argued that Margaret Sanger's ideas would harm the moral fabric of society. In response, she would say, "Throughout the ages every attempt women have made to strike off the shackles of slavery has been met with the argument that such an act would lower the moral standards." Sanger would ask, "Are we satisfied with present-day morality? Are we satisfied with the results of present-day standards of morality? Are these so satisfying that they need no improvement?"[26]

Margaret Sanger expected that many groups, such as the Industrial Workers of the World and Socialists, would support her cause. While these groups supported the birth control movement, it was limited to philosophical and moral advocacy:

> She realized that her only hope lay in the educated women of the upper and middle classes, many of whom had worked for causes like civil service reform, pure food and drug laws, better public libraries, and stricter child-labor laws. These women were searching for a new cause, since most of what they had struggled for had been achieved.[27]

In a 1917 supplement prepared for a judge hearing a case involving the Comstock Law, Sanger argued that a woman's health must be considered paramount:

> Is woman's health not to be considered? Is she to remain a producing machine? Is she to have time to think, to study, to care for herself? Man cannot travel to his goal alone. And until woman has knowledge to control birth she cannot get the time to think and develop. Until she has the time to think, neither the suffrage question nor the social question nor the labor question will interest her, and she will remain the drudge that she is and her husband the slave that he is just as long as they continue to supply the market with cheap labor.[28]

ADVOCATE OF CIVIL DISOBEDIENCE

Margaret Sanger believed her movement would benefit from an open challenge to the Comstock Law. Hence, she published the *Woman Rebel* and said that the main reason for doing so "was to feel out the authorities on the federal law . . . "[29]

Sanger's next venture in civil disobedience was the publication of a birth control pamphlet. She wrote that, "During all these months while *The Woman Rebel* was doing the window dressing for me—attracting attention and creating public discussion—I was hard at work writing a little practical pamphlet called 'Family Limitation.'"[30] Sanger had hoped to distribute one million copies of the pamphlet throughout the United States.

Margaret Sanger claimed she "was not afraid to go to jail for an ideal," but, she added, jail was not her goal.[31] After being indicted, however, Sanger fled the United States for nearly one year, traveling under an assumed name.[32] Upon her return, Sanger contacted the National Birth Control League in an attempt to garner its support. Not only was support denied, but the League's leaders said they disagreed with her tactics and, according to Sanger, with everything she had done.[33]

Undaunted, Sanger and her followers continued in their acts of civil disobedience:

> We know of some thirty-five arrests of women and men who have dared entrenched prejudice and the law to further the cause of birth control. The persistent work in behalf of the movement, attended as it was by danger of fines and jail sentences, seemed to puzzle the authorities. Sometimes they dismissed the arrested persons, sometimes they fined them, sometimes they imprisoned them. But the protests went on, and through these self-sacrifices, word of the movement went constantly to more and more people.
>
> Each of these arrests brought added publicity. Each became a center of local agitation. Each brought a part of the public, at least, face to face with the issue between the women of America and this barbarous law.[34]

On October 16, 1916, Sanger opened an illegal birth control clinic in the Brownsville section of Brooklyn, New York. Primarily a Jewish and Italian area, Brownsville is the site of the first birth control clinic opened anywhere outside of the Netherlands.

Arrested after opening the Brownsville clinic, Margaret Sanger was released on bail. She reopened the illegal clinic. Sanger was sentenced to 30 days in the Queens County penitentiary. In further defiance, Sanger "refused to have her fingerprints taken, and spent the last two hours of her sentence getting her arms bruised by struggling successfully with two officers to stop their forcing her fingers down on the inkpad."[35]

Upon release from jail, Margaret Sanger traveled throughout the United States urging the establishment of birth control clinics "where women—regardless of their economic situation—could obtain the help they need to save their lives, preserve their health and make it possible for them to fulfill themselves as wives, as mothers—and as citizens."[36] The opening line of her speech in virtually every town was, "The first right of every child is to be wanted, to be desired, to be planned with an intensity of love that gives it its title to being."[37] Sanger was successful in establishing local Birth Control League's in many cities. In some cities more than one was established.

One of Sanger's most unusual speaking engagements was to the women's branch of the Ku Klux Klan. "Always to me any aroused group was a good group . . . ,"[38] she wrote to justify accepting the invitation. Sanger was happy she had accepted. "In the end," she wrote, "through simple illustrations I believed I had accomplished my purpose. A dozen invitations to speak to similar groups were proffered."[39]

Sanger was met with significant opposition in some areas, particularly because of her "the law be cursed" approach. "I defined a woman's duty," Sanger wrote,

"To look the world in the face with a go-to-hell look in the eyes; to have an idea; to speak and act in defiance of convention."[40] Her attitude was often espoused:

> I remember almost innumerable instances of crude and usually unsuccessful attempts to silence me in those days: hotels boycotted by such organizations as the Knights of Columbus because the managers have purveyed luncheons to birth control advocates; halls, contracted and paid for, barred at the last minute on account of Catholic Church pressure brought to bear upon their owners; permits to hold meetings withdrawn by mayors or other officials in cities having powerful Roman Catholic constituency. Priests denounced me in churches and warned those who came to hear me of hell fire and the Devil! Few politicians, though they have sworn to uphold the Constitution, dare jeopardize their future as office holders by incurring the displeasure of the clerical authorities who often control the vote of their adherence.
>
> Papers would not take articles stating the facts. "News" was what they wanted—"news," "fights," "police," "controversy," "arrests." Only in this way could my voice reach the millions. Innocently my enemies helped to make this possible.[41]

Sanger continuously reminded herself of what she claimed to be the reason for her civil disobedience:

> Over and over she made her point: birth control had long been practiced by the upper classes and the well to do. Only the poor had been forced to breed without control. Margaret, like many of the social philosophers of the day, felt that it was no accident that this double standard had been maintained since an automatic by-product of the workers' large families was a self-perpetuating surplus-labor market which could be counted on to bid against itself for the always too few jobs. As long as there were more workers than jobs for them to do, they could not be choosy about wages or working conditions.[42]

It was in January 1918 that the New York Court of Appeals relaxed the interpretation of the Comstock Law, but the decision, having come from a state court, applied only to New York. It was much later when the Comstock Law was repealed.

Sanger did not let unexpected situations work against her. For example, on the last evening of the First National Birth Control Conference, Sanger had planned on opening the meeting with the question, "Birth Control: Is It Moral?"[43] Upon her arrival at the Town Hall, Sanger was met by police who were blocking the entrance. The police informed Sanger that the meeting could not take place. Sanger managed to get into the building where she announced to the crowd that the meeting would take place. The police had received their complaint from a Roman Catholic monsignor. Though Sanger was arrested, she was not about to let the incident become one which she did not use to her advantage:

> Margaret quickly turned the blunder of the church and the police into an important victory with press and public. The archbishop, intent on crushing the birth control movement, had ignored the Bill of Rights. Margaret cleverly seized the broader issue. She fought back as the defender of free speech and assembly. This approach brought hundreds of headlines and favorable editorials in the next few days, many in conservative papers that had never been friendly to birth control.[44]

In addition to the results of civil disobedience, Sanger felt that the birth control movement was aided by what she considered to be blunders on the part of those who opposed the cause:

> The growth of the movement had to a considerable extent thrived and depended on the skill of taking advantage of the stupid tactics of our bullying enemies. This skill had been called forth in our earliest battles: in the challenging defiance of *The Woman Rebel;* in every step of that legal conflict with the Federal authorities; in the founding of the Browns-

> ville Clinic; in Mrs. Byrne's [Sanger's sister]; in the tremendous aftermath of the Town Hall raid of incalculable educational value for the American public; in the long drawn out and finally victorious skirmish with the Japanese Government; in the establishment of the Clinical Research Bureau and the subsequent raid by the police; in challenging laws and defending aggressively our rights. These and other battles had been precipitated without the permission of any board of directors.[45]

Sanger's writings with regard to breaking the law were a source of division within the birth control movement. She "emphasized the historical role" of those who broke the law for a cause. In her articles, she cited Moses, Jesus Christ, George Washington, John Brown, Henry David Thoreau, and William Lloyd Garrison as examples.[46]

Margaret Sanger once wrote that she had "discovered [that] human beings must test their truths on the battlefield of this world . . ." She believed it was necessary to "fight for them [the truths] through the derision of the press, the prejudices of the courts, even through the ordeal of prison."[47] A Sanger biographer writes, "From Margaret's point of view, the law had always been the chief enemy of the movement, and with such examples she tried to inspire a revolutionary ardor in her followers. Despite these efforts, the source of inspiration for most of the activists in the movement was Margaret herself."[48]

THE CAUSE OF ALL MAN'S ILLS

Margaret Sanger was emphatically opposed to World War I. Her strong position created disharmony in the birth control movement. This was made worse because Sanger used the *Birth Control Review*, her newest publication, to express anti-war feelings.

> Margaret was neither pro-German nor pro-ally. She thought the war outrageous and refused to take any stand on any of its issues. She considered it an unnecessary slaughter of human life.[49]

Sanger's views regarding World War I did not coincide with those of the vast majority of the American people. She wrote that the American people feared those who expressed unpopular opinions which "gradually helped to impose censorship and further intolerance."[50]

Margaret Sanger's ideas became more radical as she got older. Sanger believed that overpopulation was the underlying cause of all wars. She believed that birth control would serve not only to prevent war, but it would correct most of the problems facing society. "Birth control must save the world from another and more devastating holocaust," she said. Sanger began to think more about population control in general than she did birth control.[51]

"Children," Sanger wrote, "must be brought into this strange little planet of ours by choice, not by chance." She said it was not coincidental that "both [Benito] Mussolini and Hitler encouraged the breeding of large families, while at the same time using the excuse of overpopulation to justify extraterritorial claims."[52] As evidence, Sanger pointed to the "overpopulated" countries of Japan,

Italy, and Germany which had started wars with their neighbors. She considered World War II to have more to do with overpopulation than anything else.[53]

FAMILY VERSUS THE CAUSE

Margaret Sanger put absolutely nothing ahead of her cause, including her family. She divorced William Sanger in 1920. Their sons were most often left with servants, neighbors, or in boarding schools. While Sanger was closest to Grant, communication was often through the mail. She wrote to her youngest son on his birthday from Europe:

> Darling Granty. I am in Paris and broke! So I came to the most exclusive hotel!! I sent you a (birthday) cable, trusting it reaches you on time . . . Your birthdays bring back to me always how much you were wanted and loved before you came. So *so* long before!! Also how dear Stuart was at the time, and how he too looked for your arrival. It's something to study in the future—how the wanted child differs, if he does, from the casually conceived and unwanted child.[54]

Sanger often sent her sons money and, as with many families, they occasionally exchanged rhetoric riddled with frustration. In one letter to his mother, Grant Sanger wrote, "From the tone of your last letter, it seems you should have practiced what you now preach by not having any children!"[55]

Margaret Sanger had many lovers, but she understood that as a "sexual reformer she could not afford to be labeled promiscuous."[56] One of her affairs was with H. G. Wells. Sanger was also sexually involved with Havelock Ellis, whom she met in England. Author of *Psychology of Sex*, Ellis was essentially the Dr. Ruth Westheimer of his day. "I have never felt about any other person as I do about Havelock Ellis," Sanger wrote. "To know him has been a bounteous privilege; to claim him friend my greatest honor."[57] Though numerous, Sanger's affairs usually ended without animosity.

Another sexual liaison was with J. Noah Slee, who became Margaret Sanger's second husband. As president of the Three-In-One Oil Company, Slee was quite wealthy. Slee courted Sanger for many months, even before divorcing his first wife. Sanger finally consented to marrying Slee in 1923, after he followed her on a worldwide speaking tour. Slee had given Sanger many gifts, but he "soon learned that the way to Margaret's heart was not through the florist or the jeweler—but through the movement." Slee contributed $64,000 to the Birth Control League in direct donations and much more in indirect donations.[58]

J. Noah Slee was a member of the Episcopal Church and superintendent of its Sunday school. He was a member of the Union League Club in New York and "his only hobby was trying to make more money than the nine million he already had."[59] Slee was an unyielding man who was politically and financially conservative.

Margaret Sanger, on the other hand, was an atheist with revolutionary political thoughts. Consequently, as a condition for marriage, it was agreed that Sanger would keep her own name. It was also agreed that they would live in the same house, but Sanger would have a separate apartment with separate keys. Sanger and Slee would telephone each other to make appointments and they would keep their own friends, interests, and "amusements."[60] For Sanger, this included her sexual "amusements."

Slee was useful to Margaret Sanger in that his fortune helped to finance her movement. Sanger "wanted the money just as she wanted Mr. Slee's respectable and conservative image and his considerable business ability, for what it would bring to the movement."[61] In fact, without Slee, the movement would likely not have seen success to the extent it has—at least not nearly as quickly.

While Margaret Sanger married twice, keeping in mind that one marriage was arguably for somewhat unorthodox reasons, she spoke and wrote negatively of the institution. One edition of *Woman Rebel* includes an article which reads, "The marriage-bed is the most degenerating influence of the social order . . ." It is asserted that "the marriage bed is a decadent institution—a reactionary development of the sex instinct—an institution that arrays itself against the two great fundamental principles of life—self-preservation." (The second "fundamental principle of life" is not specified.) A clear suggestion is made regarding how women should view marriage. "Let this institution then, be anathema to all thinking minds," Sanger wrote.[62]

Viewing marriage as an outdated institution, Sanger supported a "voluntary association" between sexual partners.[63] She wrote that, "It is within the marriage bonds, rather than outside them, that the greatest immorality of men has been perpetrated. Church and state, through their canons and their laws, havee encouraged this immorality."[64]

Sanger's enthusiasm "sometimes outweighed her judgment."[65] Her decision to be one of the first woman to smoke in public was "originally simply for its shock value."[66]

REALIZING THE CAUSE

In March 1915, while Margaret Sanger was out of the country, America's first birth control organization, the National Birth Control League, was formed in New York City. "The Birth Control League of America, which Margaret Sanger had prematurely announced in the *Woman Rebel,* 'never had more than a nominal existence,' according to one of Mrs. Sanger's associates."[67] The National Birth Control League was run by Mary Ware Dennett and had as its focus changing the laws regarding birth control.

When Margaret Sanger returned to the United States, Dennett told her that the National Birth Control League "did not approve of her tactics, and the two women began a competition for leadership of the birth control movement that lasted for ten years."[68] In 1919, Dennett decided to challenge federal legislation and formed the Voluntary Parenthood League which Sanger declared was founded on "an erroneous attitude."[69]

Margaret Sanger founded the American Birth Control League in November 1921 and became its first president. The official publication of the American Birth Control League was the *Birth Control Review*. Its aim was "to enlighten and educate all sections of the American public in the various aspects of the dangers of uncontrolled procreation and the imperative necessity of a world program of Birth Control."[70] Ellen Dwight Jones took control of the organization while Sanger traveled overseas.

The Clinical Research Bureau, a birth control clinic affiliated with the American Birth Control League, was founded by Sanger in 1923. Its first medical director was Dorothy Bocker, M.D. Sanger was not satisfied with Bocker and replaced her with Hannah M. Stone, M.D. Under Stone's leadership, the Clinical Research Bureau collected data and, in 1928, she published her findings which "at last provided documentary evidence that safe and effective contraceptive means existed."[71]

In 1928, due to disagreements with Jones, Sanger left the American Birth Control League and no longer worked on the *Birth Control Review*.[72] She founded a rival organization, the National Committee on Federal Legislation for Birth Control, the following year.[73]

In 1939, the American Birth Control League and the Clinical Research Bureau merged to form the Birth Control Federation of America.[74] Sanger reluctantly agreed to the merger and was named honorary chairman of the new organization.[75] D. Kenneth Rose of the John Price Jones fund-raising and public relations agency was named acting director.[76] In January 1942, over Sanger's "loud protests," the name was changed to Planned Parenthood Federation of America.[77] The change was necessitated by the programs of the Nazi regime in Germany. Population control was seen as unacceptable. Consequently, a public relations consultant recommended changing the name to something not using the words "birth control."

The formation and subsequent elimination of the various birth control organizations during the early years of the movement could be described as turbulent:

> For all her altruism and humanitarianism, one of Mrs. Sanger's goals was complete and exclusive control of the birth control movement. However hard others might work for the cause, she nevertheless insisted on the major part of the glory. She spurned any organization she could not dominate; she relentlessly maneuvered to displace her rivals within the movement. And for her enemies outside the movement, however useful she knew them to be for her ultimate purposes, she had irreconcilable scorn.
>
> The organization of the birth control movement, then, and the tactics it employed, were shaped by the movement's changing sources of support, its responses to opposition, its intramural rivalries, and above all by the imposing personality of the movement's principal figure, Margaret Sanger.[78]

In 1952, Planned Parenthood became an international organization when Margaret Sanger helped found the International Planned Parenthood Federation,[79] which is currently based in London, England. Sanger served as the honorary president of the International Planned Parenthood Federation.

Many famous and powerful men and women have served on Planned Parenthood's advisory board including American presidents Dwight D. Eisenhower and Lyndon B. Johnson. Presidents Harry Truman and Herbert Hoover supported Margaret Sanger's organization. John D. Rockefeller, III and Adlai E. Stevenson also supported Planned Parenthood. It is believed that most of the world's wealthiest families support Planned Parenthood. After all, Planned Parenthood is the charity that makes all others unnecessary—and that saves money.

IT TAKES ALL KINDS

Margaret Sanger was, to put it mildly, a peculiar woman. Telling the truth was one problem. While one biographer acknowledges that Sanger did not always tell the truth, the writer theorizes it was out of a need to deceive herself more than out of a desire to deceive others.[80]

The most pervasive untruth that continues to be perpetuated is that Margaret Sanger was a registered nurse. As previously noted, Sanger did not graduate from nursing school. Nevertheless, she repeatedly claimed to have been a nurse:

> The chief fault of the book [Sanger's autobiography], however, was her insistence on the fact that she had been a registered or trained nurse. She had been accepted, she said, as a "probationer at a hospital in Westchester," where "the work was trying because of the long hours. But these years of training now seem a period that tested character, integrity, patience, and endurance." There had of course been no "years of training," only a few months. Still, she hammered home the point of "years" by describing a vivid fantasied scene in "a New York hospital where I was taking a post-graduate course," a scene that implied she had graduated from White Plains. But a careful check by the White Plains Hospital found no record of her ever entering their nursing school, much less graduating from it and being traditionally "capped." And the unnamed New York Hospital (actually The Manhattan Eye and Ear) found no record of her ever being there at all. At most, they say, she could have worked occasionally as a nurse's aid, but so many thousands of these come and go that no records are kept.[81]

There are other examples of Sanger's untruths and deception. She claimed to have spent "almost a year" in major libraries in an unsuccessful attempt to learn about contraception:

> The *Index Catalogue of the Library of the Surgeon-General's Office* . . . listed nearly two full pages of books and articles on "prevention of conception. . . ."
>
> Yet Mrs. Sanger insisted that she had to travel to France in 1913 to find reliable contraceptive information. Again, that account served to establish her historical uniqueness and to dramatize the dedication she brought to her work. By making birth control seem an innovation she personally had imported from France, she conveniently suppressed some historical facts: that contraception was widely practiced among certain social groups in the United States as early as the nineteenth century; that the medical profession did have some, admittedly undiffused, contraceptive knowledge available; and that Emma Goldman had been advocating contraception for more than ten years. Mrs. Sanger usually used the myth of the year's fruitless search to advance her position in relation to the medical profession, which balked at her nonmedical leadership in a medical area. Claiming that before her researches in France doctors knew little or nothing about contraception was one way to establish her legitimacy with regard to organized medicine.[82]

Part of Margaret Sanger's zeal for birth control was related to her own needs, which were associated with a near obsession with sexual freedom. According to biographer David M. Kennedy, "Sanger intended birth control not simply to reduce the suffering of the poor and the number of the unfit, but also to increase the quantity and quality of sexual relationships."[83] As previously mentioned, Sanger had many love affairs but stressed the "conscious, careful selection of a lover, that is the mate, if only for an hour, for a lifetime maybe."[84]

Sanger was a determined woman who stopped at nothing to achieve her goals. Anyone Sanger believed to be threatening her position in "her movement," even if the fear was unfounded, was dealt with in a decisive manner:

> She [Sanger] was ruthless. Once she got into birth control, she wanted to be No. 1. As one of the old birth control workers I met told me, Margaret could only count one, three, four, five. Anybody who got to be No. 2 or close to her, she would knife her and manage to get her out of the movement. It was an ego trip, there's no question.[85]

Sanger had other "personality quirks." She had a fear of constipation and, consequently, had frequent colon irrigations—on at least one occasion using ten gallons of salt water. Writes one biographer, "Just as she needed to control others, just as she craved the role of leader and found it painful to compromise, impossible to follow, so did she apparently need to control her own body, to command through force of will the functions of the merely physical self."[86] Correspondence between Sanger and J. Noah Slee also referenced this behavior. Slee requested that Sanger "[b]ring the high enema tube" when she traveled to visit him.[87]

Addicted to Demerol (a pain killer and sedative) in her later years, one biographer writes that Sanger had "tried to dispel depression by sex, travel, Rosicrucianism, numerology . . . [and] astrology. She subscribed to a personal daily horoscope by Evangeline Adams."[88]

Rejecting Christianity, Margaret Sanger had other ways in which she sought direction. "Margaret had always had a strong sense of the mystical," writes another biographer. Sanger "consulted psychic researchers, graphologists and astrologists throughout her life. She placed great importance on the analysis of dreams."[89] These were not Sanger's only spiritual interests. "To ease her various aches, Margaret began toying with a new religious cult called *Unity* . . . Unity described itself as a 'mental treatment that was guaranteed to cure every ill the flesh is heir to.'"[90] Sanger remained in Unity for the remainder of life.[91]

Sanger's *Woman Rebel* included an article titled, "The Pauline Ideas vs. Woman." It is one of the most savage attacks against Christianity. The article begins by quoting Scripture. Conclusions are then drawn about Christianity and its impact on the world:

> "Wives, submit yourselves unto your husbands, as it is fit in the Lord." Col. III, 18.
>
> "Let the woman learn in silence with all subjection." Tim. II, 11.
>
> "But the younger widows refuse, for when they have begun to wax wanton against Christ, they will marry."
>
> ["]Having damnation because they have cast off their first faith.
>
> And withal they learn to be idle, wandering about from house to house, and not only idle but tattlers also, and busybodies, speaking things which they ought not.
>
> I will therefore that the younger women marry, bear children, guide the house, etc." I Tim. V, 11–14.
>
> "Let your women keep silence in the churches, for it is not permitted unto them to speak; but they are commanded to be under obedience." I Cor. 14, 34.
>
> A glance at the foregoing texts affords a glimpse of the elevating principles of Christianity, and what that religion has done for women.
>
> SUBMISSION, SILENCE, and SUBJECTION are the chief tenets of the system of religious ethics that has been imposed upon suffering women for nearly two thousand years. "Saint" Paul, officially canonized by "Holy Church," was that truly great and good man who started out with the ambition of massacring the bodies of a handful of Christians; became converted and massacred their intellects, their individual liberties and their opportunities for social, industrial, and spiritual progress instead. Filled with the Spirit of God he deprived woman of the comparative freedom and equality which she enjoyed with man under the patriarchal system, and imposed upon her the infamous serfdom of sexual, intellectual, personal and spiritual bondage which has deprived the world of the results which

should have accrued from the free and proper development of her divine potentialities, for upwards of twenty centuries. . . . Christianity, based upon the Pauline doctrines, allowed woman a soul—begrudgingly—and deprived her of personal liberty, and further denied her the opportunity of developing her spiritual attributes.[92]

As previously noted, Margaret Sanger opposed the institution of marriage. She used the *Woman Rebel* article to attack marriage as an institution designed to keep women oppressed. An alternative understanding of marriage is suggested:

Marriage, which in its Edenic purity should be the voluntary association of two individuals for just so long as they can contribute to each other those necessary qualities of mutual sympathy, respect, encouragement, and support, as shall maintain a complete unity and affinity physically, mentally and spiritually, has been seized upon by Church and State as the mightiest instrument wherewith to enforce the three cardinal principles referred to.

And Church and State co-operate to enforce SUBMISSION by taking no cognizance of the sexual relations between married people. They co-operate to enforce SILENCE by depriving woman of her very name, submerging her identity in that of her husband. They co-operate to enforce SUBJECTION by TURNING WOMAN INTO A MERE INCUBATOR. "I will therefore that the younger women marry, bear children, guide the house, etc." Woman's place in a nutshell! An incubator and the motive power of the wash tub![93]

Like today's press, the *Woman Rebel* included attacks on religious leaders:

The daily press teems with the records of ministers who have fallen from grace, and of priests who have come to grief thru their mistresses, both, to the amazement of their faithful followers to whom they stood in the place of Deity. . . . But the main point is, that under this godly system, WOMAN IS THE ONE WHO SUFFERS. She is the one to blame for tempting as did her historic ancestor Eve. And when man seeks to find a convenient instrument on which to saddle his own shortcomings WOMAN is the creature selected.

Woman demands and COMMANDS the rights over her own body. Let man remember that the ancient philosophers who lived much nearer to Nature and who had far greater inspirations and conceptions than our present wrangling schoolmen and academicians, TAUGHT THAT THE DEITY WAS THE FEMALE PRINCIPLE OF THE COSMOS.[94]

Such direct attacks against Christianity were most often not so blunt. Instead, the *Woman Rebel* often included articles attacking those things sacred to Christians. Marriage was a primary target. Witchcraft was also addressed in the *Woman Rebel*. It had been argued that those beliefs espoused in the publication, and some of the women themselves, were "obscene." The *Woman Rebel* suggested otherwise:

It is computed from historical records that 9,000,000 persons were put to death for witchcraft after 1484. The opponents of witch-belief were denounced just as the disbelievers in the "obscene" are now denounced. Yet witches ceased to be, when men no longer believed in them. Think it over and see if the "obscene" will not also disappear when men cease to believe in it.[95]

Is it any wonder that the *Woman Rebel* summarized its purpose as, "THE WOMAN REBEL: A MONTHLY PAPER OF MILITANT THOUGHT."[96]

CHARITY, EUGENICS, AND THE UNFIT

Margaret Sanger was active in the eugenics movement—the science which seeks to "improve" races through the control of hereditary factors. Eugenics was a popular philosophy in the early twentieth century. Sanger saw birth control as a principal way to limit the numbers of people she considered to be "defective." She sought to protect the freedom and power of those believed to be a superior breed capable of ruling over the impure masses.

One special editorial printed in the *Birth Control Review*, identified as being the view of "American Medicine," alleges "More children from the fit, less from the unfit—that is the chief issue in Birth Control."[97] The November 1921 edition of *Birth Control Review* was headlined, "Birth Control: To create a race of thoroughbreds."[98] Sanger also wrote, "Many, perhaps, will think it idle to go farther in demonstrating the immorality of large families, but since there is still an abundance of proof at hand, it may be offered for the sake of those who find difficulty in adjusting old-fashioned ideas to the facts. The most merciful thing that the large family does to one of its infant members is to kill it."[99]

In her autobiography, Sanger explains that the eugenics movement could not succeed without birth control:

> I accepted one branch of this philosophy, but eugenics without birth control seemed to me a house built upon sands. It could not stand against the furious winds of economic pressure which had buffeted into partial or total helplessness a tremendous proportion of the human race. The eugenists wanted to shift the birth control emphasis from less children for the poor to more children for the rich. We went back of that and sought first to stop the multiplication of the unfit. This appeared the most important and greatest step towards race betterment.[100]

Sanger viewed birth control as the primary method for achieving "racial progress":

> Birth control itself, often denounced as a violation of natural law, is nothing more or less than the facilitation of the process of weeding out the unfit, of preventing the birth of defectives or those who will become defectives. So, in compliance with nature's working plan, we must permit womanhood its full development before we can expect of it efficient motherhood. If we are to make racial progress, this development of womanhood must precede motherhood in every individual woman. Then and then only can the mother cease to be an incubator and be a mother indeed. Then only can she transmit to her sons and daughters the qualities which make strong individuals and, collectively, a strong race.[101]

In Margaret Sanger's *Pivot of Civilization*, the plan for birth control to play a major role in the eugenics program is defended:

> Birth Control which has been criticized as negative and destructive, is really the greatest and most truly eugenic method, and its adoption as part of the program of Eugenics would immediately give a concrete and realistic power to that science. As a matter of fact, Birth Control has been accepted by the most clear thinking and far seeing of the Eugenists themselves as the most constructive and necessary of the means to racial health.[102]

Mark H. Haller, author of *Eugenics: Hereditarian Attitudes in American Thought*, writes:

> . . . Margaret Sanger began increasingly to speak like an orthodox eugenist. From the beginning she had urged birth control for those with presumed heredity ailments like insanity and epilepsy. By the 1920's she advocated sterilization for the unfit, pointed to the Jukes as the sort of tragedy that birth control might halt, and stated that "it is a curious but neglected fact that the very types which in all kindness should be obliterated from the human stock, have been permitted to reproduce themselves and to perpetuate their group, succored by the policy of indiscriminate charity of warm hearts uncontrolled by cool heads."
>
> Birth control and eugenics, then, were two closely related movements. Birth control advocates used eugenics as a source of arguments and as a method of attracting scientific

support; eugenists, on the other hand, became aware that in birth control they had a weapon with which to manipulate the birth rate for eugenic purposes.[103]

Sanger sought to control the reproduction of several primary groups: the poor, immigrants (especially people of color), and religious groups which were proving to be a hindrance to her goals (primarily Catholics and fundamentalists). Sanger viewed these groups as reckless breeders who were "unceasingly spawning [a] class of human beings who never should have been born at all . . . "[104]

Sanger felt that giving charity to the poor, especially immigrants who were often people of color, served only to expand the problem, for they would cease to exist without help. She believed that charity, in the long run, is more cruel than letting nature take its course. Besides, allowed to breed unchecked, the "defectives" would eventually produce enough people to rise up and take over the world. As a result, the world would face "biological destruction." Sanger feared "the gradual but certain attack upon the stocks of intelligence and racial health by the sinister forces of the hordes of irresponsibility and imbecility. . . ."[105]

Philanthropists believe efforts to support the poor, handicapped and others less fortunate will bring about a better world. Sanger believed that philanthropy itself to be the problem:

> It [charity] reveals a fundamental and irremediable defect. Its very success, its very efficiency, its very necessity to the social order, are themselves the most unanswerable indictment. Organized charity itself is the symptom of a malignant social disease.
>
> Those vast, complex, interrelated organizations aiming to control and to diminish the spread of misery and destitution and all the menacing evils that spring out of this sinisterly fertile soil, are the surest sign that our civilization has bred, is breeding and is perpetuating constantly increasing numbers of defectives, delinquents and dependents. My criticism, therefore, is not directed at the "failure" of philanthropy, but rather at its success.[106]

Sanger wrote that those who provide free maternity care to the poor and others deemed unfit do nothing but encourage "the healthier and more normal sections of the world to shoulder the burden of unthinking and indiscriminate fecundity of others; which brings with it, as I think the reader must agree, a dead weight of human waste. Instead of decreasing and aiming to eliminate the stocks that are most detrimental to the future of the race and the world, it tends to render them to a menacing degree dominant."[107]

Margaret Sanger believed that spending fewer tax dollars on the needy would appeal to taxpayers. Her concept was especially pushed during the Great Depression. This appeal to the taxpayers would help lead to the acceptance of her programs and to the eventual success of her agenda.

On August 5, 1926, Margaret Sanger spoke before the Institute of Euthenics [sic]. She noted that England's House of Lords had passed a resolution in support of giving contraceptive training in government-supported maternity centers:[108]

> It now remains for the United States government to set a sensible example to the world by offering a bonus or a yearly pension to all obviously unfit parents who allow themselves to be sterilized by harmless and scientific means. In this way the moron and the diseased would have no posterity to inherit their unhappy condition. The number of the feeble-minded would decrease and a heavy burden would be lifted from the shoulders of the fit.
>
> Such a bonus would be a wise and profitable investment for the nation. It would be the salvation of American civilization. It would enable thousands of parents to get a firm footing on the path of life and enable them to give some care to those children they have already borne.

> It would mean facing our debts today, here and now, instead of passing them on and piling them up for future generations to pay.[109]

Sanger believed that tax relief would allow the rich and intelligent to produce more children. She wrote, "There is only one reply to a request for a higher birth rate among the intelligent, and that is to ask the government to *first* take off the burdens of the insane and feebleminded from your backs. Sterilization for these is the remedy."[110]

Sanger's comments about those she considered "unfit" were not reserved for just one or two segments of society. During World War I, American soldiers were forced to take the Stanford-Binet IQ (intelligence quotient) test. Administered on the basis of ethnic group, the results showed that the average American soldier was essentially an idiot. African-Americans and those of southern European ancestry fared even worse. The test spurred Sanger to increase her attacks on those she considered less intelligent. Sanger referred to those who were "glib and plausible, bright looking and attractive, but with a mental vision of seven, eight or nine years . . ."[111] Of the American soldier, Sanger wrote that 47.3 percent of drafted men "had the mentality of twelve-year-old children or less—in other words that they are morons."[112]

Sanger continued her analysis of the American soldier by quoting Robert M. Yerkes who wrote, "Assuming that these drafted men are a fair sample of the entire population of approximately 100,000,000, this means that 45,000,000, or nearly one-half the entire population, will never develop mental capacity beyond the stage represented by a normal twelve-year-old child, and that only 13,500,000 will ever show superior intelligence."[113]

Sanger wrote that we are "face to face with a serious and destructive practice."[114] She expanded upon her remarks:

> [O]ur failure to segregate morons who are increasing and multiplying—I have sufficiently indicated, though in truth I have merely scratched the surface of this international menace—demonstrate our foolhardy and extravagant sentimentalism. No industrial corporation could maintain its existence upon such a foundation. Yet hard-headed "captains of industry," financiers who pride themselves upon their cool-headed and keen-sighted business ability are dropping millions into rosewater philanthropies and charities that are silly at best and vicious at worst. In our dealings with such elements there is a bland maladministration and misuse of huge sums that should in all righteousness be used for the development and education of the healthy elements of the community.[115]

Margaret Sanger seemed obsessed with fear that those of lesser intelligence would have children. To avoid such progeny, she was a vociferous proponent of sterilization:

> The emergency problem of segregation and sterilization must be faced immediately. Every feeble-minded girl or woman of the heredity type, especially of the moron class, should be segregated during their reproductive period. . . . Moreover, when we realize that each feeble-minded person is a potential source of an endless progeny of defect, we prefer the policy of immediate sterilization, of making sure that parenthood is absolutely prohibited to the feeble-minded.[116]

The *Birth Control Review* often included the writings of Margaret Sanger's "voluntary sexual partner," Havelock Ellis, who wrote that, unless they agreed to be sterilized, the poor should not be given charity by the government.[117] Ellis was also a strong supporter of euthanasia—the killing of the aged and infirm.[118]

The *Birth Control Review* refers to the effect of religion on birth rates and compares the birth rate of "high grade people" to those of the "borderline class":

> It is the people of the slums, the poorest, and usually the most stupid who hear the utmost denouncement of birth control from their pastors and priests. Within their own denomination, the poor Roman Catholics have the largest families. . . . They don't have large families because they are Roman Catholics but because they are stupid like their stupid Protestant neighbors.[119]

Included in the same article is a discussion of religion:

> [T]here is another way in which religion can effect, negatively, the quality of the people by influencing the birth rate of a class. That is by organized opposition to eugenical sterilization legislation . . . Instead of sterilization, they would have clergymen tell imbeciles, low grade morons, and other defectives who can often breed if they can't do anything else, "You must practice marital continence [abstinence]," which is equivalent to pouring water into a sieve, telling it not to run through and expecting results.[120]

Margaret Sanger often linked birth control and eugenics. In a *Birth Control Review* article titled "Birth Control and Racial Betterment," Sanger suggested that eugenists should support her cause:

> Before eugenists and others who are laboring for racial betterment can succeed, they must first clear the way for Birth Control. Like the advocates of Birth Control, the eugenists, for instance, are seeking to assist the race toward the elimination of the unfit. Both are seeking a single end but they lay emphasis upon different methods.[121]

Sanger compared the two movements:

> We who advocate Birth Control, on the other hand, lay all our emphasis upon stopping not only the reproduction of the unfit but upon stopping all reproduction when there is not economic means of providing proper care for those who are born in health. . . . We hold that the world is already over-populated.[122]

Sanger believed eugenists would benefit that by giving women the right to decide whether or not to have children:

> We further maintain that it is her right, regardless of all other considerations, to determine whether she shall bear children or not, and how many children she shall bear if she chooses to become a mother. . . . We believe that if such information is placed within the reach of all, we will have made it possible to take the first, greatest step toward racial betterment and that this step, assisted in no small measure by the educational propaganda of eugenists and members of similar schools, will be taken.[123]

More than two years later, Margaret Sanger wrote a *Birth Control Review* article titled, "The Eugenic Value of Birth Control Propaganda." Her views had not changed:

> The eugenic and civilizational value of Birth Control is becoming apparent to the enlightened and the intelligent.
>
> In the limited space of the present paper, I have time only to touch upon some of the fundamental convictions that form the basis of our Birth Control propaganda, and which, as I think you must agree, indicate that the campaign for Birth Control is not merely of eugenic value, but is practically identical in ideal with the final aims of Eugenics.[124]

Sanger wrote that until parents are given "control over their reproductive faculties," it will not be possible "to improve the quality of the generations of the future . . ." In fact, Sanger argued, it is necessary "even to maintain civilization even at its present level."[125] She suggested that, "Birth Control propaganda is thus the entering wedge for the Eugenic educator."[126]

Sanger did not believe one could count on the "fit" to produce more children than the "unfit." This was of great concern to Sanger:

> As an advocate of Birth Control, I wish to take advantage of the present opportunity to point out that the unbalance between the birth rate of the "unfit" and the "fit," admittedly the greatest present menace to civilization, can never be rectified by the inauguration of a cradle competition between these two classes. In this matter, the example of the inferior classes, the fertility of the feeble-minded, the mentally defective, the poverty-stricken classes, should not be held up for emulation to the mentally and physically fit through less fertile parents of the educated and well-to-do classes. On the contrary, the most urgent problem today is how to limit and discourage the overfertility of the mentally and physically defective.[127]

Sanger argued that supporters of birth control must support eugenics. "[W]e shall best be serving the true interests of Eugenics," she wrote, "because our work will then have a practical and pragmatic value."[128]

Havelock Ellis and Margaret Sanger shared the same point-of-view with regard to eugenics and the birth control movement. Ellis wrote in the *Birth Control Review* that a major problem is that too many people cling to an "old morality" regarding procreation:

> In comparatively modern times it [the religious command to procreate] has been re-imposed from unexpected quarters, on the one hand by all the forces that are opposed to democracy and on the other by all the forces of would-be patriotic militarism, and both alike clamoring for plentiful and cheap men. . . .
>
> According to the ideas of the old morality, which placed the whole question of procreation under the authority (after God) of men, women were in subjection to men, and had no right to freedom, no right to responsibility, no right to knowledge, for it was believed, if entrusted with any of these she would abuse them at once. That view prevails even today in some civilized countries and middle-class Italian peasants, for instance, will not allow their daughter to be conducted by a man even to Mass, for they believe that as soon as she is out of their sight, she will be unchaste.[129]

Consider these words:

> In view of the large families of the native population, it could only suit us if girls and women there had as many abortions as possible. Active trade in contraceptives ought to be actually encouraged . . . as we could not possibly have the slightest interest in increasing the . . . population.[130]

These are not the words of Margaret Sanger, but those of Adolf Hitler. Like Sanger, Hitler emphasized that it was harmful to have many children as each birth endangered the mother's life and that voluntary sterilization is desirable. Adolf Hitler opposed abortion only for those of the Aryan "superior stock." As part of his plan to "preserve the race," he advocated abortion for all others. The Third Reich made effective use of propaganda about birth control and abortion.[131] The similarities between Hitler and Sanger prompted one newspaper columnist to refer to Sanger as "Hitler in a skirt." Conversely, Hitler was referred to as "Sanger with a mustache."[132]

Shortly after the German military invaded Poland, an article in *Birth Control Review* compared Italy's birth control policies to those of Nazi Germany. The article supported the German program because it had been "much more carefully worked out. The need for quality as well as quantity is recognized."[133]

Early in her career, Margaret Sanger claimed to oppose abortion. Sanger wrote that "abortion is a disgrace to a civilized community."[134] Sanger believed abortion to be a "disgrace" due to the dangers involved for women.[135] She even said that abortion "was the wrong way—no matter how early it was performed it was taking a life . . . "[136] Yet it has been argued that this was done "as a way of claiming a moral impulse for her work . . ." Sanger sought "to draw a sharp line between contraception and abortion," but only "for tactical purposes."[137] Americans were certainly not ready to accept abortion when they had not even accepted contraception. Advocating legal abortion from the start would have seriously damaged Sanger's public image and her movement.

In 1917, Margaret Sanger wrote that, "It is only through applied eugenics that the vast volume of disease and degeneracy which flows through the channels of heredity can be prevented. Obviously this can be accomplished only through education and legislative restriction upon the procreation of the unfit." Sanger argued that, "We have thus come to recognize the dominate influence of the mother's relation to the health, as well as the life of the race." She conceded, however, that, "It is not probable that the scientific methods which have been successfully applied to plants and the selective breeding of animals will ever replace the haphazard methods of human reproduction. There is no fact better established than that a man can transmit only that which he is."[138]

Sanger wrote frequently in many publications. In one magazine article she outlines her plan for improving the human race. Titled, "A License for Mothers to Have Babies: A 'Code to Stop the Overproduction of Children'—Based on Common Sense Instead of Sentiment," the article lists several steps that would help Sanger to quickly achieve her goals:

> Article 1. The purpose of the American Baby Code shall be to provide for a better distribution of babies, to assist couples who wish to prevent overproduction of offspring and thus to reduce the burdens of charity and taxation for public relief, and to protect society against the propagation and increase of the unfit.
>
> Article 2. Birth control clinics shall be permitted to function as services of government health departments or under the support of charity, or as non-profit, self-sustaining agencies, subject to inspection and control by public authorities.
>
> Article 3. A marriage license shall in itself give husband and wife only the right to a common household and not the right to parenthood.
>
> Article 4. No woman shall have the legal right to bear a child, no man shall have the right to become a father, without a permit for parenthood.
>
> Article 5. Permits for parenthood shall be issued by government authorities to married couples upon application, providing the parents are financially able to support the expected child, have the qualifications needed for proper rearing of the child, have no transmissible diseases, and on the woman's part no indication that maternity is likely to result in death or premature injury to health.
>
> Article 6. No permit for parenthood shall be valid for more than one birth.
>
> Article 7. Every county shall be assisted administratively by the state in the effort to maintain a direct ratio between the county birth rate and its index of child welfare. When the county records show an unfavorable variation from this ratio the county shall be taxed by the State . . . The revenues thus obtained shall be expended by the State within the given county in giving financial support to birth control clinics . . .
>
> Article 8. Feeble-minded persons, habitual congenital criminals, those afflicted with inheritable diseases, and others found biologically unfit should be sterilized or in cases of doubt should be isolated as to prevent the perpetuation of their afflictions by breeding.[139]

EUGENICS AND PEOPLE OF COLOR

It is clear from her writings that Margaret Sanger did not care for people not of her race. In an October 1939 letter, Sanger wrote of her desire to neutralize any opposition that might be posed by African-Americans. Sanger and her supporters were interested in hiring three or four "colored Ministers, preferably with social-service backgrounds, and with engaging personalities" to travel throughout the South and propagate the birth control philosophy.[140] The "Negro Project," as it was called, is described by Sanger in a letter to an associate, Dr. Clarence J. Gamble. Sanger had supported hiring a "Negro physician" to do her organization's bidding among African-Americans, an idea Gamble initially opposed:

> It seems to me from my experience . . . that while the colored Negroes have great respect for white doctors they can get closer to their own members and more or less lay their cards on the table which means their ignorance, superstitions and doubts. They do not do this with the white people and if we can train the Negro doctor at the Clinic he can go among them with enthusiasm and with knowledge, which, I believe will have far-reaching results among the colored people. His work in my opinion should be entirely with the Negro profession and the nurses, hospital, social workers, as well as the County's white doctors. His success will depend upon his personality and his training by us.
>
> The minister's work is also important and also he should be trained, perhaps by the Federation as to our ideals and the goal that we hope to reach. We do not want word to go out that we want to exterminate the Negro population, and the minister is the man who can straighten out that idea if it ever occurs to any of their more rebellious members.[141]

Dr. Clarence J. Gamble had written of a "great danger" that Sanger's efforts would be in vain because "the Negroes think it a plan for extermination." Gamble suggested a solution to this problem. He argued that Sanger's legion should "appear to let the colored . . . run it . . . "[142]

In a 1941 letter, Sanger argued that her plan was to "carry on a personal educational program" and that it be done "by a Negro minister or sociologist and a Negro physician to follow up the former's activities." Sanger wrote that, "Only when this type of work is done, will the Negro problem ever be solved, as far as our objectives are concerned. They still believe—large numbers of them—that God sends them children."[143] In 1944, to appease and entreat African-Americans, Planned Parenthood hired a full-time "Negro consultant."[144]

Sanger's racism eventually led to her dream of creating a "new race." She wrote of this dream in her 1920 book *Woman and the New Race*:

> If we are to develop in America a new race with a racial soul, we must keep the birth rate within the scope of our ability to understand as well as to educate. We must not encourage reproduction beyond our capacity to assimilate our numbers so as to make the coming generation into such physically fit, mentally capable, socially alert individuals as are the ideal of a democracy.
>
> The intelligence of a people is of slow evolutional development—it lags far behind the reproductive ability. It is far too slow to cope with conditions created by an increasing population, unless that increase is carefully regulated.[145]

Sanger offered a solution to what she viewed as a major problem. She also stated what benefits would be attained if her plan were adopted:

> We must, therefore, not permit an increase in population that we are not prepared to care for to the best advantage—that we are not prepared to do justice to, educationally and

economically. We must popularize birth control thinking. We must not leave it haphazardly to be the privilege of the already privileged. We must put this means of freedom and growth into the hands of the masses.

We must set motherhood free. We must give the foreign and submerged mother knowledge that will enable her to prevent bringing to birth children she does not want. We know that in each of these submerged and semisubmerged elements of the population there are rich factors of racial culture. Motherhood is the channel through which these cultures flow. Motherhood, when free to choose the father, free to choose the time and the number of children who shall result from the union, automatically works in wondrous ways. It refuses to bring forth weaklings; refuses to bring forth slaves; refuses to bear children who must live under the conditions described. It withholds the unfit, brings forth the fit; brings few children into homes where there is not sufficient to provide for them. Instinctively it avoids all those things which multiply racial handicaps. Under such circumstances we can hope that the "melting pot" will refine. We shall see that it will save the precious metals of racial culture, fused into an amalgam of physical perfection, mental strength and spiritual progress. Such an American race, containing the best of all racial elements, could give the world a vision and a leadership beyond our present imagination.[146]

Possibly because Sanger's point of view with regard to people of color was not made public, the birth control movement split the African-American community. Some African-American leaders considered, and still consider, the movement to be "a form of race suicide."[147] One Sanger biographer writes, "With an infant mortality rate 90 percent higher for blacks than for whites, it is not possible to ignore such an argument." Several African-American groups opposed birth control, including delegates to the Newark Black Power Conference and a group called Efforts to Increase Our Size.[148]

The birth control movement did receive the support of several influential African-Americans including W. E. B. DuBois who argued that African-Americans who oppose birth control "must learn that among human races and groups, as among vegetables, quality and not mere quantity really counts."[149] The Reverend Martin Luther King, Jr., also supported birth control. In his speech accepting the Margaret Sanger Award (see chapters 6, 10, and 16), King compared the movement for civil rights to that for birth control:

There is a striking kinship between our (civil rights) movement and Margaret Sanger's early efforts. She, like we, saw the horrifying conditions of ghetto life . . . Negroes have no mere academic nor ordinary interest in family planning. They have a special and urgent concern . . . For the Negro, therefore, intelligent guides of family planning are a profoundly important ingredient in his quest for security and a decent life. There are mountainous obstacles still separating Negroes from a normal existence.

Yet one element in stabilizing his life would be an understanding of an easy access to the means to develop a family related in size to his community environment and to the income potential he can command.[150]

King also said that there is "scarcely anything more tragic in human life than a child who is not wanted."[151] Today, Planned Parenthood enjoys the support of most African-American organizations, but not necessarily that of most African-Americans (see chapter 10).

Sanger was unsuccessful at convincing one influential person of color to support her cause. Mahatma Gandhi opposed the use of artificial birth control, but his successor approved of it.[152]

In January 1940, the American Birth Control Federation held a symposium called "Race Building in a Democracy." The luncheon speech was presented by Henry Pratt Fairchild, president of the American Eugenics Society. "One of the outstanding features of the present conference," Fairchild said, "is the practical universal acceptance of the fact that these two great movements [eugenics and birth control] have now come to such a thorough understanding and have drawn so close together as to be almost indistinguishable."[153]

BROADER POLITICAL VIEWS

Sanger strongly opposed the republican form of government. She believed it foolish that every person has one vote. Why should the vote of an intelligent, wealthy person be equal to that of a feeble-minded beggar? She referred to the system as "rule by mere number."[154] Sanger wrote, "We can all vote, even the mentally arrested. And so it is no surprise to find the moron's vote as good as the vote of the genius. The outlook is not a cheerful one."[155] Sanger preferred that government be run by an aristocracy—a privileged minority or upper class.[156] A socialist for a time, Sanger leaned more toward anarchy.[157]

After they decided against an amendment suggested by Margaret Sanger, which would have allowed for distribution of birth control information, Sanger attacked members of the New York State Legislature:

> These lawmakers at Albany may have exposed themselves as incapable of unprejudiced and clearsighted thinking concerning the problem of population, but the representatives of our cause were given an excellent opportunity to study State legislators at close range. The pessimistic observer of such democratic institutions as the New York Assembly might cite our experience in the legislative halls at Albany on April tenth as an example of the utter hopelessness of effecting any beneficial change in our statute books through the medium of such a body. . . .
>
> A State Legislature represents the last bulwark of prejudice, superstition and ignorance. The task of battling against these forces is one that demands all that we possess of courage and faith in our convictions. To be discouraged because the Codes Committee, a small group of adolescent minds, expresses its disapproval of a doctrine which has won the adherence of the finest intellects in the world, would be a confession of our own lack of faith. The battle for a better race and a greater America must go on, because our final triumph is inevitable.[158]

Sanger's attack on New York lawmakers was based on their unwillingness to give her what she wanted:

> One great truth lifts its head above all the interesting facts thrust upon us during our recent pilgrimage to Albany. This is the immediate and pressing need for *intelligence tests for legislators*. American schools have begun to test the intelligence of school children. Likewise, employers examine applicants for work as to their capability to fill the jobs they are seeking. There are mental as well as physical tests for recruits in the American army. Even the poor immigrant is refused admission to this country if he cannot show that his intelligence is equal to the complex problem of gaining a livelihood in these United States. Yet with a serene and bland indifference to the social well-being of the state and nation, American voters send to Congress and legislative halls noisy and ill-mannered politicians whose one outstanding talent seems to be their shrewd ability to catch votes. To understand the importance, the implications and the organic relationship of Birth Control to public health and racial strength, these men are apparently mentally and constitutionally unfit. This truth our Albany "hearing" has irrefutable demonstrated.

> We enclose the word "hearing" in quotation marks, because most of the members of that august committee refused us even the courtesy of listening to our arguments. Their attitude was that of schoolboys impatient to return to their game of marbles.[159]

LATER YEARS

Margaret Sanger is credited as the author of several books. Some of the most notable works include:

- *The Case for Birth Control*
- *Woman and the New Race*
- *The Pivot of Civilization*
- *Woman, Morality and Birth Control*
- *Motherhood in Bondage*
- *My Fight for Birth Control*
- *Margaret Sanger: An Autobiography*

Margaret Sanger had an unconventional lifestyle until her death. In a 1979 interview with Sanger biographer Madeline Gray, a *Washington Star* reporter asked, "She [Sanger] retired to Tucson [Arizona]. What was her life like there?"[160]: Gray replied:

> The wild life at the end . . . When her [Sanger's] husband died he left her $5 million and she said I'm going to blow it all, and she did her best to blow it all. At the end, I went to Tucson and she had all sorts of young men hanging around and I met them all. They looked like homosexuals to me. But anything to flatter her and have men around her and she gave them money. Ooooh, what a gang.[161]

Stuart and Grant Sanger both became physicians. Grant Sanger later served on the board of directors of the Margaret Sanger Research Bureau.[162] Margaret Sanger retired from the birth control movement in the late 1950s.

Margaret Sanger was named "Humanist of the Year" by the American Humanist Association in 1957. As the Association put it, "Contemporary Humanists find singularly appropriate channels for action in the Planned Parenthood movement which she founded. Here is one means by which they work to better man's future destiny."[163]

Sanger retired to Tucson, Arizona, where she resided until her death on September 6, 1966. Buried in the family plot in Fishkill, New York, under the name Slee, Sanger's eulogy ended with the words, "And so a stormy day ends a stormy career."[164]

More than 25 years after Sanger's death, an effort was made to admit her into the Arizona Hall of Fame. Several conservative lawmakers opposed the induction on the grounds that Sanger was a racist. Sanger's supporters argued that she should be admitted into the Hall of Fame because she founded the Tucson Medical Center and her personal beliefs should have nothing to do with it.[165] Sanger was eventually admitted into the Arizona Hall of Fame.

On January 1, 1991, Sanger's grandson, Alexander C. Sanger, became president and chief executive officer of Planned Parenthood's largest affiliate. Upon taking over at Planned Parenthood of New York City, Alexander Sanger said, "With all her success, my grandmother left some unfinished business and I intend to finish it."[166]

Born to Margaret Sanger's youngest son, Alexander Sanger graduated from Princeton University and Columbia Law School. He holds two master's degrees. Alexander Sanger was a partner at the Wall Street law firm of White and Case and later became chief executive officer of plastics manufacturing firms. He served for seven years on the board of directors of Planned Parenthood's New York City affiliate before becoming its leader.[167]

At 43 years of age when he accepted his most recent post, Alexander Sanger admits that his name has been "invaluable and recognizable and important to many people." Alexander Sanger says he hopes to increase the number of Planned Parenthood clinics in New York City from three to ten. He emphasizes that his first priority is to change the Planned Parenthood office in central Harlem into a clinic.[168]

SEEKING THE TRUTH

Now that many books have been written about the life of Margaret Sanger, it is important to remember that not all of them can be taken completely seriously. This is particularly true of Sanger's autobiographical writings. Keep in mind that not everything written by Margaret Sanger is accurate. The same is true of most of those who have written about her. Some authors, such as Joan Dash, Lawrence Lader, Milton Meltzer, Virginia Coigney, Emily Taft Douglas, Joan Marlow, and Elyse Topalian, overlooked Sanger's seedy side in favor of creating a heroine.

As David M. Kennedy notes in a biographical essay in *Birth Control in America: The Career of Margaret Sanger*, at least two of Sanger's books, *My Fight for Birth Control* and *Margaret Sanger: An Autobiography*, "were ghost-written and have the flavor (and reliability) of campaign biographies. Most biographical writing about Mrs. Sanger," Kennedy continues, "has suffered from close reliance on these two books." Kennedy cites *The Margaret Sanger Story: And the Fight for Birth Control*, by Lawrence Lader, who co-founded the National Association for the Repeal of Abortion Laws (now called the National Abortion Rights Action League; see *Aborting America*, by Bernard N. Nathanson, M.D.), as one of the worst offenders, and *The Birth Controllers* by Peter Fryer as one of the least.[169]

Three authors, Kennedy, Fryer, and Madeline Gray, though they do not appear to be anti-Sanger, are careful to include both the positive and negative aspects of her life. As Kennedy essentially states, this kind of neutral writing is rare where Margaret Sanger is the subject.

DEFENDING THE FOUNDATION

A 1954 Planned Parenthood Federation of America newsletter encourages supporters to subscribe to a journal on eugenics:

Eugenics Quarterly, a new journal published by the American Eugenics Society, carries material of interest to Planned Parenthood supporters. The following articles, written for the layman as well as the scientist, appear in the June 1954 (Vol. I, No. 2) issue:

"Effect of Birth Control on the Character and Intelligence of Succeeding Generations," by F. Osborn.

"Sex Education and Eugenics," by Jacob Goldberg.

"Heredity Counseling," by Sheldon Reed.

"Heredity and the Eye," by Conrad Berens, M.D.

"Female Sterilization in Puerto Rico," by M. Stycos.

"Genetic Studies of Population," by Bruce Wallace.

"Congregational Ministers' Birth Rate," by C. Tietze.

"The Burgess-Wallin Report: A Contribution to Eugenics Through the Improvement of Marriage," by Joseph Folsom.

A sample copy of *Eugenics Quarterly* will be sent free upon request to the American Eugenics Society . . .

(Since Eugenics depends on planned parenthood, and planned parenthood has a considerable effect, genetically, on the human race, this journal should be of considerable interest to PPFA friends and supporters.—W.V.[William Vogt, then-national director and executive vice president of the Planned Parenthood Federation of America])[170]

A 1955 Planned Parenthood newsletter advertises autographed copies of Lawrence Lader's biography of Margaret Sanger, *The Margaret Sanger Story: And the Fight for Birth Control.* The text of the advertisement refers to Sanger as "a great crusader for human rights." The advertisement quotes the Rev. John Haynes Holmes as saying, "Mrs. Sanger is one of the great and noble women of our time. Already she has achieved immortality."[171]

A Planned Parenthood affiliate newsletter notes that a party was held "honoring Margaret Sanger." The party was held in 1965 and sponsored by Planned Parenthood of Phoenix and Tucson, Arizona.[172] Another newsletter states, "The revolutionary philosophies of the compassionate, caring women who quietly met the desperate need for family planning in 1937 now are integral to the American way of life."[173]

In a foreword to a 1969 biography of Sanger, Mary Steichen Calderone, M.D., then-medical director of the Planned Parenthood Federation of America, writes that Margaret Sanger is, indeed, a heroine whom, "without question, millions of people already on earth or yet to be born will, without ever knowing it, owe her a debt without measure."[174]

Calderone, who later founded the Sex Information and Education Council of the United States (SIECUS), writes that "it wasn't the development of modern medical methods of birth control that is her greatest achievement, for many people contributed to this, but rather the concept, the infinitely basic and universal *human* concept, of *the right of every woman to total sovereignty over her own person.*"[175] For Calderone, this is the most important point of all:

Margaret Sanger recognized the right of the woman in regard to her own body, and also the right of the child to be wanted. She also clearly recognized the terrible dangers of overpopulation and its effects on human beings in terms of wars and antisocial behavior. She certainly must have foreseen, because this is what she worked for, how freedom from fear of unwanted pregnancy would serve to strengthen and deepen the sexual relationship between husband and wife and therefore the well-being of the whole family.[176]

In 1975, a publication of the Planned Parenthood Federation of America included an article concerning the intellectually challenged. "We agree," one paper reads, "that most retarded are not able to carry the burden of parenthood and that the unassailable right of the child to have a fair chance in life supercedes the right of the retarded to procreate."[177] The same article refers to the intellectually challenged as "mentally defective." As surprising as this may be, the authors also separate the "mentally defective" from "the other defectives, such as the blind, the epileptic, the criminal and the sex offender . . . "[178] Effectively, then, Planned Parenthood leaders believe that since "mentally defective" individuals cannot be good parents and, as parents, could not give their offspring a "fair chance in life," such "defective" people should not be allowed to have children.

Planned Parenthood continues to hail Margaret Sanger as a heroine and the pioneer of reproductive rights. One would think that any organization founded by Sanger would attempt to eradicate her memory and escape any association with her ideas. To the contrary, Planned Parenthood eulogizes Margaret Sanger.

In a Planned Parenthood fund-raising letter signed by actress Katharine Hepburn, Sanger's name is mentioned twice. "Over fifty years ago, my mother helped Margaret Sanger found a new, controversial organization called the American Birth Control League. That organization later became Planned Parenthood," Hepburn writes. Sanger's name is again mentioned near the end of the letter when Hepburn writes, "Planned Parenthood is not losing sight of Margaret Sanger's original goal . . ."[179]

Another fund-raising letter, signed by Faye Wattleton, then-president of the Planned Parenthood Federation of America, spoke of Sanger with adulation:

> . . . PLANNED PARENTHOOD was founded by a determined woman who was jailed many times before she saw her dream become reality.
>
> Margaret Sanger, an American pioneer in the truest and noblest self-sacrificing sense, was committed to seeing that the poor women in 1916 did not have *their* "right to life" destroyed by a cycle of oversized families and poverty. And she dedicated her own life to freeing these helpless women from a succession of unwanted pregnancies, which often led to early deaths in childbirth. And she launched her courageous crusade: To educate American parents on how to control the size of their families—*how to plan parenthood.* For this "crime" she was arrested and jailed time and again. Yet, on each release from imprisonment, Margaret Sanger with quiet determination returned to her just cause: *freeing women the world over from the slavery of uncontrolled reproduction.*
>
> Today, her dream—PLANNED PARENTHOOD—is a reality with over 100,000 supporters, 20,000 active volunteers, over 700 clinics in the United States, and with programs in 111 foreign countries. And now, more than 100 years after her birth, Margaret Sanger's memory is honored throughout the world by men and women who understand her monumental achievements for humanity.
>
> Yet, the same kind of thinking which sent Mrs. Sanger to jail is still with us.[180]

Wattleton called upon Sanger's memory toward the end of her letter as well:

> In 1916, Margaret Sanger suffered unrelenting ridicule, arrests and jail sentences before she saw her unfailing belief in the right of all men and women to intelligently plan their parenthood become a reality in PLANNED PARENTHOOD. . . .
>
> Now, we at PLANNED PARENTHOOD do not ask that you make such a personal sacrifice. We only ask that you look to your conscience and then contribute what you can. Every dollar you send us will be immediately put to full use . . . [181]

Faye Wattleton had eulogized Margaret Sanger on many occasions. Wattleton said, "I believe that Margaret Sanger would have been proud of us today if she had seen the directions that we have most recently in this organization taken."[182]

Wattleton appeared on the "Home Show" on the 75th anniversary of Planned Parenthood. She said that Margaret Sanger's "dream perhaps is mostly fulfilled, but there is still a long way to go, ah, and it's interesting that 75 years later we're using a lot of the same methods that she taught and promoted and we certainly are fighting the same political battles that she fought." Wattleton claimed Sanger "was jailed nine times for her efforts."[183]

During his campaign for president of the United States in 1988, Republican R. G. "Pat" Robertson, speaking before a legislative committee in New Hampshire, commented on Planned Parenthood's founder. Robertson claimed Planned Parenthood's long-range goal is to create a "master race" and that its founder "wanted to sterilize blacks, Jews, mental defectives and fundamentalist Christians."[184]

Robertson, host of "The 700 Club," said Sanger "was an advocate of what was called eugenics" and that "some of her literature undergirded the genetic experiments of Adolf Hitler."[185] Robertson charged that, in fact, it was Hitler who copied Sanger's philosophy, not visa versa.[186]

Robertson was attacked for his comments, especially by Faye Wattleton, who said, "All the charges are unfounded and, frankly, ridiculous." She said Robertson's allegations are "without any basis, any substance or even any remnants of facts." Sanger's philosophies, Wattleton claimed, "were not based on eugenics" but rather "on people being allowed to choose for themselves."[187]

Wattleton took the opportunity to attack Robertson's credibility. She said, "It is truly amazing that he should speak with such inadequate information on such a serious subject . . . It makes me wonder what other issues of significance he is ill-informed about."[188] The opportunity was surely welcomed as the election of Pat Robertson would certainly have been Wattleton's worst nightmare.

In a 1984 interview, however, Wattleton conceded that Sanger held views based on "eugenics and the advancement of the perfect race . . ."[189] Either Wattleton has a short memory or she was willing to employ deceitful character assassination to masque her organization's legacy and agenda.

When Kay Lindley was a California radio program host, she prepared a report on Planned Parenthood for "Focus on the Family," a popular program heard throughout North America. Lindley asked Janice Sinclair, a Planned Parenthood spokeswoman from Los Angeles, to comment on the organization's founder. Sinclair said, "We're definitely proud of our heritage and proud of our founder, Margaret Sanger, and we continue to keep fighting the good fight in her honor because she laid the groundwork for family planning, for legal abortion for American women, and many of her ideas that were seen as being radical back then would be considered commonplace today."[190]

To this day, no major leader of Planned Parenthood has repudiated Margaret Sanger's heinous comments and beliefs.

2

A NEW DIRECTION

There are many reasons for Planned Parenthood's astounding prosperity and influence. Planned Parenthood is known for its articulate leaders, most of whom are women. The selection of good spokesmen is one of the most important advantages enjoyed by the organization. The past president of the Planned Parenthood Federation of America did more for the organization than virtually all of its present and former employees combined.

EARLY YEARS

Alyce Faye Wattleton was born in St. Louis, Missouri, on July 8, 1943. Her father, a factory worker, passed away in 1970. Wattleton's mother, the Reverend Ozie Wattleton, is a minister at East Atlanta Church of God. Her grandmother was also a minister. Ozie Wattleton disagrees with her daughter on abortion.[1] Nevertheless, Faye Wattleton calls her mother "a woman of very high integrity."[2]

Faye Wattleton was raised on a "strict fundamentalist creed." Wattleton describes her mother, who had wanted her only child to become a fundamentalist nurse and missionary, as her role model. This is not because of the Reverend's beliefs, but because her mother had been a strong example. As Wattleton puts it, "I come from a long line of women who are quite dignified, quite proud, and are hardly intimidated by anything."[3]

Faye Wattleton earned a bachelor of science in nursing degree at Ohio State University. She received a master's degree in maternal and infant health care, with certification as a nurse-midwife, from Columbia University.[4]

Wattleton claims that her fanatical support of legal abortion is based on having witnessed a teenager die from a botched abortion:

> She just went into renal failure and died.
>
> I believe everyone should have a chance to live.
>
> That teenager was coherent to the end and when her heart stopped and long after she grew cold all I could think was "what a waste."[5]

Faye Wattleton says seeing "sickness, death, birth, [and] trying to live" first-hand caused her to break with her family's morality.[6]

Wattleton divorced Franklin Gordon, a jazz pianist and mental health social worker, in 1981. Frederick C. Smith, a Wattleton friend and colleague for many years, says he asked her if she could hold the marriage together. Smith says he asked Wattleton where she put the marriage on her list of priorities. "Well, it's pretty clear, looking back, where she put it," Smith said.[7]

Faye Wattleton has one child, a daughter, named Felicia Wattleton. They attended Marble Collegiate Church, where Norman Vincent Peale has been the pastor for many years, when they lived in New York.

A LITTLE TO THE LEFT

Faye Wattleton became president of the Planned Parenthood Federation of America in 1978. She had served as executive director of Planned Parenthood's Dayton, Ohio, affiliate since 1970.

Wattleton immediately made history upon her ascension to the top of the organization. According to one writer, "Wattleton's election to the presidency of Planned Parenthood was an effort to answer some of the organization's critics . . . "[8] She is the first woman since Margaret Sanger to head Planned Parenthood. Wattleton is also the first African-American to lead the group. She became president at the age of 34 which also makes her the youngest person to lead Planned Parenthood.[9] Until Wattleton became president, the organization was described as a "largely white"[10] or "upper middle class"[11] charity.

One national business magazine notes that soon after being hired as president, Wattleton sought the most skilled employees and launched a high-incentive salary program:

> She [Wattleton] also recruited top talent and installed novel incentive-pay arrangements. Without clear profit-and-loss responsibility, how does a nonprofit pay people for performance? At Planned Parenthood, all employees must set personal objectives every year. Each goal is assigned a percentage weight to determine its importance. Managers evaluate progress against each goal, grading them from 1 for unsatisfactory to 5 for superior performance. Pay hikes are dished out based on the overall grade.
>
> "If you work for a nonprofit, you shouldn't have to commit yourself to self-denial, poverty, and self-sacrifice," says Wattleton. "I don't subscribe to the fruit-and-flower philosophy of the nonprofit world."[12]

In a major policy shift, Faye Wattleton turned Planned Parenthood from simply a contraceptive provider into the strongest defender of unrestricted abortion. As one writer observes, "Since it took the role as a standard-bearer in the crusade to keep abortion legal, Planned Parenthood has become far richer and more famous than ever before." In fact, Planned Parenthood places "slightly ahead of more mainstream health charities like the American Lung Association and the Easter Seals . . ." in fund-raising.[13]

The *New York Times Magazine* published a feature story about Wattleton in 1989. The article points to the change in direction made by Wattleton:

> For most Americans, Planned Parenthood remains a provider of gynecological examinations, Pap smear tests and birth-control counseling. . . . But it now brings its considerable heft to a pro-choice coalition that includes the National Organization for Women (NOW), the National Abortion Rights Action League, the Fund for the Feminist Majority and the American Civil Liberties Union.[14]

Before Wattleton, Planned Parenthood was careful not to offend donors and potential donors:

> "When Faye first came, Planned Parenthood wouldn't use the word *abortion* in its mail," recalls Roger Craver, a direct-mail consultant whose many clients include Greenpeace and Planned Parenthood. "It wasn't polite to use that word. The organization's most vocal critics at the time—five years after *Roe*—were not right-to-lifers, they were civil rights groups, which accused Planned Parenthood of practicing a form of genocide, and feminists, who viewed the organization as a male-dominated effort to control women's reproductive lives."[15]

Not everyone approves of Wattleton's new direction, the main component of which is her decision to fight hard for unrestricted abortion:

> Some of the group's longstanding members are unhappy with the policy shift under Wattleton. "We have always been a contraceptive-services health-care provider," says a former executive director, stressing each syllable. "I think it is very damaging for the organization to be associated in the public mind so completely with abortion."[16]

Internal struggles regarding Planned Parenthood's role in abortion were common when Wattleton first became president of the organization. Such struggles continued throughout her reign, but each battle usually ended quickly:

> There have been heated debates within the organization over just how much energy and resources Planned Parenthood should devote to abortion rights—debates that Wattleton has usually won. Over the objections of some of her own board members, Wattleton has launched explicit pro-choice mail campaigns and spent hundreds of thousands of dollars on full-page newspaper ads. Two year ago she pressed—successfully—for the creation of a special lobbying arm to allow Planned Parenthood to engage directly in the political fight over abortion. Although Planned Parenthood has decided not to endorse specific candidates, through its political arm it can—and Wattleton frequently does—urge women to vote pro-choice.[17]

Wattleton's establishment of a more corporate image for Planned Parenthood has also not been met with total enthusiasm:

> When she first assumed leadership of Planned Parenthood, Wattleton had to battle on two fronts: one, predictably, against the anti-abortion forces and the other against those within her organization who resented the corporate structure she imposed on the New York [national] office. Wattleton brought in the media consultants and the pollsters. She established a Washington lobbying office. She created nine vice presidencies, responsible for matters ranging from legal affairs to international programs and medicine, that now constitute a hierarchic layer between the president and staff members. In the course of this corporate makeover, 60 to 70 percent of the New York staff resigned or were dismissed.[18]

While some claim Wattleton harmed the organization she once led, few seem willing to speak publicly:

> Staffers at the Planned Parenthood affiliates—and the other organizations in the pro-choice coalition, for that matter—show a marked reluctance to speak on the record about either Wattleton or the organization in general. Once voiced, any criticisms are quickly retracted. Caution seems to be rooted in a healthy respect for Wattleton's powers of righteous indignation, and her reputation for having a very long memory.[19]

While some within Planned Parenthood may have opposed Faye Wattleton's changes, the fact remains that during her tenure, she was in firm control of the organization. This control seemed to increase when Wattleton appeared in public.

Wattleton's success in turning Planned Parenthood into a powerhouse has been recognized even by those not directly involved in the abortion debate. *Business*

Week named Wattleton one of the best "social service agency" managers in the United States. "In terms of public recognition, Faye Wattleton may be the non-profit equivalent of Lee Iacocca," the magazine reads. "As president of Planned Parenthood Federation of America, she is widely known as the nation's leading pro-choice advocate."[20]

Business Week points to the growth of Planned Parenthood under Wattleton's leadership, and no wonder. Donations to Planned Parenthood's national office alone increased from $4.7 million to between $44 million and $50 million per annum, depending on the year, and the overall budget more than tripled.[21] In 1990, Planned Parenthood had at least 911 clinics, 172 affiliates, 26,000 staff and volunteers, and 480,000 donors throughout the United States.[22] Following restructuring and consolidation which took place in 1991, the number of Planned Parenthood affiliates at the end of the year stood at 170.

Other publications recognize Wattleton's success:

> Showing a keen understanding of the underdog's advantage, Wattleton has used each loss to rally pro-choice sympathizers, organizing speaking tours and demonstrations and launching aggressive advertising campaigns. As a result, in the last few years, she's managed to almost double the size of Planned Parenthood's contributor list. . . .
>
> Today there is almost no one who would question Wattleton's ability to oversee Planned Parenthood or its . . . budget. But in the course of proving herself, Wattleton has generated a new set of anxieties about her leadership style. Much of the controversy is about just that—style. Many Planned Parenthood staff members and volunteers are uncomfortable with Wattleton's distant—some call it imperious—manner; others are dismayed by her $184,000-a-year salary [later increased to $200,000] and her glamorous, and obviously expensive, taste in clothes and jewelry. A statuesque five foot eleven [some sources say six feet], Wattleton doesn't fit most people's image of a crusader; Florence Nightingale in a starched blouse or Mother Teresa in a shapeless habit.[23]

One Wattleton colleague says, "If she were an ax murderer, no one would tell you."[24]

Wattleton claims to have considered, and rejected, all objections to her emphasis on abortion:

> "What this criticism suggests," she says, "is that the fight for legal abortion is something that is unpleasant and unattractive and negative. I think that it comes out of the same genre as those people who believe that the only women who get abortions do so with gnashing of teeth and wringing of hands and who do not realize that for a lot of women this is a positive decision—the only decision—and they don't have to gnash their teeth and feel horrible guilt."[25]

Wattleton did not simply insist that Planned Parenthood play the leadership role in defending legal abortion. She changed her strategy from one of acknowledging the moral dilemma involved with abortion to one of approving it as a positive decision:

> "It's not," she concedes, "that I don't understand the philosophical and ethical dilemmas"—but she insists that such moral questions lie outside her purview. "We're talking about women having a choice—a choice to be left alone with their personal decisions."[26]

Wattleton apparently believes that emphasizing personal choice over the moral questions can mean greater success for her cause. "I am very positive about this being a choice for women," she says.[27]

While Wattleton shaped a new course for Planned Parenthood, it is not vastly different from that envisioned by the organization's founder. In her speech accepting the Humanist of the Year Award, Wattleton spoke of how proud she was to be walking "in the footsteps of Margaret Sanger" and she was "truly honored" to receive the award.[28] "It means that I have one more thing in common with a woman who was a sister nurse and the first leader of Planned Parenthood—Margaret Sanger, the founder of the family planning movement in this country and the recipient of the Humanist of the Year Award in 1957," Wattleton said.[29] As noted in chapter 1, Sanger was not a nurse.

It is clear that Faye Wattleton moved Planned Parenthood even further into the forefront of the battle for unrestricted abortion. This decision, whether best for the organization or not, will have a long-lasting impact on the group's public image. Additionally, the decision will significantly impact the kinds of services Planned Parenthood will offer in the future.

"For better or worse," states Warren Pearse, executive director of the American College of Obstetricians and Gynecologists, "Planned Parenthood has become identified in the popular mind as an organization that has a primary emphasis on abortion." Even though Pearce's organization actively supports legal abortion, he says that if it "were to form a coalition to deal with unintended pregnancy," its leaders "would probably not choose, first off, Planned Parenthood."[30]

Wattleton was paid $200,000 per year and received $7,736 per year in benefits at the time of her departure from Planned Parenthood.[31] The salary is up from the $70,000 per year received when she became president.[32] Wattleton had said she wanted to remain president of Planned Parenthood as long as it takes to see the introduction of the abortion pill RU 486 into the American market.[33] However, on January 8, 1992, Wattleton announced her resignation effective in March 1992.

The resignation of Faye Wattleton was a surprise to most people on both sides of the abortion issue. Wattleton said she was quitting to host a one-hour television talk show in Chicago, Illinois. It was developed by the Tribune Entertainment Company and will be a "serious, issues-based program."[34] "While it is very difficult to leave Planned Parenthood after 14 exciting and rewarding years as its president," Wattleton said, "I am looking forward to this challenging new venture."[35]

Phil Donahue, an active supporter of legal abortion, says Wattleton will be a good addition to the long list of talk show hosts. "I must not tell a lie—I'm crazy about Faye Wattleton. She's a woman of extreme courage. I think she's going to be a real presence in the increasingly crowded talk show field."[36]

"Among the things I learned to appreciate was the enormous power of the media to shape the debate," Wattleton told one writer, "to focus on individuals, to really provide channels for voices." The show will start on a few stations and eventually go national. All topics will be considered for discussion on the show, except for one—abortion.[37] The Pro-Life Action League launched a campaign to keep Wattleton off the air soon after plans for the program were announced.

It has long been my view that Wattleton will eventually run for public office. "I would not make a good politician," Wattleton says. "The art of compromise is the substance of politics, and I'm not very good at compromising principles."[38] Maybe so, but that does not exactly mean she is absolutely ruling it out.

STAR QUALITY

The February 1990 edition of *Glamour* states that Wattleton had been "emerging as the leading" spokesman for legal abortion and she is "articulate, strikingly telegenic, bright, and most importantly, messianic on this subject."[39] She has also been described as tough, rational, cool, glamorous, and shrewd.

Comparing Wattleton's public speaking abilities to those of Demosthenes, one newspaper describes her as an "urbane woman" and a "woman of intellect."[40] A "PrimeTime Live" correspondent referred to Wattleton as "one of America's most beautiful women and even in a crowd of Hollywood personalities, it's Faye Wattleton who is the star."[41] A *Detroit News* article states that Wattleton "looks like a Hollywood version of a corporate queen" and refers to her "passionate rationalism and measured indignation."[42]

Some in the media note Wattleton's relative calm on the outside, even though she is angry on the inside:

> In the face of the most provocative, even personal, attacks, Wattleton can always be counted on to remain poised and articulate, her calm reinforced by her striking good looks. "Faye," Eleanor Smeal, the former president of the National Organization for Women, says with admiration, "simply radiates confidence."[43]

The August 1989 issue of *National Geographic* named Wattleton one of the nation's most influential African-Americans. A summer 1990 special issue of *People* featured Wattleton as one of the "50 most beautiful people in the world." In the summer of 1989, *Harper's Bazaar* named Wattleton one of eight "Over-40 and Sensational" women. She was listed as one of the "twenty coolest women" by *Sassy*, the largest readership of which is young women, primarily teenagers.

In an interview with the *New York Times Magazine*, a supporter of legal abortion refers to Wattleton's race as a plus:

> "She is stunning," says Molly Yard, [then-] president of NOW [National Organization for Women]. "She is also black. And she is a mother. She makes a pretty picture."[44]

While Faye Wattleton may want little more than to see unrestricted abortion the law throughout the world, there may be other reasons for her zealous involvement in the abortion debate. Wattleton's "stardom," combined with her work for legal abortion, led to other opportunities and she may have planned to capitalize on it:

> [A]s she crisscrosses the country, speaking in her powerful rhythms, she not only advances the cause but advances herself as well.
>
> "It's not only what she says," explains Ann F. Lewis, a political consultant who is the former political director of the Democratic National Committee. "It's how she's saying it that has made her such a force. We yearn for a woman's voice speaking with authority. And she is emerging as a role model, an individual viewed as courageous and committed by a society that is hungry for heroes."
>
> "Listen, most politicians spend their entire careers in search of an issue," says Robert Squier, media consultant for Democratic candidates, "and here we have a situation in which a person and an issue have perfectly come together. Suddenly we have this woman who comes center stage . . . and she has to be taken seriously as a political force."[45]

FRAMING THE DEBATE

Wattleton is a master at using rhetoric and techniques of persuasion to frame the abortion debate in a manner which serves her cause, though it could be argued that it avoids the real issues. Her most common technique was to argue that the issue being debated has nothing to do with abortion:

> [T]his is not a debate about abortion. . . . This is about a fundamental right to make choices about our sexuality—without the encroachment of a president, the Supreme Court and certainly without the encroachment of politicians! . . .
>
> This is an issue about what American women will be able to do with their lives.[46]

The strategy was used time and time again. When Congress considered allowing Washington, D.C., to spend locally raised funds on abortions for poor women, Wattleton would frame the debate as one of "home rule." When Congress considered reversing the Title X (pronounced "title 10") regulations, the debate was framed as one of "free speech" (see chapters 4 and 9). When state legislators considered requiring parental consent or notification for abortions performed on minors, the debate was framed as one of "child abuse" and "broken homes."

While this strategy seems to be universally employed by supporters of legal abortion, others believe it should be carried even further. Laurie Belin writes that Planned Parenthood should frame the debate by rejecting such phrases as "abortion rights" and slogans like, "Keep abortion safe and legal." Belin explains:

> Planned Parenthood is not completely blind to the power of rhetoric. The phase "right to life" does not appear anywhere in the organization's literature; opponents are labeled "anti-choice." Not bad. "Anti-free choice" would be better still.
>
> But strangely, free-choice advocates seem unable to apply this principle to themselves. Last April [1989], hundreds of thousands of free-choice supporters marched in Washington. Unfortunately, the march was billed as an "abortion rights rally." A plea for abortion rights may have been enough to inspire those who marched, but it distorted the true goal of the rally: to preserve personal freedom, not to preserve abortion.
>
> Two weeks ago I marched in Washington as free-choice supporters mobilized again. Many carried signs advocating "Choice for Women" or "Abortion on Demand." But for every person who carried a placard with the critical word "freedom," dozens waved official Planned Parenthood signs with the slogan, "Keep Abortion Legal."
>
> The free-choice movement needs more than the support of the already converted. Planned Parenthood's leaders must urge free-choice supporters to change the terms of the debate.
>
> "Keep Abortion Safe and Legal" is a counterproductive slogan. Even the label "pro-choice" fails to convey the central idea. Framing the argument in terms of "free choice" addresses the real issue at stake. Who maintains the right to choose, the individual or the state?[47]

Wattleton used other techniques. She strategically used the fact that she is African-American, often referring to it in debates as though her opponents are not aware of it and implying that because of her race, her opinions should not be questioned. Similarly, in a televised debate with Operation Rescue founder Randall Terry, Wattleton declared, "I do not need you to tell me what my choices are about my life and my body because I am a black person. I can make that choice for myself, just as every black woman can make that choice for herself."[48]

Wattleton claims it is Terry and his ilk who make use of rhetoric instead of logic:

> "I have not tried to counter the emotional rhetoric [of Randall Terry], because I don't think this is a battle about rhetoric," she says. "That's why it is not hard for me to maintain a level of dignity and decorum while he is yelling and pontificating. Because it's not about that. It's about women's lives, it's about our value.
>
> "I really go quite berserk at those people who write that the anti-abortion people—I am always loath to call them pro-life—have won the rhetoric battle," Wattleton continues. "The women that [sic] I saw who were injured and died were not victims of rhetoric."[49]

Another Wattleton pattern was to make it appear as though a question had been answered when in reality she was evading its point. When asked a question by a reporter or at a public gathering, she would often twist it into something else. For example, NBC's Tom Brokaw posed a question to Wattleton:

> [A] recent Boston Globe poll indicated that 75 percent of the American women who were having an abortion said the baby would interfere with their work or with their school, with other responsibilities. Are you beginning to lose that argument, do you think, with the American public, because the same poll indicated that that wasn't sufficient reason for an abortion?[50]

The question posed to Wattleton is not complex. A simple answer would do. Planned Parenthood opposes *all* restrictions on abortion. A strong majority of the American people believe that most reasons given for having an abortion are not good enough. Is Planned Parenthood losing this argument? Wattleton responds by saying, "Well, I think what we've seen is that the American public believes that there are increasingly more reasons why abortion is legitimate."[51] A direct answer does not appear to be in Wattleton's response. Moreover, she denies the facts of the situation.

The poll showed even more. Wattleton continues:

> There's no question that there is a good deal of conflict and ambiguity among Americans for the reasons that people give in having abortions, but I think that poll also showed that while some women feel that the time may be wrong for them to, in terms of their being best suited, to have a baby, they also desire in the future to have children and feel that they can be better prepared to give a child a better life and a better family if they forego a pregnancy at this time and I think that's a very best environment to bring a child into the world.[52]

The poll does not show a "good deal" of "conflict and ambiguity" regarding the reasons for having an abortion. It said 75 percent of the American people oppose most abortions. The poll is not the least bit unclear, yet Wattleton convinces her audience that "conflict and ambiguity" are reflected in the results. In addition, look for the logic in the remainder of the answer. Wattleton starts to say what the poll "also showed," but the remainder of the answer does not relate to the poll at all. Her supplementary remarks have nothing to do with the poll and nothing to do with the question. Without close examination, however, it seems to many listeners that a good response has been given. In reality, Wattleton turns a question, which is void of a pro-Planned Parenthood answer, into a fragmented speech entirely independent of the question. It must be noted that listening to the manner in which the non-answer is given, it sure *sounds* like a good response.

The case cited is not an isolated example. There have been many other situations in which Wattleton succeeded in avoiding an uncomfortable issue. In the televised debate with Terry, Margaret Sanger's eugenic philosophy was raised. Terry charged that, "Margaret Sanger, the founder of Planned Parenthood, was an avowed racist. She wanted to eliminate the black community." While a brief part at the end of Wattleton's response is drowned out by audience reaction, she begins by saying, "I think it is outrageous that you have chosen to use my race to exploit your . . . "[53] Bottom line: Wattleton used supposed indignation over a perfectly legitimate issue to duck the point raised by Terry. She never did respond to the point raised. Instead we heard only a "how dare you raise that point" type of response.

Linda Layton, who authors a weekly column for the *Rockford Register Star*, makes several observations about Planned Parenthood:

> I always thought Planned Parenthood was the advocate of women, allowing them the freedom to choose if and when they have children—without government interference. The reality is, from the beginning Planned Parenthood has sought mandatory control measures. Over the years, it has proposed that our government implement:
>
> - Compulsory abortion for out-of-wedlock pregnancies.
> - Federal entitlement payments to encourage abortion.
> - Compulsory sterilization for those who have already had two children.
> - Tax penalties for existing large families.[54]

Keeping the issue in mind, examine Wattleton's response:

> Planned Parenthood's mission has always been to provide the information and options that allow individuals to make their own decisions about sexuality and fertility. We have never at any point in our 75-year history, advocated any sort of compulsory reproductive behavior—including contraception, sterilization, abortion or childbirth. For example, in recent months we have spoken out repeatedly against potential abuse of Norplant, the newly approved contraceptive implant. In one case a California judge conditioned a woman's probation on her agreement to use Norplant; in other cases there have been calls for financial inducements to encourage poor and minority women to use Norplant. Planned Parenthood vehemently opposes these and all other attempts to coerce women not to have children.[55]

How does Wattleton define "coercion"?:

> We oppose any effort to coerce women to bear children against their will. Coercion is present whenever disadvantaged people are robbed of their choices by poverty, youth, ignorance or any other reason. This is why Planned Parenthood advocates expanded access to, and government funding for family planning and safe abortion services. Basic rights must not be the privilege of the rich. Freedom of speech, freedom to vote and freedom of religion must not be based on one's ability to pay. Neither should the fundamental right to control one's own fertility.[56]

Wattleton is surely aware of the suggestions (see chapter 11) printed in the October 1970 issue of *Family Planning Perspectives*. This is probably the source of the specific measures of coercion listed by Layton. There are many more which Layton did not list including encouraging "increased homosexuality" and limiting childbearing to "a limited number of adults."[57]

Instead of dealing with the measures of coercion made in Planned Parenthood's publication, Wattleton declares fertility control a "fundamental right" which, of course, makes it supreme over other rights. It is tied to freedom of speech, the right to vote, and freedom of religion. While arguing that these rights should not be based on the ability to pay, Wattleton does not suggest that the government pay for loud speakers, printing presses, and transportation to polling booths for the poor. The argument is ridiculous on its face, but at least it filled newspaper space in a manner which made it *appear* that Wattleton addressed the issue. As usual, she turned one point into a license to discuss several unrelated matters.

Wattleton declares that Planned Parenthood has "never" advocated "compulsory reproductive behavior." While Norplant is mentioned (a poor example), she ignores Planned Parenthood's support of the forced abortion and sterilization policies of the People's Republic of China (see chapters 6, 11, and 15). Only time will tell whether Planned Parenthood's new-found "non-advocacy of" (not the same as "opposition to") coercion will remain intact.

Layton has other reasons for her concern about Planned Parenthood:

> I believed that Planned Parenthood served the needs of low income families, and especially, poor women. The reality is Planned Parenthood has always targeted minorities, the unwanted and the disadvantaged. Its goals for these groups? Limit the family, contraception, abortion and finally, sterilization. Planned Parenthood founder Margaret Sanger's idea of charity was to "eliminate the stocks (minorities)" because she felt they were detrimental to the future of the race and the world.[58]

Wattleton uses the charge as an opportunity to plug Planned Parenthood. She eventually gets to the point. This technique is used many times in the guest column:

> Planned Parenthood is America's oldest, largest and most trusted provider of voluntary family planning care. That's why nearly three million women and men turn to us each year for high-quality, confidential reproductive health services. And, contrary to Layton's claim, we do serve the needs of low-income families. In 1989, 68 percent of our contraceptive patients had incomes at or below 150 percent of the poverty level. We do not, however, "target" the poor, minorities or anyone. Our goal is to make services available to all who want and need them.[59]

Did Wattleton respond to the Sanger issue? Did she mention that the reason 68 percent of Planned Parenthood's clients are "at or below 150 percent of the poverty level" is because a teenage girl from "Beverly Hills 90210" could go to a Planned Parenthood facility, honestly write that she has no income (though her parents are worth millions), and receive free care?

Did Wattleton mention the official Planned Parenthood plans which specifically target the groups mentioned? Maybe the word "target" is the problem. The Planned Parenthood Federation of America 1989-1993 strategic plan states, "The following are the areas to be evaluated . . ." The first area mentioned is "Increasing access to services especially for the underserved, low-income, adolescent and minority populations."[60] This is not much of a change from the organization's 1975-1980 five year plan: "Emphasis shall be put on services to: Persons with low and marginal incomes; Teenagers and young adults." What services? Contraception, sterilization, abortion, "educational counseling," and venereal disease screening and diagnosis.[61] No, Wattleton does not mention these points. Did she forget? Does she think these are unimportant details, or did she intend to mislead?

Wait. It gets worse. Layton writes:

> I held the belief that Planned Parenthood was a nonprofit family planning organization. The reality is that with over 300 separate organizations in the world, a vast amount of its funding comes from you. Title X appropriations (Public Health Service Act) provide over $100 million from American taxpayers, as well as funds from 18 other federal statutes.[62]

Wattleton's responses become even more slippery:

Layton's implication that Planned Parenthood is not a legitimate nonprofit organization verges on libel. Our not-for-profit status is confirmed each year by independent audit, and any failure to meet IRS regulations would surely have been exploited by our opposition.[63]

The point is being ignored. Being a nonprofit or not-for-profit organization merely means the group does not have to pay taxes, allows a tax deduction for those supporting the "educational" aspects of the group, and implies that making a profit is not the *goal* of the organization. This does not mean the group does not make a profit. Funds left in the treasury after the fiscal year remain in the organization for increasing support of its programs, an emergency fund, or similar purposes. Of course, there are no regulations regarding how much a person working for such a group may be paid. The fact is that Planned Parenthood has an astoundingly large budget and millions of dollars are left in reserve at the end of the year. The issue has nothing to do with Internal Revenue Service regulations.

Later in the column, Layton refers to the Nuremberg Trials which followed the Nazi Holocaust.[64] Wattleton offers this response:

Layton's equation of abortion and the Holocaust is vicious and vile. There are 1.6 million women each year who make thoughtful, humane, personal decisions not to continue a pregnancy; it is monstrous to suggest that those women are the equivalent of Hitler. Moreover, in the words of the Religious Coalition for Abortion Rights, this comparison "trivializes the immensity of the Hitler government's deliberate and systematic attempt to annihilate the entire Jewish population and other groups deemed 'undesirable.'"[65]

Layton's point concerns dehumanization. She never equates Hitler with women who choose abortion. Layton does not even equate Planned Parenthood's abortion facilities with Hitler's ovens. What Wattleton seeks to do is paint Layton as "vicious," "vile," and "monstrous" in an effort to discredit her real points. Moreover, keeping in mind that Hitler is believed to be responsible for the deaths of approximately six million Jews, all of whom were innocent human beings, and that abortion in the United States has taken the lives of approximately 30 million innocent human beings, can these tragedies be compared? Are the deaths of 30 million human beings "worse" than the deaths of six million human beings? Only if we look exclusively at numbers, but a tragedy is a tragedy.

The point is that such a tragedy—a holocaust, if you will—is deplorable, period. Furthermore, when one considers that Nazi disrespect for human life allowed for unimaginable horrors, it is not hard to imagine how such a massacre could occur. People were convinced of what they knew in their hearts to be untrue: that Jews are less than human and the source of national problems.

Is it the term "holocaust" that bothered Wattleton? Would Hitler and his supporters have called what happened to the Jewish men, women, and children, a holocaust? Of course not. They would have chosen another word or phrase, such as "termination of post-placental tissue."

Wattleton uses another paragraph to refer to the "narrow, dogmatic beliefs" of the "self-righteous zealots who presume to have all the 'right' answers . . . "[66] A comparison is not made between these personal attacks and those used by slaveholders against abolitionists in the South of old.

Wattleton participated in a televised debate with John Hale, an attorney and advisor to New York's Catholic Archdiocese. She would speak at length and when Hale did get to speak, Wattleton would interrupt him. To politely suggest that

Wattleton should let him finish, Hale, a slight, gentle man, who speaks slowly and deliberately, lightly touched her forearm. Wattleton rapidly and definitively jerked her forearm away,[67] apparently in an attempt to make Hale look abusive or aggressive. It had a clear "How dare you touch me! You abusive *man!*" implication.

Faye Wattleton is skilled at controlling time in those speaking situations where she has an opponent. Virtually every answer includes unrelated material. This is a useful skill as it forces people to hear points not raised by the questions or issues posed. The debate becomes centered on Wattleton's issues, not the questions.

One of Wattleton's most intriguing techniques is to avoid questions about Planned Parenthood itself. Her response to such questions is similar to "I don't believe this is a discussion about Planned Parenthood" or "I don't think this is a program about Planned Parenthood." Of course, Wattleton would never have agreed to participate in a debate "about" Planned Parenthood.

Wattleton would insult her opponents whenever possible. This not only serves as a "red herring," it also casts doubt on the integrity of anti-abortion speakers. In addition, she liked to trap her foes into saying they oppose abortifacient methods of birth control. Throughout the remainder of the debate Wattleton notes that the abortion foe opposes "most" methods of birth control which "prevent the need for abortion." Wattleton would also use the demeaning, "I have had a baby and I don't believe you have . . ." when she debates men.[68]

Wattleton would seldom defend abortion itself. Instead, she relied on rhetoric or secondary related issues such as "freedom of choice," "back-alley abortions," and "preventing the need for abortion." (See Appendix D and E for more examples of Wattleton's techniques.)

DODGING DEBATES

Faye Wattleton has appeared on countless television and radio programs. She was the most often quoted spokesman for the pro-legal abortion movement. The National Right to Life Committee, however, says Wattleton carefully picked programs. It says she refused to debate women who are equally or more articulate. Wattleton "bullied" television networks, refusing to participate if "unacceptable" persons were scheduled to oppose her. For example, Wattleton refused to debate Mildred Jefferson, M.D., and Kay James, both of whom are intelligent, articulate, and attractive African-Americans.[69]

Other abortion foes are seeing similar tactics on the local level. Assistant Professor Gary J. Gillespie, an expert in communication, says it is understandable that Planned Parenthood spokesmen would refuse to debate articulate opponents. He argues that pro-legal abortion activists have been winning the media war because of superior strategy, style, and technique, not substance:

> The [Supreme Court's] *Webster* decision has pushed pro-choice leaders onto uncomfortably defensive territory. We've recently seen them adopt a strategy of nullification that goes like this: Don't be seen on camera with an articulate pro-lifer. Apparently, these leaders fear the positive media exposure inadvertently given to the very groups they seek to discredit. As public sentiment shifts against them, they don't want to do their cause more harm than good.[70]

Gillespie believes Planned Parenthood's philosophy is essentially that it is better to refuse a debate than to be destroyed in one:

> In short, rule number one, don't agree to public debates. Rule two, if you must debate, insist on an opponent who is inarticulate. When we think of what the pro-abortion mentality actually requires of a person, this strategy of hiding from the truth is not at all surprising.[71]

Gillespie notes that he knows several articulate abortion foes who "cannot get someone from Planned Parenthood to debate them—no matter how hard they try." According to Gillespie, "They [Planned Parenthood leaders] have too much to lose."[72]

Planned Parenthood leaders on the local level, while generally not as articulate as their former national president, are also known for their persuasive public speaking. This skill is surely one of the most important components of the hiring process at Planned Parenthood. The national office provides training and imposes limits on what can and cannot be said in public.

Abortion foes, on the other hand, are most often untrained or poorly trained volunteers. Many of those working full time to outlaw abortion are also weak at persuasive public speaking. Many abortion opponents seem uninterested in improving in this area. Many do not see a problem, thinking they are quite effective, even though they are not. The fact remains that, generally, abortion foes are destroyed in speaking situations by supporters of legal abortion. This is due exclusively to a style and technique advantage enjoyed by supporters of legal abortion.

Abortion foes must learn that not everyone is gifted to be in front of a public audience. Not everyone is gifted to debate the abortion issue on television, be it a national or local program. Not everyone is skilled to speak at a press conference. Those who oppose legal abortion, sometimes self-appointed leaders and spokesmen, tend to address audiences in a way that is pleasing to them but they are ignored (or worse) by the listeners. The end result is that the audience is not motivated to change and, sometimes, the stereotypes about abortion foes are reinforced.

It should be noted that skills of persuasion often, but not always, are attainable by those who are properly trained. This is one area, and a critical area, where supporters of legal abortion are generally dominant. This is not to say that the movement working to outlaw abortion has no skilled speakers. The best speakers are those who know that speeches and debates should be done with only two considerations in mind: Who am I trying to convince and how can I best do so? Some of my personal, well-known favorites include: Bernard N. Nathanson, M.D., Carol Everett, Michael Schwartz, George Grant, Ken Connor, J.D., Greg Schlueter, Janet Folger, Mildred Jefferson, M.D., and Kay James.

Nathanson and Everett are extremely difficult to debate given that they were once intimately involved in the abortion industry. Both are cool under pressure, articulate, knowledgeable, and have a high degree of credibility.

Schwartz, who is with the Center for Social Policy at the Free Congress Foundation, is exceptionally knowledgeable and skilled. Grant is not only an expert on Planned Parenthood, he is also an excellent speaker.

Connor, with Florida Right to Life, is handsome and articulate. More importantly, it is difficult to dislike him. Even some of Connor's most ardent opponents like him. As a correspondent with ABC said, "If the anti-abortion movement needs a poster boy, it could do worse than Ken Connor."[73] That is probably the best compliment an anti-abortion activist ever publicly received from a network correspondent.

Schlueter and Folger are young and articulate. Schleuter's specialty seems to be with young anti-abortion audiences as he is a great motivator. Folger, who is with Ohio Right to Life, is an intelligent and attractive woman who has a tremendous sense of humor which she uses during her speeches.

Dr. Jefferson, the first African-American woman to graduate from Harvard Medical School, has a lot in common with James. Both are beautiful, intelligent, and glib African-Americans. They would likely have given Wattleton the most trouble.

All of the speakers noted above, as well as some not mentioned, could surely have done well against Wattleton. The only problem is they will never have the chance.

One of the most common strategies to "train" speakers opposed to abortion is for "experts" to hold speaking and strategy seminars across the country. Those who attend largely leave with a greater knowledge of the issues and techniques. They also often feel they are prepared to take on the world. Knowledge does not mean an ability to apply the required techniques. Unfortunately, most techniques taught are not learned. This is because they require three important elements which cannot be attained at a seminar: a certain kind of personality, a quick mind which can immediately analyze an argument and come up with an appropriate response, and, most importantly, many years of practice. While the seminars are good for examining the issues of concern, they cannot "train speakers" per sé.

ATTITUDE

Not surprisingly, Faye Wattleton has strong opinions regarding her race and gender. She believes that those who oppose public funding of abortion are essentially anti-poor, anti-woman, and anti-African-American. Questioned about the Hyde Amendment, which bans federal funding of abortion except when necessary to save the mother's life, Wattleton says the law "is a reflection of this country's tremendous anger and resentment toward poor people."[74] However, Wattleton does not just see the law and other restrictions on abortion as anti-poor:

> I see the attacks on abortion and family planning as fundamentally antiwoman, and the attacks on poor women as being primarily antipoor and antiblack, because poverty conjures up images of black women on welfare. So they punish them by cutting off certain health services.[75]

Wattleton did not comment on the fact that approximately one-third of all abortions are performed on African-Americans while they only make up about 12 percent of the entire population. Therefore, by percentage, anti-abortion laws would protect more African-American lives than those of other races.

Planned Parenthood should wake up and smell the genocide. Wattleton's comments are especially interesting considering Margaret Sanger's reasons for advocating birth control and abortion. For Sanger, they were tools to advance her eugenic philosophy because she was anti-poor and anti-African-American. For Wattleton, they are somehow tools to "free" the same groups (see chapter 10).

Similarly, Wattleton sees anti-abortion laws as attempts to control women in general. She refers to the historic exploitation of women:

> I have always seen it [abortion] as an issue of choice and an issue of self-determination. Make no mistake—the double standard is still alive and well in our society. The imposition of male values, the exploitation, the statistics on rape, and date rape in particular, all point to the perception that women are there to be used, that women's choices and desires are not to be honored and respected. . . .
>
> We're out of the kitchen and it is unlikely that we're going to go back; so, how do you maintain control over a major segment of the community that has always been controlled? The strong, overarching message is that the best way is by maintaining sexual control. . . .
>
> If we can't take charge of this most personal aspect of our lives, we can't take care of anything.[76]

A comment about Wattleton's emphasis on "choice" is important. *New Dimensions* puts the tactic in perspective:

> "Planned Parenthood does not advocate abortion," insists David Hass, Planned Parenthood of Wisconsin's board president. "We advocate the right of women to make choices."
>
> Choices.
>
> It's a magic word. "Choice" is the sacred mantra whose utterance excites supporters and silences critics; it is the "Open Sesame" that mysteriously opens up the congressional treasure cave. Across the country, from major cities to small towns, Planned Parenthood's thousands of clinic workers are able to hold their heads high in the face of constant criticism over their abortion advocacy, and to look children, parents, school boards, and presidents straight in the eye. How? By intoning the magic word, of course. "We believe in informed choice. We offer unbiased, accurate, complete information and let women choose for themselves. We believe women have the right to choose when to have children."[77]

"Choice" is cherished by abortion opponents as well, but they claim that no civilized society has unlimited choice. Choice cannot be used as an excuse or license to kill.

The new direction established by Faye Wattleton is here to stay. Due to the composition of the board of directors of the Planned Parenthood Federation of America, which is strongly supportive of the changes, Wattleton's successor will hold to the same philosophical positions. The only difference may be in personal style, not public commitment and strategy.

3

TARGETING YOUTH

Planned Parenthood is increasing its efforts to pick up a new clientele—teens. As noted in chapter 2, Planned Parenthood's five year plan states that all clinics should include "a choice of all methods of fertility management including . . . Abortion Services (or local referral) . . ." with emphasis on, "Persons with low and marginal income; Teenagers and young adults."[1]

Planned Parenthood has used multiple methods for reaching teens, including placing advertisements in movie theaters and speaking in public schools. Fewer than one-fourth of all American communities and school districts are not directly affected by Planned Parenthood programs.[2]

REACHING FOR YOUTH

More than 50 Planned Parenthood affiliates have teen drama groups which perform skits designed to teach young people about issues addressed by Planned Parenthood. The group in Phoenix, Arizona, is called the Positive Force Players. A group in Massachusetts is called Youth Expression Theater. In Washington, D.C., the group is called the Washington Area Improvisational Teen Theater. The New Image Teen Theatre is based in southern California. In Nashville, Tennessee, the group is called the PG 13 Players and in Northeast Texas, the name used is Teen-Age Communication Theatre. While the groups have different names, the goals are the same.

The newsletter published by Planned Parenthood of Metropolitan Washington, D.C., details the role of its teen troupe, which has performed more than 10,000 times:

> The troupe of about a dozen aspiring young actors and actresses is made up of student volunteers from area schools . . . In addition to their theatrical talents, each has trained to become a peer educator and is qualified to answer questions from other teens about family planning, sexually transmitted diseases and AIDS [Acquired Immunodeficiency Syndrome].
>
> The group acts out "slice of life" scenes that have to do with teen pregnancy prevention, AIDS, and teenage fatherhood.[3]

It is important to remember that these young people, trained by Planned Parenthood, are providing guidance to others.

Connie Youngkin, a parent who has researched the teen drama groups, is appalled by the skits performed at schools. She cites a "condom demonstration" done by a Planned Parenthood sponsored teen drama group "which includes one scene of girls that had flesh covered garbage bags over them and they represented the penis . . . They would move up and down and act like they were ejaculating and then they would spray whip cream up on the top hole . . . Another person would run out 'to the rescue' and then they'd put a big, giant condom over one of them and then the whole group would applaud." Youngkin initially became interested in Planned Parenthood when she visited a San Diego, California, office to get literature she could use to teach her 12-year-old son about sex.[4]

Much to the surprise of abortion foes, the PG 13 Players received a merit citation as part of the 1989 President's Volunteer Action Awards. The group's coordinator states that those who perform skits and counsel their peers are trained in drama and sexuality issues.[5] Richard C. Mock, deputy executive director for communications of the National Volunteer Center, defends its role in honoring the group, calling it "a model program."[6]

The PG 13 Players have also been honored by the Tennessee House of Representatives. A proclamation, dated December 16, 1988, recognizes and honors the group for its "many worthwhile achievements."[7] The proclamation takes a strong view with regard to teen pregnancy:

> WHEREAS, Tennessee children, aged seventeen and under, who become pregnant create and perpetuate a wide range of difficult and complex social, educational, health, and economic problems; and
>
> WHEREAS, pregnancy not only hampers the quality of life and financial well being of Tennessee adolescents and their babies: it negatively impacts all the citizens of the state . . .[8]

Planned Parenthood has implemented a program called Campus for Choice. Intended for college students, the program calls for the creation of campus groups which work to defend legal abortion:

> You, the college student of today, are the future leaders of this country.
>
> Many student movements in this country and elsewhere have redirected repressive public policies and moved society in more positive directions—if not at first, then in the long run.
>
> Your Campus for Choice group, as part of a nationwide campaign on college and university campuses, has the same potential.[9]

The campus group is given an opportunity to be associated with Planned Parenthood's pro-legal abortion advocacy campaign:

> You have the option of identifying your Campus for Choice group as being affiliated with Planned Parenthood and its National Campaign to Keep Abortion Safe and Legal. Many students believe wholeheartedly in what Planned Parenthood stands for and feel comfortable with the type of action it recommends. Many students, in fact, use Planned Parenthood's services.[10]

Suggested projects for Campus for Choice groups include setting up a table in a public place featuring literature and other materials, voter registration drives, campus canvassing, holding forums and rallies, building coalitions, and organizing letter writing campaigns.[11]

Some of North America's youth have embarked on a mission to convince their peers that Planned Parenthood's educational approach is not good for them and abortion should not be legal. Many students develop lifelong views on sexual matters and political issues during their post secondary education years.

Several leaders have emerged among America's anti-abortion youth movement including Eric Kennerk, Ron O'Leary, Emily Colehower, Moses Remedios, Nathan and Greg Schlueter. There are many other young people who are also making a difference.

Some young people take a stand against Planned Parenthood and its agenda long before entering a postsecondary educational institution. Conor Gallagher, a 14-year-old who will likely be a future candidate for president of the United States, argues that Planned Parenthood is "abusing women just to get money." He asserts that the only way to be completely safe from pregnancy and sexually transmitted diseases, including acquired immunodeficiency syndrome, is "through abstinence or monogamy."[12]

Gallagher, an honorary member of the board of directors of the Christian Action Council of Western New York, has little regard for polls which state that most teenagers are sexually active. "That depends on whom you poll," he states. "I think that's twisted. . . ." He believes that most teenagers who have sex are pressured into doing so.[13]

Why should teenagers reject the Planned Parenthood message? "What they're saying may seem great right now," Gallagher says, "but in the long run it's going to hurt you and you'll end up in one of their abortion clinics giving them money."[14]

Young Americans are not alone. Many young Canadians have spoken out. Leaders such as Kevin Koopmans, Denise Funke, Wayne J. Ottenbreit, Coby Vandenberg, Greg McNeely, Jodean Wohlgemuth, Rebecca Morcos, and Michael Shane Lambert have spoken eloquently against the Planned Parenthood philosophy. While these leaders will not be part of youth anti-abortion groups forever, the foundation established early in their education will likely last throughout their lives.

Some college and university campuses have student groups opposed to abortion. Unlike those associated with Planned Parenthood, however, most are poorly organized and receive little attention, direction, and other assistance from national organizations. This could prove to be a critical error on the part of anti-abortion leaders. Despite these disadvantages, many campus groups have strong leaders. Leadership seems to be the key in running an active and effective student organization.

SAYING "NO" TO SEX

Amid criticism that its programs promote teenage sexual activity, Planned Parenthood points to its pamphlet, *Teen Sex? It's Okay to Say: No Way!*. The pamphlet states it is not true that "everybody's doing it," as some would claim.[15]

"It may be true that nearly half of today's young people have had intercourse," the pamphlet states.[16] This is odd since an analysis of Planned Parenthood's own surveys show that only 20 to 28 percent of teens have had sexual intercourse.[17] Many of these teenagers had intercourse one time, regretted the decision, and chose not to do so again until a later time in their lives. Many of the girls report being pressured into sex. A poll conducted by *Seventeen* states that almost 50 percent of females and, interestingly enough, 20 percent of males, report being pressured into sex.[18] Nevertheless, for statistical purposes, teens who have had sexual intercourse one time are labeled "sexually active" by Planned Parenthood. These inflated statistics translate into financial gain.

A national magazine reports that, "Fully 50 percent of college women 18 to 25 years old are virgins . . . A Canadian investigation puts the figure even higher—53 percent of 18-19-year-old women have never had sexual intercourse."[19] These statistics call into question the motive behind those statistics gathered with the involvement of Planned Parenthood.

As far back as 1969, Planned Parenthood and others were reporting that teenagers are really looking for love, not sex. "Teen-agers and young adults are increasingly following a love ethic and are willing to be open about their activities and needs," the October 1969 edition of *Family Planning Perspectives* reports. It is also acknowledged that what teens do not need are mixed messages:

> The girls we see have replaced society's confused messages about premarital chastity with their own group code, often that of a love ethic. We feel that these girls will be more responsive to a straightforward discussion about responsible contraception than to a mixed message such as "don't do it, but if you do do it, do it with this."[20]

A more recent study shows what many people have always known. Teenagers "pay close attention only to what their friends say, even when the subject at hand is as deadly as AIDS." This is particularly true among minority teenagers.[21]

Teen Sex? It's Okay to Say: No Way! continues, "It's just as true that MORE THAN HALF HAVE NOT [had sexual intercourse]."[22] So, if teens are to believe Planned Parenthood leaders when they say it is about 50-50, what should young people think about sexual activity at a young age? Moreover, these statistics vary depending on which Planned Parenthood publication is being read. One 1987 publication declares that between 70 and 80 percent of teenagers are sexually active.[23]

The *Seventeen* poll shows that 49 percent of 14- to 21-year-olds have not had sexual intercourse. It is important to emphasize that the survey includes 18- to 21-year-olds, which surely increases the figure when considering "teenage" sexual activity. Interestingly enough, of those who have not had intercourse, 57 percent of the females said they simply did not want to do so, and 56 percent said they were worried about becoming pregnant. For males, 56 percent say they have not met the right person, and 46 percent report fear of getting someone pregnant. Of course, Planned Parenthood is working to eliminate the reason for abstaining from intercourse mentioned by both males and females.[24]

Teen Sex? It's Okay to Say: No Way! states, "The only question is: What's right for you?" The pamphlet stresses that teens should make up their own minds and do what they feel is best. It does not say teen sex might be wrong, or teens might regret having sexual intercourse, or even that sexual intercourse might not be in the self-interest of teens. The pamphlet merely states that the teen might not be ready. If the teen feels he or she is ready, is it right to have sex? "Make up your own mind," the pamphlet urges.[25]

The pamphlet shows a cartoon of a teen telling her boyfriend, "Give me a break! I decided I'm just not ready." Another cartoon shows young men snickering and laughing at a young woman and calling her a "prude." The response of the young woman is, "Not being ready for sex doesn't make me a prude."[26] While this is a true statement, the implication is that a teen will be teased by her peers if she says "no" to sex. This is an even larger problem for male teenagers.

What means more to most 16-year-olds: being accepted by their peers or using good judgment? Saying, "I'm not ready" is like saying, "I'm too immature." How likely is a teen to make such a statement? Moreover, this line of reasoning makes "getting ready" the ultimate goal. If a parent tells a daughter she is not ready to wear make-up, the daughter cannot wait to do so. Wearing make up becomes her ultimate goal in life, the only thing on her mind, and her only reason for living. I should know; I have three sisters.

Some questions must be asked: What makes someone "ready" for sexual intercourse? How do they get ready? Do not most teens believe they are ready—old enough—for everything?

Making Sensible Decisions About Sex tells teenagers, "Only you can make decisions about your sexuality, because you know yourself and what's right for you."[27] One piece of advice is given to those who decide they are "ready" for sexual intercourse:

> One out of five teenagers get pregnant the first time they have sex, and five out of ten get pregnant within the first six months. Having sex without using an effective method of birth control is like asking for an unwanted pregnancy.
>
> Make a conscious choice about pregnancy. If you do not wish to be pregnant, consider an effective method of birth control.[28]

One study reported in an Alan Guttmacher Institute publication places the problem in perspective. "On average, sexually active males aged 15-19 spend half a year with no sexual partner . . . This picture contracts sharply with a common view of young men as 'sexual adventurers' . . . "[29] Moreover, keep in mind that the study includes 18- and 19-year-olds who are essentially out of school adults. This surely cannot be compared to "sexually active" 15-year-olds.

Of course, the words of Kenneth Edelin, former chairman of the board of the Planned Parenthood Federation of America, should not go unnoticed:

> We still have people who say if you teach kids about sex they'll want to do it. Come on. They don't do it now? It's everywhere, in rap songs, movies, everywhere. Even if it weren't, the biological urge is so strong. We need to tell them, "Say no if you can, but if you can't, use protection."[30]

However, the November 1991 edition of *Seventeen* includes an anonymous letter to the editor from a teenage reader:

> A majority of my generation's parents think we're sex-crazed maniacs. False! Most teenagers I know are worried and plum scared about what could happen when they become sexually active. I know I am.[31]

PUBLICATIONS FOR TEENS

Planned Parenthood distributes pamphlets and other material designed specifically for teenagers. Parental consent is not obtained.

The pamphlet *Choices . . .* outlines various methods of birth control. It also addresses several physical activities which would likely prevent pregnancy:

> You can have mutual masturbation, or self-masturbation, or interfemoral intercourse (penis between the legs). This last may be dangerous. Sperm swim, and if between the legs is anywhere near the vagina, it may be too close. Panties are not protection—sperm can go right through.
>
> You can have "petting to climax", which is just fooling around until you come. Just keep the penis away from the pubis or vagina.[32]

In *Ten Heavy Facts About Sex . . .* , fact number four addresses the category of "perversions." Teens are told that "no one has the right to condemn a person on the basis of that person's manner of sexual expression."[33] It is not explained how certain behavior can be labeled as perverse if "no one has the right to condemn a person on the basis of that person's manner of sexual expression." It is noted that, "Obviously, if one person forces another to engage in any sexual act, or if an adult has sex with a child, that is not good."[34]

The Great Orgasm Robbery discusses sexual standards:

> Sex is fun, and joyful, and courting is fun, and joyful, and it comes in all types of styles, all of which are OK. Do what gives pleasure and enjoy what gives pleasure and ask for what gives pleasure. Don't rob yourself of *joy* by focusing on old-fashioned ideas about what's "normal" or "nice." Just communicate, and enjoy.[35]

The Planned Parenthood pamphlet *You've Changed the Combination!!!*, tells teenagers that, "There are only two basic kinds of sex: sex with victims and sex without. Sex with victims is always wrong. Sex without is always right."[36]

In a pamphlet called *Planned Parenthood: A Strong Voice for the Most Personal of Human Rights*, the authors write about the consequence of little sex education. They write, "Accidental pregnancies [are] leading to hundreds of thousands of unintended births. All because young people don't *know* about their own bodies."[37]

Sex Facts addresses many issues for young people including marriage, sex, birth control, and abortion:

> Married couples usually want to have sex together. Many people believe that sex relations are right only when they are married. Others decide to have sex outside of marriage. This is a personal choice.[38]

One section of *Sex Facts* says condoms "are made in different colors and choosing a color can be part of the fun. The man may enjoy putting the foam in the woman; the woman may enjoy putting the condom on the man." It is noted in another section that abortion is legal. "A woman does not need a husband's nor parent's consent," the document tells teenagers. "Abortion is a matter between a woman and her doctor"[39] (see chapter 6).

Sex Facts discusses various types of sex and sex in general:

> By sharing their bodies intimately they [couples] can show deep feelings without words. When both want to please each other and can say what feels good to them, sex can be deep communication. How the couple feel about each other may be very important. Sex is different every time. There is no right way to have sex or place to have sex or time to have sex. All these things depend on the couple.[40]

The publication discusses oral sex:

> Many people enjoy having backs, legs, and other parts of the body rubbed. Many people enjoy oral intercourse when one partner's mouth and tongue stimulate the other partner's sex organs. A man may like to have a woman rub his penis. A woman may like to have a man rub her breasts.[41]

Sex Facts continues its discussion of oral sex and also includes detailed information about anal sex:

> Some people like to do this. Others don't like it. Personal choice is the most important. For those who enjoy it, it is not harmful and there is certainly nothing wrong with it. Of course, being clean is important in all sexual relations.
>
> Often oral intercourse is included as a part of the sex play during sex which also includes vaginal intercourse.
>
> The anus (the hole for making bowel movements, often called a—hole) is one sensitive part of the body. Couples sometimes enjoy touching each other's anus. Anal intercourse means that the penis is inserted into the anus. Sometimes this is pleasurable for the partners. Sometimes the anus is uncomfortable and the partners may choose not to include this activity in their sex play. Since the anus may hurt during anal intercourse, the inserting partner must use care in attempting this. As with all sex relations, the couples can discuss their likes and dislikes and make choices.[42]

The discussion of homosexuality is consistent with other Planned Parenthood literature. An illustration of two homosexual men is included on the same page:

> Sometimes, people are sexually attracted to others of the same sex. This happens to many teens. Lots of people have had sex experiences with someone of the same sex. When adults choose to have most of their sex experiences with such a person, the activity is called homosexuality. The people are called gay or homosexual. All homosexuals are different. They do not all look alike or act alike. Nobody knows why some people want same-sex partners.
>
> Unfortunately, many homosexuals feel they must keep their private lives secret to avoid losing a job or losing friends. Even religious groups are not completely understanding about homosexuality. Laws are beginning to guarantee basic rights to gay people. The society has a long way to go before discrimination against homosexuals is gone. People of good will are working to make life just as fair for homosexuals as for heterosexuals (those who choose to have sex with partners of the other sex). Female homosexuals are called lesbians. People who choose sex partners of both sexes are called bisexual.[43]

The statement regarding homosexuality should not surprise anyone considering Faye Wattleton's comments on the subject. "The most positive approach," Wattleton argued, "is to remember that same sex relationships may be equal to heterosexual relationships in their capacity for loving and caring . . . "[44] She continued:

> Young children will need guidance to avoid developing prejudices, which could become burdens later on, when they have urgent questions about their own sexual identities. Girls and boys need especially to be reassured that sexual play with a friend of one's own gender is fairly common and that it is not an indication of future, adult homosexuality.[45]

Sex Facts concludes with a question and answer section. One question is, "Is abortion safe?" The answer is, "Yes, legal abortion is safer than childbirth. If a woman decides to have an abortion as soon as she knows she's pregnant, it is easier and cheaper than later."[46]

Another question concerns sex education. "Who should tell children about sex and when?" The answer given is, "Children learn a lot about what their parents feel about love and sex just by being with them. Parents teach children about sex—sometimes by not answering questions or by saying sex is nasty or bad."[47]

Planned Parenthood has a number of ways to help teenagers learn more. It recommends books such as *Changing Bodies, Changing Lives*, authored by Ruth Bell. It also recommends *Our Bodies, Ourselves*, and *The New Our Bodies, Ourselves*, by the Boston Women's Health Book Collective.[48]

In *Changing Bodies, Changing Lives*, young people are taught about several sexuality related issues, including sexual exploration. The authors go into an extensive discussion of oral sex. Other topics include homosexual sex, petting, and abortion. Much of the book includes comments from teens who, in most cases, have had positive experiences with sexual intercourse, homosexual sex, and abortion:

> For you, "exploring sex" might mean kissing and hugging someone you're attracted to. It might mean staring at each other a lot, or touching each other's bodies, or taking your clothes off with each other. Later, it might mean giving each other orgasms, or even making love. This chapter makes no assumptions about what you have and haven't done![49]

The authors write that it is their hope that the chapter "will help increase the pleasure and make the painful times less frequent."[50]

A subsection of *Changing Bodies, Changing Lives* discusses sexual fantasizing. "Fantasies are mostly fun," the authors write:[51]

> Fantasies are a safe way to explore your feelings. Fantasies are thoughts—they are under your control. You don't have to act them out unless you want to.[52]

Several fantasies are given as examples. They come from interviews conducted with young people throughout the United States. One example is, "I dream about being covered in whipped cream and some stranger comes and licks it all off."[53]

It is noted that there are several kinds of sexual fantasies:

> A fantasy may be about someone of your own sex (a "homosexual" fantasy). This may mean that you are trying out feelings and possibilities that you will never choose to act on. It could also mean that you would like to have a sexual relationship with someone of your own sex—anything from kissing and hugging to making love. . . . Many people have a homosexual relationship at some point. For some it is a brief experience; for others it is a way of life.
>
> Having same-sex fantasies, however, doesn't predict one way or the other whether you will have a homosexual relationship in the future.[54]

Regarding masturbation, this Planned Parenthood recommended book states, "Many teenagers told us that masturbating lets them enjoy their sexuality when they aren't in a relationship with someone or if they don't want their relationship to be sexual." There is a subsection titled, "How People Masturbate." Young people are further told, "Masturbating doesn't hurt you, and you can't really do it 'too much' unless you make yourself sore, or unless you find yourself doing it so much that it interferes with other things you want to be doing."[55]

One young man interviewed by the authors of *Changing Bodies, Changing Lives*, says he received inaccurate information regarding consequences of masturbation when he was younger so he stopped doing it. The authors response is, "It's too bad that he feels he has to fight his natural sexual urges." The book's authors do not specifically state the degree to which people should not have to fight their "natural sexual urges."[56]

The book's authors suggest that masturbation is actually a good idea. "In fact," the authors write, "if and when you decide to make love with someone else, you may find that having masturbated helps you enjoy lovemaking more. It teaches you what makes you feel good, and you can communicate that to the person you are making love with."[57]

Parents are urged to respect the privacy of their children when sexual exploration or intercourse is taking place:

> Teenagers have such a hard time getting privacy that often they end up making out or even having intercourse in a car (if they can get one) or in a public place at night, or with a relative in the next room. This is unfair.[58]

It is important to know that some parents fully concur with this philosophy. At least two daytime talk shows, "Donahue" and "The Oprah Winfrey Show," have done programs featuring parents who allow their children to have sex in their home. The rationale:

- at least the parents know their children are safe;
- their whereabouts are known, pressure is diminished;
- parents can help obtain birth control and urge the children to use it;
- parents can get to know the sex partner(s); and
- if one partner gets too rough, parents will be home—likely in the next room—to do something about it.

Few people in each audience opposed the practice.

One part of *Changing Bodies, Changing Lives*, discusses incest:

> The most common type of incest is between brother and sister, while they are growing up. This may not be harmful or upsetting to children, especially if they don't continue as they get older. It is more like experimenting with sex with your brother or sister before you begin to have sexual relations with other people. What is harmful, however, is to have sexual contact with an older family member.[59]

A large amount of space in *Our Bodies, Ourselves*, a book intended more for females, is devoted to the discussion of sexual fantasies. It is argued that such fantasizing is healthy. Many examples are given. One of the more shocking is from a teenage girl who says, "I fantasize about sleeping with my brother, who is nineteen . . . I fantasize sleeping with him because he's the person most like me. I acted on it by sleeping with his best friend."[60] Additional examples are provided:

> I imagined I was sitting in a room. The walls were all white. There was nothing in it, and I was naked. There was a large window at one end, and anyone who wanted to could look in and see me. There was no place to hide. There was something arousing about being so exposed. I masturbated while having this fantasy. . . .
>
> I used to have a recurring fantasy that I was a gym teacher and had a classful of girls standing in front of me, nude. I went up and down all the rows feeling all their breasts and getting a lot of pleasure out of it. . . .
>
> I had the fantasy of making love with two men at once. I pictured myself sandwiched between them. I acted on this one, with an old friend and a casual friend who both liked the idea. It was fun. . . .
>
> I fantasize making love with horses, because they are very sensuous animals, more so than cows or pigs. They are also very male animals—horse society is very chauvinist.[61]

One chapter in *Our Bodies, Ourselves* is titled, "In Amerika They Call Us Dykes." Sections include "The Bars," "Loving," "Blessed Are The Poor," "Lesbian Mothers," and "Out of the Closet and Into the Frying Pan." Another chapter is titled, "Sex With Ourselves—Masturbation." Much of the book is too crude to quote. Slang is used to describe sexual acts and organs. There are illustrations, with descriptions, of a nude couple in various sexual positions.[62]

The New Our Bodies, Ourselves follows the same path as that laid by its predecessor. It includes a paragraph regarding the education of children about sexual organs:

> The other day I was taking a bath with my almost-three-year-old daughter. I was lying down and she was sitting between my legs, which were spread apart. She said, "Mommy, you don't have a penis." I said, "That's right, men have penises and women have clitorises." All calm and fine—then, "Mommy, where is your clitoris?" Okay, now what was I going to do? I took a deep breath (for courage or something), tried not to blush, spread my vulva apart and showed her my clitoris. It didn't feel so bad. "Do you want to see yours?" I asked "Yes." That was quite a trick getting her to look over her fat stomach and see hers, especially when she started laughing as I first put my finger and then hers on her clitoris.[63]

With regard to masturbation, one female expresses her reason for doing so. "I have tried masturbating because I learned about it, not out of natural desire," she states.[64]

The New Our Bodies, Ourselves states that, "As we come to understand that most people have some homosexual feelings, we begin to accept a lot of things we were taught to fear."[65] The authors suggest that women who assume they are heterosexual should consider lesbianism:

> Some lesbians today are asking their heterosexual sisters to reconsider the "naturalness" of heterosexual preference. Can heterosexuality be a free choice when we are taught such a deep fear of loving women? Can we comfortably assume that women are "naturally" drawn to men when we consider the many cruelties which drive us to seek protection from men and punish us for being alone: rape and sexual harassment, consistently lower pay for women workers, the lack of economic protection for widows, the derision of "old maids," the fact that prostitution is often the only available work which pays enough to support a family? If it is unsafe to be a woman anywhere without a man, then heterosexuality is not so much natural as compulsory.
>
> Compulsory heterosexuality may make us feel desperate when we're not with a man, and cause us to jump into the arms of men who are available but not good for us. It means we never have a chance to make a real choice, to ask ourselves whether we would be happier with a man, a woman or alone. Free to ask these questions, we might well end up choosing to be with men, but we would be responding to what we genuinely want and not to what society tells us we ought to want.[66]

A footnote states that, "Homophobia is politically useful for those who want to preserve the traditional forms of family life and to suppress any alternatives."[67] The tenth chapter in *The New Our Bodies, Ourselves* is titled, "Loving Women: Lesbian Life and Relationships."[68]

All three books include extensive sections on abortion, including a long diatribe in support of legal abortion. It is important to remember that these books are recommended for teaching adolescents and they are made available to teenagers without parental knowledge. Graphic sexual material is often included as part of Planned Parenthood's comprehensive sexuality education.

A Planned Parenthood *Resource Guide* recommends *Our Bodies, Ourselves,* and *Changing Bodies, Changing Lives*. They are offered for sale at a price below most retail outlets.[69] The publication also recommends *Abortion: For Survival,* a production of the Fund for the Feminist Majority (see chapter 15 and appendix E). *Personal Decisions*, which features several women explaining why they chose to have abortions, and *Committed to Choice: Women of Faith Speak on Reproductive Freedom,* a film which highlights a Baptist, Roman Catholic, and other people of "faith" who discuss how "abortion can be a moral decision made in the context of religious beliefs," are also recommended.[70]

Another Planned Parenthood publication recommends the *You're Having My Baby*, described as a film featuring "the Paul Anka hit song with a disc jockey interrupting to give statistics on teen pregnancy, consequences, and other appropriate remarks to the unrealistic lyrics of the song." *It Happened to Us* is described as a film in which women "speak candidly about their abortion experiences. Their stories reveal the problems of illegal versus legal, medically safe abortions." *Seasons of Sexuality*, recommended for junior and senior high school students, adults, church groups, and counselors, is a film which discusses "touching, loving, privacy, friendship, body image, fantasies, decisions and values." *Miracle of Life*, which shows fetal development, is recommended only for "professionals."[71] .

The recommended film list of at least one Planned Parenthood affiliate includes *About Sex*, which is "for and about teenagers." It addresses issues such as "sexual fantasies, homosexuality, masturbation, abortion, etc." *What About McBride* is about homosexuality. The film is described as good for discussion groups for "raising and questioning all the cliches [sic] and myths about people with a same sex preference." *What About McBride* is "designed for use in schools and with adolescents."[72]

AUDIOTAPE EDUCATION

"Start Smart," an audiotape by Berlex Canada Inc. and Planned Parenthood of Manitoba, includes dialogue between two teenage girls, interspersed with information on several subjects including sexually transmitted diseases and birth control. Some of the dialogue is worth studying. For example, one teenage girl says to her friend, who is considering having sexual intercourse with her boyfriend, "If you do it with Dan, I'm going to be the only girl left at school that's [sic] a virgin." It is noted that about 50 percent of teens are sexually active.[73] This dialogue, however, is comparatively tame:

Teenage Girl #1: *Hi. Remember that guy we met at the dance last week?*

Teenage Girl #2: *Rob?*

#1: *Yah, he called me Saturday and we went to a movie Saturday night.*

#2: *Ahh.*

#1: *Man, is he good looking. Sort of like Tom Cruise. (giggling) And Tom Cruise is who I was thinking of while we were doing it in the back seat.*[74]

A conversation ensues regarding the level of sexual activity a teenage girl is having with her boyfriend:

#1: *Well, how far do you go?*

#2: *We do everything but [have vaginal intercourse]. Like, we have oral sex which we both like and that way I don't have to worry about getting pregnant. And we have a really good time just touching each other. You know, masturbation.*

#1: *Does it work?*

#2: Well, it does for us. It's great! One of our sex ed teachers told us about low risk, no risk and high risk. No risk things like massaging, body-to-body rubbing, hugging and kissing. That sort of thing.

#1: Oooooun.

#2: Don't knock it. It can be really wonderful. Oral sex and making love with a condom is low risk and making love without a condom whether its regular or anal intercourse is high risk and stupid.

#1: Well, from now on I guess I'm not going to fool around with guys I just met, unless I meet Tom Cruise.[75]

The second teenage girl later suggests that, "For a partner that you know, masturbation and oral sex can add a lot to sexual enjoyment as well as reducing the risk of pregnancy."[76] Another conversation:

#1: I know it's pretty bizarre, but I have heard of some people having anal sex as a way of avoiding pregnancy.

#2: Really.

#1: I think I would rather take the Pill.[77]

The announcer states that, "It's true that some people do have anal sex. Obviously, people's sexual preferences vary."[78]

Planned Parenthood's feelings regarding parental involvement are made clear in another conversation between two teenage girls:

#1 . . . I was talking to Laura and she's on the pill and she goes, "Look, if you're not ready to tell your Mom, you don't have to. Just go to this clinic where I go and they will give you the Pill." I found one in the blue pages under Health. It's a good thing because I really didn't want to have to go to my family doctor.[79]

It is later suggested that a teenage girl "should carry her own condoms. That way she doesn't have to rely on a guy to remember." As one teenage girl says, "I'm learning that an erect penis has no conscience (laughing)."[80]

Birth control is discussed on the tape in some detail:

#1: I was reading this book the other day and it said to make using condoms and foam a part of sex. You know, like a girl putting the condom on a guy in a romantic way. Like a guy putting the foam into the vagina. They made it sound pretty exciting really. I mean fun!

#2: Have you tried that?

#1: Actually we tried it that night and it was a lot of fun, and the things you can do with the foam! But you have to remember that after you or he puts the foam in it's only effective for one hour and if you want to do it again you put the foam in again.[81]

There is no way Canadian Planned Parenthood officials can claim they are less controversial than their American counterparts. Tobi Klein, a Montreal sexual counselor, has traveled throughout Canada promoting "Start Smart."[82] Her personal views are consistent with those espoused in the program:

> Teenagers should be told about the other methods of sexual love that do not involve intercourse, Klein says.
>
> "Hugging, kissing, mutual masturbation, pleasing each other's bodies—there's no reason to rush things, if they can enjoy doing the preliminaries."[83]

While Klein says abstinence is acceptable,[84] it seems unlikely that those who choose to participate in the behaviors she suggests will actually delay sexual intercourse.

JUST FOR YOUNG MEN

While the pamphlet is titled *A Man's Guide to Sexuality*, the language is designed more for those who are young males (teenage through early twenties). The pamphlet states that, "Being your own man is your birthright. It means doing what you know deep down is right for you." Young males are told that masturbation is the "only kind of sex that has no serious consequences."[85]

The pamphlet puts men on notice with regard to pregnancy:

> If your partner gets pregnant, she can choose to have an abortion, whether you like it or not. If she chooses to have the baby and raise it, you can be legally responsible for helping to pay the expenses. Whether you want it or not.
>
> Few teenaged men and women are financially ready for parenthood. Having a baby can short-circuit their plans for the future, like completing school and pursuing a career.[86]

In other words, if the woman decides to have an abortion, the young man is totally left out. If the woman chooses to give birth, he can be held financially responsible. What kind of advice is the young man likely to give if his opinion is sought?

The pamphlet discusses sexual orientation. Note that in the second paragraph quoted below, parents are not listed, despite Planned Parenthood's claim that parents are the "primary," as opposed to only, source of sexuality information:

> It may be you're not interested in sexual relationships with women. Most men will become interested sooner or later. Some won't. About one out of ten men is gay (homosexual) and is interested in sexual relationships with other men. No one knows for sure what makes men or women gay or straight. We do know that people don't decide their sexual identities. Our sexual identities develop as naturally as the rest of what makes us who we are. Gay men do not usually have to deal with pregnancy as a consequence of sexual intercourse. But everything else is pretty much the same for them—except for the prejudice.
>
> If you want to talk with someone about your sexuality, whether you're gay or not, try a trusted friend, teacher, counselor, or someone at Planned Parenthood.[87]

The last section of *A Man's Guide to Sexuality* includes a true/false quiz for readers. Question number two reads, "Even if you don't have sex often, you should carry condoms just in case?" The answer given is true. "People who don't have sex often are more likely to do it on the spur of the moment, without being prepared. Always be prepared."[88]

Question number five reads, "The right time to start going with girls is when you start high school?" The answer is false. "There's no right age or right time. You must decide for yourself. Some men may never feel it's right for them."[89]

A Planned Parenthood advertisement intended for young men depicts a teenage male who receives a telephone call from his girlfriend. She tells the young man that she is pregnant:

> "The worst part is I wake up in the morning and it just rushes at me. Quit school. Get married. Run away from it. I don't know.
>
> "I didn't know then and I don't know now."
>
> Nobody has all the answers about sex. But keep in mind that a million teen girls get pregnant every year. Which means a million guys don't hear the end of it. Here's your choice. You can take responsibility when it's easy or you can wait until it's impossible. Don't make a big mistake. Buy a condom. You can get them at any drug store or from your local Planned Parenthood. If you need help or information, call us. That's what we're here for.[90]

Planned Parenthood has used several techniques to give men "responsible sexual attitudes and behavior." These efforts did not always target young men:

> [I]t was found that presentation of factual information would not necessarily change the attitudes of some males toward family planning, as evidenced by the following example: A six-session presentation aimed at men over 25 was developed and offered at a local YMCA; it was heavily promoted through local newspapers, neighborhood stores and barber shops and through mailings to residents of the "Y." At least 15 participants were expected. Surprisingly, only six males showed up at the first two sessions and all were over age 50. The other sessions were canceled because of lack of interest. Interviews of potential participants revealed they had felt embarrassed at the idea of attending or believed they already possessed sufficient knowledge.
>
> This was one of numerous failures in attempts to reach men over age 25. Even such inducements as beer, sandwiches, free condoms and stag movies failed to build audiences. There were a few queries, far fewer enrollments. As a result, the decision was made to focus recruitment efforts toward the under-25 male population in the belief that a younger group would be more open to the family planning educational effort because of their involvement in other educational activity.[91]

ACTIVITIES

The *San Francisco Examiner* reports that a Planned Parenthood staffer, Daniel Walsh, urged high school officials to suggest that students participate in a condom couplet contest:

> The invitation—issued by an enthusiastic employee without the knowledge of officials—urged students to take part in the contest as part of "National Condom Week . . . "
>
> Prizes included a gold condom for first place, a bronzed wallet with a condom imprint for second place, and a gross of condoms (that's 144) for third place.[92]

The suggestion that high school students enter the contest, which was sponsored by the Population Institute of San Francisco and the Pharmacists Planning Service, generated many telephone calls from concerned school administrators. Bonnie Simler, director of Marin Planned Parenthood, issued an apology, claiming neither she nor other Planned Parenthood officials had approved of the letter which included the recommendation. Simler did add, however, that Planned Parenthood supports "the goals" of the contest[93] (see chapter 4 for more activities recommended for teenagers).

POOR TEENAGERS

With Planned Parenthood targeting teenagers and the poor, what happens to poor teenagers? Planned Parenthood commonly paints a bleak picture of poor teenagers who give birth. They will not be able to finish school. They will face greater economic hardship. The pregnancy and birth will tear the family apart, if a family exists in the first place. The child's life will be miserable and the baby will end up making the same mistakes in his or her teenage years.

Are these results necessarily accurate? Consider an article from the *Lansing State Journal*:

The stereotype goes something like this:

A 15-year-old girl from a low-income family becomes pregnant, drops out of school to have the baby and goes on welfare.

In a single stroke, the pregnancy ruins her future and that of her child.

Because of this stereotype, many states spend millions of tax dollars on programs to prevent teen-age pregnancy.

Now, however, a new study at the University of Michigan suggests states might be throwing money at the wrong part of a complex problem.

Preliminary findings in an ongoing study by Dr. Arline Geronimus, assistant professor in the U-M School of Public Health, shows that among the poorest teen-age girls, pregnancy is not a disaster, but a relatively benign event.

It usually causes the girl's family to rally around her with support, Geronimus says, and makes little difference to her economic future. In addition, for these very low-income mothers, the teen years may be the healthiest ones in which to bear a child, the study suggests.

Geronimus' conclusions are alarming state officials and counselors.[94]

The *Journal* quotes Pat Belasco, director of Wayne County Children and Youth Services, as saying, "We do need to try to prevent unwanted pregnancy . . . But the real evil is not pregnancy, but the lack of available health care for young women . . ." She also argues that, "What we really need . . . are health services available for all people at the same level of quality and quantity, safe housing for all, increased education and equal opportunity for all our children."[95]

Dr. Arline Geronimus claims that other studies conducted on this subject have reached erroneous conclusions which, in turn, have generated unsuccessful programs because "they compare poor teen-age mothers with older mothers from a broader economic group, including some middle-class women." In order to avoid the same error, Geronimus examined national economic statistics and compared pairs of poor teenage sisters, one of whom became pregnant and one who did not.[96] The results were surprising:

In such cases the figures showed that both sisters remained poor, says Geronimus, but the one who became a teen-age mother was no worse off than her nonpregnant sister. Nor was the teen mother more likely to go on welfare or stay on welfare longer than her nonpregnant sister.

Furthermore, Geronimus found that the infant mortality rate in the first month of life was actually lower for the low-income teen mother than for older low-income mothers. She attributes this to the poor health care available to families, pointing out that the health of low-income women often deteriorates from the teens to the 20s, and so the best chance for a healthy pregnancy for these women may be in the teen years.[97]

The University of Michigan study is not the only one of its kind. A University of Pennsylvania team followed more than 400 teenage mothers in Baltimore, Maryland, for 20 years. The study began in the late 1960s and primarily included African-Americans. As *Newsweek* reports, it "challenges the common assumption that early pregnancy means lifelong poverty for mothers and children." In fact, many of the teenage mothers returned to school. Moreover, two-thirds of the daughters of these mothers did not become teenage parents and most graduated from high school. While the teenage mothers did face hardships, the study shows "that these hurdles can be overcome and daughters do not have to follow in their mothers' footsteps."[98]

Planned Parenthood's problem is not with teenagers who are having sexual intercourse as it expects such activity. Planned Parenthood's problem is not so much with teenage females who become pregnant. Planned Parenthood's problem is with teenage females who give birth. Its leaders seem to view poor teenagers as they view the person who carries a "defective" gene which can be passed to others. This attitude ignores scientific fact and research and becomes an opinion held with an almost religious, yet political fervor.

4

CONFLICTING PHILOSOPHIES

Planned Parenthood's former leading spokesman, Faye Wattleton, was fond of asking her foes, "[W]hy don't you join us in working for better birth control technology so that people do not have to face that [abortion] problem?"[1] It is actually a rhetorical question—one designed more for the audience than to gather information.

"Can't you people agree on anything? Can't you compromise?" are questions often asked by those who interview pro-Planned Parenthood and anti-Planned Parenthood leaders. This question is heartfelt, but lacking in an understanding of the issues involved.

The answer to both questions is simple. Those opposed to Planned Parenthood and those supporting it may want to achieve one or two of the same overall goals, but the methods are completely different. Moreover, the philosophies of those who support the Planned Parenthood agenda and those who oppose it are probably more divergent than any others. With such core philosophical differences involved, it is impossible for the groups to "work together." This difference in philosophies deserves an examination.

TEEN SEXUAL ACTIVITY

In *Teen Sex? It's Okay to Say: No Way!* (see chapter 3), we learned that Planned Parenthood officials have made an attempt to placate parents and anti-Planned Parenthood leaders who claim the organization encourages teen sexual activity. Is Planned Parenthood serious when it tells teenagers it is acceptable to say "no" to sex?

In a publication called, "Is It O.K. for PPFA to Say 'No Way'?," Susan Newcomer, then-director of education for the Planned Parenthood Federation of America, argues it may not be in the best interest of the organization to tell teens it is acceptable to say "no" to sex. She writes that chastity training, teaching children to say "no" to sex, "seems to set up moral conflicts."[2] However, she says it may be necessary to include chastity training if there is no other way to get into the schools:

> Sometimes the decision to design or use a "chastity training" program is pragmatic, based on the opportunity to obtain funds and/or to get into certain schools. Sometimes the decision is more of an implicit assumption on the part of the [Planned Parenthood] staff or board at the affiliate about the value of abstinence for young people. The age at which intercourse is thought to be acceptable varies widely, though I have met few people who wholeheartedly think 12- or 13-year-olds are ready for intercourse.[3]

Newcomer opposes the definition given to "prevention services" because it emphasizes stopping sexual activity among teenagers. She writes, "I think that the definition of prevention services as 'those services necessary to *prevent* adolescent *sexual relations*' . . . is unrealistic. Teens are having intercourse, they have always done so, and no amount of exhortation will cause them to stop."[4]

Newcomer relies on an example to show the primary reason for her opposition to teaching young people to say "no" to sex:

> Consider the scenario when a person identified with the best, most confidential source of information on sexuality and birth control, usually Planned Parenthood, is seen in the schools ONLY to talk about how to say "No" to sex. I wonder if the tentative young person will then say, "Hah! If I go there for birth control, they'll give me the same kind of lecture they gave me in 7th grade. Forget it."
>
> Planned Parenthood has always presented abstaining from sex as one contraceptive option. We must remember, though, that it is *only one* of the many, and informed choice is critical. . . .
>
> By "getting into the schools" with the most limited or "acceptable" material, we may actually deprive young people of some of the information and support they need in order to make intelligent decisions about their sexual behavior.[5]

Newcomer argues that "we should not spend much of our energies on programs exclusively promulgating chastity" and Planned Parenthood should "work to assure that contraceptive services are accessible to young people." The former Planned Parenthood executive says "all people can make informed choices about whether and when to have children."[6]

Newcomer believes expecting teens to abstain from sexual relations is unrealistic. She writes, "I will agree that abstinence is safe and has an almost perfect method-failure rate, but it sure has a pretty poor user-failure rate!"[7]

Abstinence has an "almost perfect" method-failure rate? Such a statement is ridiculous, unless Newcomer is only referring to the event in Bethlehem about 2,000 years ago. The statement is less ridiculous, however, when one considers what is meant by the term "abstinence." To most people, "abstinence" has something to do with keeping your clothes on. To Planned Parenthood, anything short of vaginal intercourse, anything at all, constitutes abstinence. Therefore, since it is possible to become pregnant through other physical, sexual activities, the statement is accurate. It depends on how the term "abstinence" is defined.

During a debate on a university radio station in Illinois, I clashed with Newcomer over the issue of chastity. At the time of the debate, Newcomer was still with Planned Parenthood. When challenged on Planned Parenthood statements that it is acceptable for teens to be involved in sexual relationships, Newcomer again claimed there is no universal standard for when sexual activity should begin. With that comment the debate became more heated. I claimed it is not possible for a sexual relationship to be "right for you" when you are 16-years-old.[8]

> Newcomer: *That is your value judgment.*
>
> Scott: *No, it's not my value judgment. That's what's best for teens. That's what's best for young people, and there are certain basics I think we can say that are not a question of values but a question of what is good for teens. It is not good for teens to be involved with drugs. It is not good for teens to be involved with alcohol. It is not good for teens to be involved in sexual activity. It is just not good for them—psychologically, physically, emotionally, and there is no positive aspect of that.*
>
> Newcomer: *[I] can't say as I can be as categorical about sexual behavior as I am about the use of [cigarettes and] illicit substances.*[9]

This last comment is consistent with Newcomer's document. Newcomer argues that, "Abusing drugs or alcohol and smoking are *never* healthy, unlike having intercourse."[10]

On the one hand, when seeking government and corporate funding, Planned Parenthood argues that young people cannot be expected to say "no" to sex. On the other hand, a 1977 Planned Parenthood publication says teenagers can control their sex drive:

> Nature also gave humans a big wonderful brain. We control our own actions. People are able to love and care about others. People are able to be responsible for their own lives—including their sex lives. This isn't always easy but it is possible. People can learn. People don't have to repeat mistakes. People can plan for the future. People can decide when sex relations should take place and when they should not. People can have sex relations without making babies—they can use birth control. People are not ruled by their sex drive. Normal people may have sex relations not at all, a little, or a lot. People always have choices. People can choose to make sex a good part of their lives.[11]

CHASTITY PROGRAMS

Planned Parenthood's attacks on programs that promote chastity among unmarried young people have not been limited to the publication of "Is It O.K. for PPFA to Say 'No Way'?" Most of the attacks have been against the two most widely known programs, *Sex Respect* and *Teen Aid*.

In an article titled "The Sex Respect Curriculum: Is 'Just Say No' Effective?," authors Susan W. Wilson and Catherine A. Sanderson make a point of saying that the program is endorsed "by Right to Life . . . "[12] The attacks continue from there:

> However, *Sex Respect* limits the application of these skills [assertiveness, abstinence is acceptable, self-esteem, responsible decision-making] to "always say no" situations. Experts in child growth and development recommend allowing young people to make their own decisions. But, radical programs like *Sex Respect* dictate "correct" choices and condemn alternatives. Such authoritative teaching techniques have been negatively correlated with reasoning, planning, memory, and IQ skills. . . . Young people need to learn to be assertive when they feel uncomfortable in sexual and other situations. They also need to know that their limits will change depending on the partner, the circumstance, and the level of comfort . . .
>
> *Sex Respect*, on the other hand, instructs teenagers to "say no" to all premarital sexual activity.[13]

The writers attack the "catchy phrases" used in *Sex Respect*, such as, "Don't be a louse, wait for your spouse"[14]:

> These slogans leave adolescents no choice and rob them of decision-making and responsibility. Sex education programs can empower adolescents by supporting the decision to say "yes" as well as "no." In *Sex Respect*, the adolescent's ability to make decisions is only valued when the "right" choice is made. This approach rejects information in favor of ideology . . .
>
> *Sex Respect* links sex with guilt, fear, and shame. According to the guide, there is "no way to have premarital sex without hurting someone."[15]

Some would argue that teaching young people to say "no" to sex *is* teaching them responsibility. In addition, according to the National Institute for Child Health and Human Development, 80 percent of American parents want their teens to be discouraged from having premarital sexual relations.[16]

Wilson and Sanderson even attack the part of the *Sex Respect* program which urges young people to keep their clothes on at all times during a date:

> Such negative attitudes do not discourage sexual activity, but do discourage responsible birth control . . . *Sex Respect* avoids any mention of a "sexuality of desire" . . . Intimacy, pleasure, and closeness are ignored in favor of the often inaccurate and "dangerous" details of premarital sex. . . .
>
> Studies in other countries have repeatedly shown that without accurate, available birth control information, teenage pregnancy rates increase dramatically . . . [17]

The authors have another major problem with the program which they refer to as "religious overtones." They claim that statements such as, "Many men and women still prefer to marry virgins," are examples of a "religious overtone" in the program and such overtones "are problematic for a public school sex education curriculum."[18]

It is worth noting that the United States Supreme Court, in *Bowen v. Kendrick*, ruled that programs which promulgate a position consistent with a religious belief do not necessarily violate the separation of church and state. The case directly challenged the Title XX (pronounced "title 20") program as unconstitutional because it stresses abstinence which is also the standard maintained by many religions. Thomas L. Jipping, J.D., director of the Center for Law and Democracy at the Free Congress Foundation, argues that those filing the suit "lacked any rational basis for their claim." He notes that the Supreme Court, in ruling in *Bowen*, cites several cases in other areas, going back nearly three decades, which assert the same position.[19]

A document published by the Illinois Planned Parenthood Council is titled, "BEWARE!!! 'SEX RESPECT' MAY BE COMING TO YOUR CHILD'S SCHOOL." *Sex Respect* is referred to as "the most extreme abstinence curriculum." The document also argues that "the psychological risks entailed in adolescent completion of pregnancy are substantially greater than the psychological risks of adolescent abortion."[20]

Susan Newcomer attacks *Sex Respect* specifically in an August 20, 1987, memorandum. She attacks the author of the program, Coleen (Kelly) Mast, by writing, "However, we do find it interesting that Mast has also written *Love and Life: A Christian Sexual Morality Guide for Teens* put out by the Ignatius Press of San Francisco, heavily promoted in the right wing press, and, as it says in the parent's guide, 'with ecclesiastical approval.'"[21]

Newcomer even attacks what she calls the program's "poor production quality and sloppy graphics . . ." Newcomer suggests an alternative program she calls "more balanced in its perspective." She says her alternative is "a real tool, not propaganda," because it "was designed by some of the same people who developed the first school-based clinic in the United States."[22] Newcomer includes with her memorandum a "point-by-point refutation of the curriculum," written by Marie Haviland James of the Planned Parenthood affiliate in Grand Rapids, Michigan.

Throughout Newcomer's memorandum, the Wilson/Sanderson article, and the "point-by-point refutation" of *Sex Respect*, it is never argued that the program does not achieve its objective: a decrease in the number of teen pregnancies due to a decrease in the number of teen sexual encounters. Instead, arguments are based on peripheral issues. Sure, some of the "catchy phrases" may be somewhat absurd, as far as "catchy phrases" go, but does the program work? Sure, the art work on the cover may be poor, but does the program work? Sure, there may be poor production quality involved, but does the program work? It seems that if *Sex Respect* had the financial resources of Planned Parenthood, many of the "problems" cited could be corrected. Nevertheless, Planned Parenthood is now using a more confrontational approach. Unsuccessful in getting its way with elected officials in Jacksonville, Florida, who adopted the *Teen Aid* program, Planned Parenthood of Northeast Florida filed a lawsuit against the school district demanding that a judge order that a *real* program—such as Planned Parenthood's—be instituted.

Faye Wattleton concurred with Newcomer's feelings about teaching chastity. The *Los Angeles Times* quotes Wattleton as saying, "We are not going to be an organization promoting celibacy or chastity. Our concern is not to convey 'shoulds' and 'should nots,' but to help young women to make responsible decisions about their sexual relationships."[23] Wattleton is also quoted as saying, "We've got to be more concerned about preventing teen pregnancies than we are about stopping sexual relationships."[24] Similarly, Wattleton has said, "Too many of us are focused upon stopping teenage sexual activity rather than stopping teenage pregnancy"[25] and, "Rather than focusing primarily on stopping teenage sexual relationships, we must place the highest priority on preventing teenage pregnancy."[26]

The executive director of one Planned Parenthood affiliate sums up Planned Parenthood's feelings regarding chastity. "[W]e can't totally solve the problem by telling teens to say 'no,'" argues Gloria Feldt of Planned Parenthood of Central and Northern Arizona. "And Planned Parenthood believes that one thing worse for a teenager than sexual activity is teen pregnancy."[27]

Another local Planned Parenthood leader, responding to a letter to the editor of a man who writes that "safe sex and contraception techniques are not the answer that our youth need today, yet, that is not only the 'bottom line' of Planned Parenthood, it is their active philosophy," first suggests that the writer "step out of their fantasy world and start dealing with realities of the world we live in today."[28] This ridicule is intended to cast a shadow of ignorance on the writer. In other words, Planned Parenthood leaders live in the real world so only they know best.

The Planned Parenthood leader writes that the organization "does in fact stress abstinence as your only 100 percent effective method of birth control and prevention of sexually transmitted diseases." However, she also writes that she has "a great deal of respect for the teen-age girls who do choose to come to Planned Parenthood. It shows great maturity and responsibility on their part to protect themselves."[29]

A distinction must be drawn between "information-based" and "value-based" approaches when educating young people about sexual matters. Schools have used the information-based approach for many years without any discussion of values. Information is easy to teach, but it is values that have the greatest influence in determining behavior. Simply giving students information has little impact on teen sexual activity and, subsequently, rates of teen pregnancy and sexuality transmitted diseases. This is true even when considering something as deadly as acquired immunodeficiency syndrome.

Ralph DiClemente, Ph.D., research psychologist at the University of California at San Francisco School of Medicine, reports that knowledge of AIDS and its transmission is "not associated with positive behavior change." Strangely enough, "those adolescents with lower levels of knowledge about disease transmission and prevention reported slightly less sexual risk-taking behavior."[30]

A comment about the "pro-life view" of sexual behavior is in order. While Planned Parenthood officials claim that those opposed to abortion are anti-sex, the fact is that most see sex as a gift from God and, as such, is something to be used appropriately. Abortion foes are quick to point out that the natural result of sexual behavior (called "contraceptive failure" or "product of conception" by Planned Parenthood, and "children" or "babies" by abortion opponents) should not result in the death of anyone based on the choice of someone else. When not practiced as it was intended, sexual activity leads to several problems of a physical, emotional, and spiritual nature. In short, lifestyle choices have cried out for the legal right to abort. If sex took place only inside of marriage, the number of people crying out for legal abortion would be minuscule. Those opposed to abortion argue that sex, when practiced between married couples, leads to comparatively few problems, including few dead offspring.

The Family of the Americas Foundation runs a program called *Fertility Appreciation for Families*. A comparison between programs run by the Alan Guttmacher Institute, a Planned Parenthood program, and the Family of the Americas Foundation program shows interesting results. The resulting teen pregnancies for the Alan Guttmacher Institute program were 96 per 1,000. Planned Parenthood's result was 113 per 1,000. The Family of the Americas Foundation program had a rate of five pregnancies per 1,000.[31]

In testimony before the Select Committee on Children, Youth and Families, Mercedes Arzu Wilson of the Family of the Americas Foundation makes some interesting observations:

> With all this evidence before the American people and before this committee, I strongly recommend that the government stop isolating the parents in this critical challenge of raising their children as responsible adults. It is a strange society indeed, where we teach that killing and stealing and drug abuse are wrong for teenagers, but that sexual promiscuity is permissible so long as they are protected. Protected from what, may I ask—venereal disease? rape? violence? AIDS? abortion? The fact is—none of the above![32]

Wilson claims there are three groups benefiting from teen sexual behavior and three which are being harmed. Those benefiting are the pharmaceutical industry, the mass media, and the makers of pornography. The losers are parents, children, and taxpayers. Wilson suggests that parents begin rejecting "the delusion that outside experts can do the job better than they can. . . . When others are permitted to serve as primary educators, parental authority is compromised and the parents' right and obligation to educate and protect their children is violated."[33]

In addition to *Sex Respect*, *Teen Aid*, and *Fertility Appreciation for Families*, there are several other abstinence-based programs worthy of consideration, including *Aanchor*, *Community of Caring*, *Postponing Sexual Involvement*, and *Values and Choices*. *Why Wait?*, a program designed by Josh McDowell, is excellent for Christian adolescents. Many abstinence-based programs are funded through Title XX, the United States government's Adolescent Family Life (abstinence) program.

A Planned Parenthood fund-raising letter, signed by Faye Wattleton, tries to make use of the problem of teen pregnancy. Wattleton said Planned Parenthood is resolved to "*STOP* the spread of teenage pregnancies which now extends across every ethnic and financial group in the nation. The only way we can curb this tragedy is by instilling in each teenager sexual understanding and responsibility, *before* he or she becomes another unprepared parent of yet another unwanted, unloved child."[34]

Planned Parenthood assumes that being an unprepared parent means the child will be unwanted and unloved. Moreover, it is implied that a continuation of the Planned Parenthood approach will help solve the problem.

WHAT IS PREGNANCY?

Why would Planned Parenthood spread such attitudes about pregnancy among young people? We get a good look at its basic philosophy by reading *Family Planning Perspectives*, a regular publication of the Alan Guttmacher Institute which is an affiliate of the Planned Parenthood Federation of America. One article is titled, "Is Pregnancy Really Normal?" Warren M. Hern, M.D., the author, writes that pregnancy "is a venereal disease treated by evacuation of the uterine contents."[35]

Willard Cates, Jr., M.D., who won Planned Parenthood's 1991 Arthur and Edith Wippman Scientific Research Award, joined with David A. Grimes, M.D., and Jack C. Smith, M.S., to write, "Abortion as a Treatment for an Unwanted Pregnancy: The Number Two Sexually Transmitted 'Disease'":

> Although rarely classed as a venereal disease, unwanted pregnancy is transmitted sexually and is also socially an [sic] emotionally pathologic. . . . As with other sexually transmitted diseases, unwanted pregnancy occurs primarily in the most sexually active age groups. Both unwanted pregnancies and other venereal diseases seem to have seasonal variations, and finally, the barrier method used to prevent unwanted pregnancy also serves to prevent the other conventional venereal diseases. Having suggested that unwanted pregnancy be considered a sexually transmitted condition, what do we know about its epidemiology?[36]

The authors argue that pregnancy is a serious problem for the country. "Therefore," they write, "figuring conservatively again, unwanted pregnancy appears to be the second most [prevalent] problem of sexually transmitted disease in our Country. What about the outcome of unwanted pregnancy? Without any treatment the natural history of unwanted pregnancy involves either a spontaneous abortion or a term delivery."[37]

The authors cleverly use statistics by comparing the safety of induced abortion to the administration of a shot of penicillin to treat gonorrhea. "Thus, abortion is 10 times more effective for treating unwanted pregnancy than is penicillin for treating gonorrhea. . . ," the authors argue. "Therefore, in terms of morbidity and mortality, the risks for the two treatments, abortion and penicillin, are remarkably similar."[38]

Other observations of interest are provided:

> Moreover . . . the cost benefit of legal abortion in the first trimester vs. the outcome of non treatment of unwanted pregnancy. It has been estimated to be between three to five years more cost beneficial. Beside putting the risk of abortion in some perspective what other benefits might be derived from considering it [abortion] as a treatment for a sexually transmitted condition? . . . If legal abortion were viewed as a justifiable treatment for a sexually transmitted condition, it would not be considered an elective or preventive procedure

> which is usually ineligible for insurance programs. Rather it would be considered a curative treatment, making it eligible for remuneration from federal and private third party insurance plans.[39]

The authors draw a conclusion based on the rational used throughout the document. They write, "In summary . . . it appears that unwanted pregnancy is the second most prevalent sexually transmitted condition in the Country. . . . Therefore, we conclude that unwanted pregnancy should be considered a sexually transmitted condition of epidemic proportion and, moreover, that legal abortion is an effective, safe, and curative treatment for that condition."[40]

In 1968, Mary S. Calderone, M.D., then-medical director of the Planned Parenthood Federation of America, said, "We are unable to put babies in the class of dangerous epidemics, even though that is the exact truth."[41]

A reporter for the *Colorado Springs Gazette Telegraph* attended a speech given by Planned Parenthood's former program director, Rachel Cressman. "The point is still under debate as to whether pregnancy is a disability, a disease, a choice or a right," Ms. Cressman said. "'Public policy is full of contradictions' which consequently punishes some and rewards other pregnant teens."[42]

BIRTH CONTROL PHILOSOPHY

The Planned Parenthood publication titled *Facts About Birth Control* begins with an introduction by Louise Tyrer, M.D., then-Planned Parenthood's vice president for medical affairs. Tyrer writes that she is "very glad to have lived during a time when women could decide when to have children."[43]

The pamphlet discusses the major forms of birth control. One assertion made by the author is that, "All prescription methods [of birth control] give reliable protection against pregnancy when used according to instructions."[44] While this assurance is given, the failure rate for each respective contraceptive method is included in the pamphlet.

"Of 100 women [on the Pill], only three will become pregnant during the first year of typical use," the pamphlet reads. If one is using the intrauterine device, about three in 100 will become pregnant during the first year of typical use. Eighteen women will become pregnant after one year's typical use of the cervical cap or diaphragm.[45] Therefore, writing that prescription birth control provides "reliable protection" is based on a comparison—especially if *you* happen to be the three or 18 out of 100. In addition, these statistics are for only one year of typical use. No statistics are given about a teen who is using birth control for two or more years.

Failure rates of over-the-counter methods of birth control are listed in *Facts About Birth Control* at 18 per 100 for the first year of typical use for the contraceptive sponge (28 per 100 for women who have had a child), and 21 per 100 for the typical use of contraceptive foam, cream, jelly, and suppositories. The condom failure rate, for typical use, is listed at 12 per 100. Fertility awareness methods are considered unreliable and one problem listed regarding such methods is that, "Frustration can result from long periods of abstinence." Advice given for the intrauterine device is that, "If a woman desires to end the pregnancy, an abortion should be done early."[46]

The most interesting advice is given to men who use condoms. "Men need to know what it feels like when a condom breaks during intercourse so they can withdraw if it happens," the pamphlet states. "To find out, they can practice breaking condoms while masturbating."[47]

Another publication, which appears to be designed more for women than for men, suggests practicing "putting condoms on objects that are shaped like a penis until you get over your embarrassment."[48]

A magazine for men includes information regarding condom failure rates as well:

> Myth—I don't have to worry [about HIV] if I wear a condom.
>
> Fact—Out of every 100 couples who use condoms for birth control, between two and ten will still conceive a child by the end of the year—because the condom breaks, slips, or wasn't put on properly to begin with. That isn't a terrible rate of effectiveness for something designed to prevent pregnancy. But it's not the sort of odds you should gamble your life on.[49]

As for contraceptive failure as it relates to pregnancy, Tyrer admits that, "More than three million unplanned pregnancies occur each year to American women; two-thirds of these are due to contraceptive failure."[50]

This essentially becomes a question of odds. Teens who see numbers as low as 18 out of 100 almost never think the number reflects 18 lives that were impacted by the decision to have sex. Instead, teens see the 18 out of 100 as odds one would find in Las Vegas, a lottery, a race track, or, even more likely, as one would see the chances of getting cancer from smoking three packs of cigarettes a day. Sure, the remote possibility of disaster is there, but the odds are on their side. Most teens see themselves as indestructible. Everything really bad, especially when it comes to enjoyable activities with such good odds, always happens to someone else. After all, it was not this teen who was killed while driving drunk. As one student notes, young people say, "We're young. This isn't going to happen to us."[51]

One teenager said that her sexual activity "sort of just happened one night in the heat of the moment. Stupidly, we didn't use protection." She became pregnant and had an abortion.[52] A 15-year-old girl had the same thought:

> We both knew that we should be using some kind of protection. But I guess I thought that if we used birth control, that would mean that we'd planned to have sex, and for some reason I thought it was better, more okay, if we were just swept away by the moment. Justin would say, "What are you going to do if you get pregnant?", and I'd just say, "Don't worry; I won't." It's not that I thought I couldn't get pregnant—I just didn't think it would happen to me.[53]

This attitude is prevalent despite statistics which show that more teenagers contract the virus which can cause acquired immunodeficiency syndrome through heterosexual contact than do adults.[54] Of course, one should keep in mind that while a female may be impregnated approximately one week a month, a carrier of the human immunodeficiency virus can pass it to his or her partner 365 days per year.

Another Planned Parenthood publication includes a suggestion that there are good reasons to take the Pill, beyond the pregnancy prevention aspects. Readers are told that "ovarian and uterine cancer are substantially *less* common among women on the Pill. What's more, Pill users are less likely to develop pelvic inflammatory disease, benign breast disease, ovarian cysts, and iron deficiency anemia—not to mention menstrual cramps."[55] Similarly, the April 1992 issue of *Self* includes a statement about the Pill which reads, "*The Pill is Safe!* The much-maligned birth-control pill may be a wonder drug for protection against certain cancers and other ills."[56] Of course, if the Pill is that great, I expect men will soon be asking their doctors for it.

While condoms are pushed by Planned Parenthood as a part of "safer sex," emphasis should be placed on the word "safer." Sex is, statistically and biologically speaking, "safer" with a condom, but it is not "safe." With a failure rate averaging about 12 percent, this means that, *on average, only* 12 percent of young people run the risk of contracting the virus that leads to AIDS or some other sexually transmitted disease. *On average, only* 12 percent of teens will run the risk of having to deal with an unwanted pregnancy. Nevertheless, Planned Parenthood continues to stick close to its insinuation that the condom will prevent every problem, and the condom will provide protection, and the condom will make you a responsible sex partner. Of course, this says nothing about moral or psychological implications of the philosophy.

While Planned Parenthood officials are urging that the United States embark on a high cost, highly concentrated birth control educational campaign, an article appearing in *Family Planning Perspectives* should not be overlooked. In comparing the situation in the United States to a study done in Sweden, a question is asked: "Can the large and heterogeneous U.S. population mobilize an effective contraceptive education program, even with the earnest encouragement of the national government?" A clear answer is given: "Sweden's experience would indicate that it cannot."[57]

It should be noted that the terms "birth control" and "contraception" are often used interchangeably. A clarification of terms would be useful. *The American Heritage Dictionary of the English Language* defines "contraceptive" as "Capable of preventing conception." The same dictionary defines "birth control" as, "Voluntary limitation or control of the number of children conceived, especially by planned use of contraceptive techniques." This latter definition is somewhat awkward since "birth" is defined as, "The passage of a child from the uterus" and "control" as, "To exercise authority or dominating influence over direct regulate."[58]

These definitions seem to leave out the most effective form of birth control—abortion. It seems that the term "birth control" includes all methods which prevent birth, for such measures would indeed *control* birth. This could include both contraception and abortion. The term "contraception," on the other hand, implies a more narrow meaning. Abortion is not a contraceptive because it does not "prevent conception." The intrauterine device is not a contraceptive as it does not prevent conception, but it is a form of birth control because it does prevent birth.

The terms "conception" and "fertilization" are also often used interchangeably. Some argue that the terms have the same meaning while others point out a slight distinction. Those who draw a distinction most often say that fertilization takes place when the egg and sperm meet. Conception, they argue, takes places when a zygote attaches to the wall of the uterus.

The dictionary defines "fertilization" as, "The process in which two gametes [the sperm and the egg] unite to form a zygote." The term "conception" is defined as, "The formation of a zygote capable of survival and maturation in normal conditions." The term "zygote" is defined as, "The cell formed by the union of [the sperm and the egg]."[59] Given these definitions, it appears that "fertilization" and "conception" really are different. A zygote exists soon after the sperm and the egg meet, but must implant to have the ability to mature.

It is interesting to note that, historically speaking, the terms "conception" and "fertilization" have always been seen as synonymous. This is still largely true outside North America. The change came when some in the scientific and medical communities sought to separate the two. It has been argued that the change was brought about by the desire to abort and experiment on those who have been fertilized but not yet implanted.

Using the definitions noted above, it is clear that the movement to stop legal abortion does not want to outlaw contraception. The movement does oppose birth control that does not also prevent conception. Nevertheless, Planned Parenthood continues to claim that those opposed to abortion also oppose contraception and/or birth control.

Roman Catholics, who have long taken a position against the use of birth control, have never moved to outlaw contraception. The Roman Catholic admonition against birth control is for those of the Roman Catholic faith and they have clearly stated reasons for their position. Roman Catholics do oppose the legality of abortifacients, however, as do Protestants who oppose abortion.

As a Protestant, I believe Roman Catholics make a point concerning artificial methods of contraception that should not be dismissed out of hand. "I am a Protestant," it is argued by many, "so I don't oppose contraception." True, but are Protestants able to support this position biblically? If yes, that is fine. If no, Protestants had better continue their research or alter their position. Either way, *no one is even suggesting outlawing contraception* for those who choose to use it. As for the use of birth control by minors, however, abortion foes do support parental notification and/or consent laws.

FALSE PROMISES

Planned Parenthood claims it is offering the best solutions for the problem of unwanted pregnancy, especially teen pregnancy. Michael Schwartz, director of the Center for Social Policy at the Free Congress Foundation, argues that the teen pregnancy problem is serious and creates countless personal tragedies. He says that out-of-wedlock births among teenagers used to be a relatively rare occurrence. Increases began to be noticed in the 1960s. However, needing a "new market," Planned Parenthood "went to work creating more public concern about teen pregnancy because they were the folks, of course, who had the answer."[60]

Schwartz explains that Title X (pronounced "title 10"), the federal government's family planning program, was to be made available without discrimination. Everyone, regardless of age or marital status, is able to get many methods of birth control free of charge and, for minors, without the knowledge of their parents. It was expected that giving a government stamp of approval for these programs would help to alleviate the "pseudo moral barrier"[61]:

> The managers, the bosses of Planned Parenthood, knew . . . that promoting contraceptives among teenagers would lead to more and not fewer teen pregnancies. They hoped that the bottom line number of babies born to unmarried teenagers would decline because more of those teenagers who became pregnant would seek abortion. That was their plan—deliberately. They knew.[62]

Schwartz points to studies which show that the existence of teen family planning programs have made the "problem" worse:

> [Teen family planning programs have] contributed to far more widespread sexual activity among teenagers . . . Those who were enrolled in family planning clinic programs tended to have intercourse 1.5 times more frequently than others. They tended to have more partners and so forth. In other words, these programs . . . subsidize and they facilitate teenage sexual activity and you don't have to be a college graduate to know that the cause of teenage pregnancy is teenage sexual activity.[63]

The standard figure disseminated by Planned Parenthood and its research arm, the Alan Guttmacher Institute, is that more than one million teenage girls become pregnant every year. It should be noted that most of these pregnancies occur to women 18 and older. The number decreases as the age drops. Therefore, the debate should be over out-of-wedlock births to females 17 and younger. However, an argument can be made for excluding out-of-wedlock females 17 and younger who wanted to become pregnant. Michael Schwartz explains:

> The problem is not pregnancies among teenage women. It is neither medically nor socially undesirable for women to have babies before their twentieth birthday. Nor is it all that unusual in American or other cultures. A generation ago, in the late fifties, teenage pregnancy was relatively more common than it is today, but it was not a social problem. The difference between then and now is that almost all of the pregnant teenagers thirty years ago were married, while today only a small minority are married.[64]

Schwartz states that the problem became significantly worse in the 1970s. This is true despite the fact that the federal family planning program was established in 1970. From 1971, the first full year of operation of the program, until 1980, the peak year for the program, enrollment of teenagers in family planning clinic programs increased 233 percent, out-of-wedlock births increased 36 percent, abortions increased 222 percent, and problem pregnancies by 113 percent (see chart below). "This is not the account of a triumph of public policy," Schwartz says.[65]

It is easy to see the relationship between appropriations to the federal family planning program and family planning clinic enrollment. As Schwartz points out, the money was intended to provide family planning services, and it has been used for that purpose:

> The normal expectation—surely the expectation of those congressmen who passed and those officials who administer the family planning program—is that the result of those expenditures and the clinic enrollments will be a decrease in the number of out-of-wedlock pregnancies among the target population. That, plainly, has not happened. On the contrary, it is my thesis that the family planning program had precisely the opposite effect to that intended, that it has contributed to worsening rather than alleviating the problem.[66]

In short, the higher the enrollment of teenagers in family planning clinic programs, the higher the level of premarital pregnancy. Schwartz provides analysis:

> [T]he factors which have been holding sexual activity down, the social sanctions, the directives from authority figures, the peer group expectations, and even the fear of pregnancy, are no longer such strongly operative motivational factors. Those who are currently sexually active are likely to have intercourse more frequently (and there is empirical evidence

Family Planning Program Effectiveness[67]					
Year	**Title X ($ mil)**	**FP Enroll (000s)**	**OW Birth (000s)**	**Abortion (000s)**	**Problem (000s)**
1970	6.0	330	190	46	236
1971	61.8	518	194	138	332
1972	100.6	718	202	183	385
1973	100.6	894	205	232	437
1974	100.6	982	210	278	488
1975	100.6	1,143	222	325	547
1976	113.6	n/a	225	363	588
1977	135.0	1,303	240	398	638
1978	135.0	n/a	240	419	659
1979	162.0	1,478	253	445	698
1980	161.0	1,726	263	445	708
1981	124.2	1,306	259	433	692
1982	124.0	1,251	260	419	679
1983	140.0	1,255	261	411	672
1984	142.5	1,270	261	n/a	n/a
1985	n/a	n/a	271	399	670
1986	n/a	n/a	281	n/a	n/a

> that this happens among teenage family planning clients). Those who are not sexually active are more likely to become so. The culture among teenagers has been altered by government intervention. . . .
>
> [I]n 1981, the funding is reduced, programs are cut back, family planning clinic enrollment falls, and instead of a new explosion of more teen pregnancies, we have, for the first time in history, a reduction in the number of premaritally pregnant teenagers.[68]

Clearly, pregnancy among unmarried teenagers is not caused by a lack of contraceptives or a lack of understanding regarding how to use them. Pregnancy is caused by sexual activity and the only way to reduce the effect is to reduce the cause. Schwartz offers two key suggestions:

1. Stop subsidizing the activity that leads to premarital pregnancy. No government-sponsored family planning program should provide services to unmarried minors. If they want contraceptives, they can buy their own; and
2. All public institutions should adopt the policy of discouraging premarital intercourse among teenagers.[69]

TEACHING THE TEACHERS

Planned Parenthood is the primary resource for those who teach children about sexual matters. Planned Parenthood of Northern New England, in cooperation with the Vermont Department of Education, scheduled "A Conference on Family Life Education: Are We Prepared?" The conference was designed to educate "school administrators and school board members, home economics, health, physical education, and science teachers, guidance counselors, mental health counselors, librarians, and resource coordinators, sexuality and family life educators, youth and recreational leaders, parent-child, [and] staff."[70]

Information provided on the conference includes an announcement for a "Special Pre-Conference Dance Party" called a "Safety Dance." The dance is billed as a "musical extravaganza guaranteed to keep you moving while learning about sexuality and safer sex!" Developed by Jay Friedman, a disc jockey and sexuality educator for Planned Parenthood of Tompkins County, New York, the dance includes "safer sex trivia . . . crazy condoms from around the world, and hot contemporary music with sexual messages." Potential participants were urged to, "Come and get ideas for reaching teens with valuable prevention information. Better yet—assign the dance to students as homework! Free and open to conference participants and the general community. Don't miss it!" The dance was to be co-sponsored by the Vermont Department of Education and VT [Vermont] C.A.R.E.S.[71]

The "Safety Dance: A Safer Sex Dance Party," targets "high school, college and adult audiences." A description and outline of the party is provided. One part of the event includes "Puttin' on the Condom"[72]:

> During the course of the evening each person receives and wears a nametag depicting a different step in condom use. During this activity, participants arrange themselves in a line (or a circle) according to how they think a condom is used (if there are a large number of participants, have several groups perform the activity at the same time, and compare results!). After the line is formed, have the participants read off their tags in order. Acting out the steps can increase the fun of this activity. The nametags are labeled as follows:
>
> - Physical attraction
> - Think about having sex
> - Talk about having sex
> - Decide to use a condom
> - Pool money
> - Go to a condom store
> - Decide what kind to buy
> - Take box off rack
> - Pay cashier
> - Decide where to store them
> - Meet your lover
> - Decide to have sex
> - Need to use a condom
> - Open package
> - Penis hard?
> - Place condom on penis
> - Fall in love (throughout, or at all?)
> - Leave space at tip
> - Roll condom down penis

- Enough lubrication?
- If no, use KY jelly . . . or, more foreplay
- Intercourse
- Ejaculation
- Hold on the rim of the condom
- Withdraw penis
- Remove condom
- Loss of erection (two of these)
- Decide where to throw condom away
- Trash it
- Wash penis
- Relax (throughout)
- Feel good? (throughout)
- Partner have an orgasm?[73]

Another suggestion for the Safer Sex Dance Party includes, "Demonstrations of fun and unusual condoms [from Amsterdam, etc.] and condom use by placing a human-sized condom over a volunteer's body." One activity is called the "Safer Sex Continum [sic] activity" which involves taping placards to a wall listing different forms of sexual activity including: french kissing, oral sex, the use of sex toys, dressing and undressing one another, skinny-dipping, showering together, masturbation, mutual masturbation, fellatio, cunnilingus, anal intercourse (with, without a condom), intercourse (vaginal, with and without a condom), rimming, phone sex, and looking at erotic films and magazines. About 20 other sexual activities are listed. Participants are asked to place the placards in order, ranking the sexual behaviors from least to most risky for becoming infected with the virus which causes AIDS. As noted previously, educators are urged to assign the dance to students as homework.[74]

It is recommended that the party include a "condom relay race." This event is described as, "A fun, 'competitive' activity enabling participants to become comfortable handling condoms." The relay requires one condom per participant and several firm (not ripe) bananas. The players are to open the package and roll the condom onto the banana. Another player rolls the condom off. This process is repeated until all players have participated. The Safety Dance is concluded following the breaking of a "condom pinada" at midnight.[75]

Naturally, many parents and others object to this kind of education being given to those who are expected to pass it on to young people, often without parental knowledge. The conference was to take place on May 12, 1989, in Burlington, Vermont, but was canceled due to public pressure. One Planned Parenthood official said that Vermont was just not yet ready for the program.

Jay Friedman is also responsible for a program co-sponsored by Planned Parenthood of Minnesota. This time, however, Friedman is billed as director of education for Planned Parenthood of Northern New England and director of the Institute on Relationships, Intimacy and Sexuality. Friedman's program is called "Countering Homophobia."[76] It has a specific purpose:

> Homophobia affects us all. Women, men, gays, straights and bisexuals experience a tremendous impact on their sex roles and self-esteem at every stage of life. It is important that we understand how homophobia can act to decrease our communication skills with others both personally and professionally. Fears and mistaken beliefs about homosexuality can pre-

vent us from effectively discussing vital information about safe and healthy sexuality with our clients, partners and children. This workshop will focus on innovative teaching techniques that increase compassion, provide alternative responses, and promote understanding of and appreciation for differences.[77]

Participants are presented with several objectives:

1. List three negative effects of homophobic attitudes and practices in families and workplaces.
2. Describe two exercises that can be used in education to promote appreciation of differences.
3. Explain how homophobia negatively affects sex roles and self-esteem.
4. List four techniques to remove heterosexism from sexuality/family life education.
5. Relate five common myths and stereotypes of gays and lesbians.
6. Explain how personal attitudes and biases relate to homophobia.[78]

The program is open to "health educators, family planning professionals, nurses, teachers and other interested community service professionals."[79]

Several items were distributed at the event including a Planned Parenthood newsletter the first article of which is headlined, "Let's Get Heterosexism Out of Sexuality Education."[80] The newsletter defines heterosexism as "The assumption that everyone is heterosexual and if they aren't they should be."[81] Another article is titled, "Out of the Closet and Into the Classroom."[82]

According to participants, it was noted at the event that the seminar was designed to increase "sensitivity to the issues of homophobia . . . the same as if it were with the disabled and hearing impaired."[83] Participants also offer the following information based on the seminar:

- It was suggested that the more heterosexuality and homosexuality are linked in casual conversation, the more natural and less of a controversy homosexuality will become. For example, if one is discussing Bob and Bonnie's wedding and honeymoon along with Ted and Frank's, people begin to accept them as intellectually indistinguishable.[84]
- Teachers were told to recognize that 10 percent of their students are homosexual. They were urged to discuss this fact with the class and explain the difference in this way: "How many are left-handed in this classroom? Do we force them to be right-handed?"[85]
- Teachers should tell students that 10 percent of their family members are homosexual. After doing so, students should be encouraged to work on bad attitudes and feelings, learn to appreciate the differences between people, and how to tolerate homosexuals.[86]
- It was suggested that heterosexual stereotypes should be eliminated in schools, particularly proms and "Sadie Hawkins Day." If proms must be held, posters should include both heterosexual and homosexual couples.[87]
- School board members and teachers should be sure that school curricula: teaches that everyone is diverse; that sexuality education curricula is incomplete if homo-

sexuality is omitted; includes same-sex couples and individuals in discussions for all subjects; teaches tolerance; and integrate homosexuality into schools.[88]

- All school employees should address homophobic behavior and comments among students and colleagues in the same way they would confront those using racist or sexual rhetoric.[89]
- Principals and librarians should add homosexual-related literature to the school library.[90]
- Health educators should include positive homosexual role models in their discussions. This may include inviting homosexual speakers to address staff and students.[91]
- Educators and others should drop language with heterosexual connotations, such as "married," and use terms such as "partners" instead.[92]
- Educators should show students that there are many positive and healthy ways of loving and being intimate, regardless of sexual orientation.[93]

Concern must be raised about that which is being taught to prospective teachers in universities. Diane Ravitch, in reviewing *Ed School Follies: The Miseducation of American Teachers*, by Rita Kramer, makes an interesting point:

> For the past half century, the most common complaint about American schools is that they try to be all things to all people. Critics have charged that schools have taken on the functions of social work agencies, health clinics, families and police, losing sight of their responsibility for developing children's intellects. . . .
>
> She [Kramer] finds few professors who recognize the importance of achievement or who stress mastery of subject matter. On the contrary, Ms. Kramer frequently encounters the attitude that competition is distasteful, standards are elitist and the content of the curriculum is irrelevant.
>
> What is it, then, that our future teachers *are* learning? They learn about the necessity of teaching children to have self-esteem and about the teacher's role as an agent for social change. . . .
>
> In one class the professor says to the future teachers, "More important than content or thinking is the students' feelings. You are not there to feed them information but to be sensitive to their need for positive reinforcement, for self-esteem." . . .
>
> Ms. Kramer describes professors with an ideological agenda, who proselytize on subjects . . .
>
> Ms. Kramer repeatedly finds evidence that the jargon of the human potential movement has become the lingua franca of ed schools, "role playing, getting involved, task-oriented, priority goals, peer interaction, feedback, role models, support groups . . ." In one class, the professor rattles on about "contributive strategies to norms of interaction."
>
> What most disturbs her is a common aversion to academic standards and substantive content. . . . The undergraduates, in particular, seem woefully uneducated . . . [94]

Soon-to-be-teachers who do happen to get a professor who stresses mastery of the subject matter are quick to "object to the professor's emphasis on tests and achievement. Their job, they argue, is to help their students 'feel good about themselves.'"[95]

TEACHING THE CHILDREN

Planned Parenthood's efforts to teach the teachers has had a profound impact on what is being taught to students. Jo Ann Gasper, former deputy assistant secretary for population affairs with the Department of Health and Human Services, summarizes Planned Parenthood's teaching philosophy.

> The Planned Parenthood movement wants the seeds of its moral relativism in sexuality planted in the youngest children, beginning even in kindergarten. These seeds of moral relativism are sown and watered until they bear the fruit of promiscuity, abortion, and homosexuality. The seeds are nicely packaged with such slogans such as "responsibility," "decision-making," "self-fulfillment," "toleration," and "compassion."[96]

Gasper provides some examples of Planned Parenthood's teaching methods. These include having young students handle "life-size models of male and female genitalia." In another exercise, "a girl fits a condom over two fingers of a boy."[97] In addition to these "exercises," students are taken on field trips:

> Field trips to the local drug store to purchase contraceptives may be organized. Names, addresses, phone numbers, and business hours of local birth control and STD (Sexually Transmitted Disease) facilities are provided. When students receive information about the facilities, they also learn that services are free and confidential.[98]

As would be expected, abortion is discussed with young people. However, according to Gasper, only the Planned Parenthood party line is presented:

> Abortion is discussed as an "option." The willful killing of a baby is treated as an equal choice to that of giving birth. Children are told how and where—including addresses and phone numbers—to get an abortion. Students are taught that no one else has to know, not even parents. They learn that it is absolutely, totally the "women's right to choose." Any rights of the unborn child, parents, or the father of the child to know about the pregnancy or be involved in the decision are ignored. Planned Parenthood's stated objective is to promote abortion. They're in business to sell sex and to lure young people into dependence on their lucrative contraception and abortion services. You can be sure that they will take advantage of the captive audience provided by a school classroom to do just that.[99]

Planned Parenthood spokesmen are usually the only persons invited to speak about matters involving sexuality, including abortion and contraception. Groups representing a different viewpoint are excluded for various reasons, the most common being that the teacher's personal belief is that Planned Parenthood's approach is the only correct and reasonable approach.

In an article titled, "Safe Sex and Teens," Planned Parenthood educator Debra W. Haffner provides a clue about the philosophy of those who teach children about sexual matters:

> Colleagues and I have fantasized about a national "petting project" for teenagers. The object would be . . . to help them learn courting behaviors and to, once again, give teens time to learn slowly about their sexuality. I am not advocating a return to the days of technical virginity, but rather to an unhurried and unpressured norm of teen sexual activity.[100]

Haffner makes specific suggestions:

> Today's teens also need to have that opportunity for unpressured discovery of sexual feelings and responses. We need to tell teens that the safest sex doesn't necessarily mean no sex, but rather behaviors that have no possibility of causing a pregnancy or a sexually transmitted disease. A partial list of safe sex practices for teens could include:
>
> - Talking
> - Flirting
> - Dancing
> - Hugging
> - Kissing

> - Necking
> - Massaging
> - Caressing
> - Undressing each other
> - Masturbation alone
> - Masturbation in front of a partner
> - Mutual masturbation
>
> Teens could surely come up with their own list of activities. By helping teens explore the full range of sexual behaviors, we may help to raise a generation of adults that [sic] do not equate sex with intercourse, or intercourse with vaginal orgasms, as the goal of sex. Rather, we can help teens understand that sex is more than intercourse and that abstinence from intercourse does not mean abstinence from all intimate expression.[101]

Planned Parenthood educators visit thousands of schools every year and provide curricula to thousands of schools. Planned Parenthood officials educate those who will educate children. School officials are happy to accept Planned Parenthood and its materials, which saves the school district from having to develop a curriculum from scratch. Since Planned Parenthood receives government funding and much of the curricula is developed with these monies, the programs essentially have a government stamp of approval. This approval, and the opportunity for a school district or state to save hundreds of thousands of dollars, is appealing. Moreover, Planned Parenthood officials are seen as experts on certain matters. Without significant public outcry, school, local, and state officials have little reason to turn down Planned Parenthood's offer.

Kate Fillion, writing for a Canadian magazine, suggests that, "If pulling condoms over bananas seems like a drastic way to teach safe sex in Grade 9, think again. By Grade 11, almost half those kids have had sex."[102] The article briefly discusses one discussion during a tenth grade class:

> It's a typical Grade 10 class, boisterous after lunch, but the teacher has no problem getting the students' attention. As soon as she displays a little white package, they're jockeying for a better view. And midway through the class, there are giggles and even a gasp when she demonstrates how to open the package, then pulls a condom over her hand with a flourish, holding it up high so everyone can see. "OK, now the penis is erect. What's the next step?["] This lesson on the ten steps of using a condom is part of a unit on human sexuality that deals with issues ranging from dating and relationships to abortion.[103]

Is this really what parents think about when they discuss sex education? Fillion notes that, "Sex education in the '90s is not for the easily embarrassed."[104] No kidding. She explains why this is true:

> In some schools, ninth graders rate condoms in terms of texture, durability and appeal, and practice putting them on bananas. Other students are lectured on the joys of "outercourse," sexually pleasurable alternatives to intercourse. Elsewhere, teens earnestly scribble notes while a container of contraceptive foam makes the rounds.[105]

At least one city health unit in Ontario uses "Sexual Jeopardy," based on the game show "Jeopardy," with high school students. The students compete in categories such as sexually transmitted diseases, pregnancy, and birth control.[106]

Surely, this is as far as it is going to go. Maybe not. According to Fillion, "many teachers feel that education about sexuality is not going far enough, fast enough." She quotes one Toronto educator as saying, "We get questions that never would have come up 15 years ago . . . One little third grader asked, 'Do people really put a man's penis in their mouth?' She's seen Daddy's video by accident." The educator suggests that we urge teenagers to abstain from sexual activity, but, "If they're going to do it, we have to give them the skills to protect themselves. The first time a kid crosses the street you don't just let him go out there without telling him how to avoid getting hit by a car."[107] This may be true, but why would one continue to cross the highway (not just some residential street), even if he knows how to do so in the "safest possible way," when he does not *need* to do so? Is "just for the fun of it" an adequate reason to take such a risk?

Fillion states that sexuality education generally starts in seventh grade in Canadian school systems, except for Alberta which begins in the fourth. Of course, "instead of innocuous drawings of the reproductive system, we're faced with condom machines in the schools and field trips to birth control clinics."[108] "Today, ignorance can be life threatening," she writes. In reality, it seems that many of those who know the most about sex are those suffering, even dying, from sexuality transmitted diseases.

Despite the gruesome statistics, some educators believe students are "better prepared to make difficult decisions about sex and sort out their values if they've been allowed to learn through trial and error that choices have consequences."[109] The reality today is that trial can lead to a deadly error.

Human Sexuality: What Children Should Know and When They Should Know It discusses age-appropriate education. The introduction is aimed at educators. Parents, it argues, are "overprotective"[110]:

> In this country, we profess great concern about protecting our children from the harm that might come to them through exposure to unsuitable information. In fact, adults often "overprotect" to the point that children and young people are denied information that will help them make responsible decisions about their actions. Nowhere is this "overprotection" more evident than in the area of sexuality. For children to make healthy and helpful choices regarding sexuality throughout their lives, they must be encouraged to make their own choices from the youngest ages.
>
> This publication was designed to help educators and those who develop curricula for schools and other teaching organizations.[111]

According to the publication, by age five children should:

Use correct terms for all sexual body parts, including the reproductive organs.

Understand the concept that a woman does not have to have a baby unless she wants to.

Know where babies come from, how they "get in" and "get out."

Be able to talk about body parts without a sense of "naughtiness."

Be able to ask trusted adults questions about sexuality.[112]

Children between the ages of six and nine should:

Be aware that all creatures reproduce themselves.

Have an awareness of the life cycle and sexuality at all ages, including those of parents and grandparents.

Have and use an acceptable vocabulary for communication about body parts, their own and those of the opposite sex.

Have a grasp of different types of caring home backgrounds, so that no single type is seen as the only possible one.

Be able to identify family members' roles and responsibilities.

Begin to be aware of non-stereotyped gender roles, and to operate within them.

Become familiar with the health care system . . . [113]

Nine to 13-year-olds should know about:

Human reproduction, including:

- an understanding of human sexuality as a natural part of life (by 12–13), . . .
- the idea that sex is pleasurable as well as the way to make a baby—the realization that sexual acts can be separated from reproductive acts, . . .
- what abortion is . . .

Contraception, including the knowledge that:

- no one has to become pregnant;
- it is possible to plan parenthood;
- having a child is a long-term responsibility, and every child deserves mature, responsible, loving parents;
- contraceptives exist (should be able to name some and how to obtain them).[114]

The Planned Parenthood publication states that 12 or 13-year-olds should be able to recognize the ways behavior "can be interpreted as sexual, and how to deal with such interpretation, including . . . recognition of male and female prostitution and its dangers." By age 13, children should have "an awareness of the differences between biological sex and socially assigned gender roles." In addition, they should know about sexually transmitted diseases including how they are transmitted and treated.[115]

Human Sexuality: What Children Should Know and When They Should Know It concludes with a list of what teenagers (between 14 and 18 years of age) should know. Human sexuality is first on the list, which includes:

- recognition of the impact of media presentations that encourage sexual involvement,
- the understanding of differences in sexual behavior, including heterosexuality, homosexuality, celibacy, marriage,
- an articulate value system about interpersonal relations, including sexual behavior,
- contraceptive alternatives,
- STD [sexually transmitted disease] causes/cures.[116]

The publication suggests that adolescents understand "values" as they relate to their "experiences, attitudes, and feelings about sexual activity." They should also understand the "problems of adolescent marriage and pregnancy" and have a "clarity of one's own values and emotional needs."[117]

By age 18 a person should have an understanding about birth control, the pamphlet states, including:

- advantages, disadvantages and effective use of contraceptive methods . . .
- comfort in asking about and asking for contraception, understanding where to obtain contraception, understanding the probability of becoming or making someone pregnant as a result of unprotected intercourse.[118]

In October 1991, Planned Parenthood Ontario sent a letter to school board chairmen noting that one of its areas of concern is "the status of sexuality education in our school system." The letter refers to the "financial burden to the province in health care costs" related to teen pregnancy as well as "welfare and social costs which tend to be higher for single and/or teenaged parents." It is also written that, "Sexually transmitted diseases (S.T.D.'s) are ravaging our teenage population. Notwithstanding the current AIDS Awareness programme, teens are still contacting S.T.D.'s in alarming numbers."[119]

The authors of the letter, Jeff Gill, president of Planned Parenthood Ontario, and Ray Tomalty, vice president of the organization, encourage school board chairmen to work with Planned Parenthood to implement "mandatory sexuality education" throughout the province.[120] Enclosed with the letter is a Planned Parenthood Ontario "policy position paper" titled "The Effectiveness of Current Sexuality Education in the Ontario School System." The document gives nine reasons why action should be taken despite the fact that "many school boards have implemented sexuality education programmes":[121]

1. There is a lack of standardized content because the Ministry of Education only sets guidelines. Studies show a wide variability in the range of topics incorporated into various school board curricula. The Orton-Rosenblatt report indicated that, because of the autonomous structure of boards of education around the province and the Ministry's "lack of leadership" in mandatory content, it is impossible to determine the adequacy of sexuality education programme content and effectiveness of delivery without a research study of each individual board to compare content, quality, and effectiveness in relation to specific objectives—e.g., reducing the teenage pregnancy rate and promoting safer sex practices.
2. The Ministry guidelines give inadequate emphasis to topics of manifest importance. The Orton-Rosenblatt report indicated that, in general, "curricula reflected the weighing of ministry guidelines, concentrating on reproduction, childbirth, and sexually transmitted diseases, to the relative neglect of the concept of family planning, contraceptive methods and information on local community resources to facilitate self-referral as needed."
3. The guidelines need to be more specific and conceptually consistent as to the timing of specific topics—e.g., at what grade level should attention be given to sexually transmitted diseases as compared to adolescent pregnancy.
4. There is a need for annual reinforcement of basic sexual health issues throughout the students' primary and secondary education.
5. School sexuality education programmes must address the differing levels of need between younger and older teens.
6. The variation in the number of students actually taking the courses and programmes is "worrisome." There is no requirement for mandatory attendance. Some studies showed that less than 50 percent of students have taken the sexuality education component presently available in the school system.
7. Classes, as are presently constituted, are too large! Studies have shown that small group discussion is necessary "to develop communication skills essential to effective relationships and to integrate content within the context of personal life education."

8. Studies have indicated that more extensive teacher training and ongoing staff development are necessary in the sexuality training and counselling area.
9. The Ministry must attempt to strengthen the link between individual school learning systems and other systems, such as parents, the Public Health Units, and other related community organizations like The Children's Aid Society, The Rape Crisis Centre, Planned Parenthood, etc.[122]

Planned Parenthood Ontario makes several recommendations, based on its view of the situation in the province:

Mission and Purpose Statement

A Mission and Purpose Statement for the sexuality education portion of the Physical Health curriculum must be clearly stated. The statement must indicate the extent to which the programme is oriented toward birth planning, toward the prevention of teen pregnancies, toward the prevention of sexually transmitted diseases, and toward the promotion of healthy sexual attitudes and values. Without clear statement of goals, the Ministry is unable to evaluate the effectiveness of its curriculum.

Standardized Content

Mandatory and standardized content in the area of sexuality education defined by the Ministry to all school boards is imperative to ensure a uniformly high standard of education for all of Ontario's youth.

No teenagers in Ontario should have to suffer the consequences of receiving inadequate education in the crucial area of sexuality health issues and birth planning.

Mandatory Attendance

Attendance should be mandatory for the Sexual Education programme. It should start in kindergarten and continue to grade 12. Students throughout their primary and secondary schooling should have yearly mandatory sexual education courses with content material appropriately targeted to the age group—e.g., early primary focusing on street-proofing, families, where babies come from, body parts, etc.; grades 4–6 focusing on changing bodies, reproduction; grades 7–9, concentrating on decision-making, relationships, sexual orientation, saying yes or no to sex, reproductive technology, birth control, options for pregnancy, etc.; and grades 10–12, focusing on further issues of human sexuality, communication, self-esteem, sexual responsibility, etc.

"Hands On" Instruction

Studies show that learning comprehension is greatly increased through the us [sic] of sensory/tactile hands-on instruction. For example, with regard to condom use, simply lecturing students is not sufficient to ensure understanding. Unless the students are actually given condoms in class, asked to open the packages and allowed to practice on an artificial model how to put it on correctly, we will be negligent in providing students with the knowledge they need to protect themselves from sexually transmitted diseases and unwanted pregnancies.

Use of Outside Resources

Sexual health and birth planning education in the school system should be complemented by outside training and resources in such key areas as safe sex, sexual orientation, birth planning, sexual abuse including rape and incest, AIDS, drug and alcohol abuse and addiction, etc.

The knowledge and resources available from community agencies should be tapped by the Ministry in order to maximize the educational benefits to its students.

We strongly recommend that the Ministry coordinate thoroughly with the Ontario Ministry of Health in designing and implementing this programme.

Trained Human Sexuality Educators

Sexuality education in the school system should be taught in a language the students understand by professionals trained in the area of human sexuality. In addition, the programme and services provided must be confidential and non-judgemental [sic] in nature.

Instructors should not be authoritarian or moralistic, but supportive, nurturing and emphathetic [sic].

It is critically important that the Ministry tailor the information and delivery model to fit the audience, and then address that audience in the language and terminology they use, no matter how our adult sensitivities to that language might be (Goldman and Goldman, 1982).

We advocate that professionals trained in human sexuality be the primary educators in this area. Studies have shown that both boys and girls are more comfortable in asking questions of their mothers and sexuality education teachers than in approaching their fathers, friends or teachers in general (Goldman and Goldman, 1982).

Sex education, to be effective, must encourage open, frank talk on very sensitive and sometimes embarrassing topics. Students are less likely to open up to teachers whom they will meet later in the day in another class. Sex education, to be effective, must be provided by trained professionals concentrating in that area and instilling confidence in their expertise and respect for confidentiality.

Health and Life Education Programme

We suggest that the Ministry of Education separate the Sexual Health Education component from the Physical and Health Education Programme as they are two distinct disciplines.

We recommend that the Sexual Health Education programme be a pass/fail course. Students should not feel academically threatened by this all-important course. Curriculum planning should have student input to ensure that the areas and topics that they are interested in and curious about are covered.

Although special care must be given to the reality of religious, cultural, racial an [sic] ethnic diversity in Ontario schools, it is imperative that all students receive basic sex education, not only for their individual benefit, but for the good of society as well.

Evaluation of Programme

A mandatory yearly evaluation by the students old enough to complete one, of both the teachers and course content, should be conducted so that the perceived needs of Ontario youth are identified and served. The evaluation form should be designed by the Ministry.[123]

This Planned Parenthood Ontario approach, which is similar to its sister organizations, ignores religious objections as well as all others "for the good of society." Not only are parents seen as incompetent, educators also cannot do a good job without Planned Parenthood's help. Planned Parenthood's miserable failure to effect true positive change is not addressed. It is true, of course, that the Planned Parenthood definition of "positive change" involves every teenager using birth control and its programs and speakers in every school—unlimited access to children.

A WASTED GENERATION

There has been an increase in the number of mainstream media questioning the rewards achieved through the sexual revolution. A remarkable article by Kathleen Parker appeared in the *Buffalo News*, in which she argues that "1991 was a banner year for bad behavior among men and women." She cites several examples including the fact that Earvin "Magic Johnson became a national hero upon announcing that he has contracted AIDS—from a woman."[124] (Actually, Johnson has contracted the human immunodeficiency virus which causes acquired immunodeficiency syndrome. At the time of the announcement he did not have the disease.) More examples of "bad behavior" are cited including the following:

- Teen-age girls were sending sexually explicit candygrams to their boyfriends and, in at least one case, slashed a boy's tires when he failed to respond in the expected manner, whatever that might have been.
- And in a politically correct episode of "Doogie Howser," the nation's prodigal son turned 18 and lost his virginity in one fell celebration.[125]

Parker states that she does not wish to be "moralistic," but "America could use a good slap" over what they have been doing:

> [S]omething is missing from our national portrait when "safe sex" is considered an antidote to AIDS . . .
>
> I suppose the so-called sexual revolution is to blame. When it was suddenly OK for people to do whatever they pleased, no one was responsible anymore.
>
> Nothing is anyone's fault these days.
>
> AIDS isn't anyone's fault. It's an accident.
>
> Pregnancy isn't anyone's fault. It's an accident.
>
> Applying our instant, fix-it ingenuity, we come up with instant solutions.
>
> Unwanted pregnancy can be "cured" with an abortion.
>
> AIDS can be prevented by using condoms.[126]

Parker suggests that another solution is available:

> Unwanted pregnancy, which occurs routinely among the teen-age population, can be prevented by abstaining from sexual intercourse.
>
> Likewise, AIDS.
>
> But, you say, those are unreasonable solutions. Teen-agers are going to keep having sex. And people are going to continue having casual sex with strangers.
>
> They are? Why, exactly, is that?
>
> Why are people going to continue to do things they shouldn't when it is clearly unwise?
>
> Because it is human nature to have sex? Indeed it is. But there have been rules of conduct and values related to sexual behavior for thousands of years.
>
> Thousands of years—and billions of human beings—can't have been all wrong.
>
> The reasons for most rules of human conduct have evolved as a direct result of plague, pestilence and other threats to survival. It would seem imperative to our survival that we develop—or at least revive—certain rules of conduct.[127]

One cannot refer to Magic Johnson without noting his comment that "the safest sex is no sex."[128] He has also stated that his lifestyle was "wrong."

A similar article appears in the *Wall Street Journal*. "If we have just lived through 25 years of the Sexual Revolution, it looks as if a lot of people might be ready for the Counter-Revolution," the commentary suggests.[129] As with the Parker article, the *Wall Street Journal* first outlines the facts:

> . . . the Census Bureau reported that one in four women who gave birth to a child in the previous year wasn't married. Since the mid-1970s, the rate among white women (actually, a lot of them are girls) had doubled and now stands at 17 percent. As a footnote, the report notes that a lot of the children were born into "two-parent families"—except that the two people weren't married.[130]

The *Journal* suggests that, "The media has served as the [sexual] revolution's tuning fork, pitching at us every conceivable modulation of these more open 'relationships.'"[131] A suggestion regarding how things have become so bad is offered:

> Sin isn't something that many people, including most churches, have spent much time talking about or worrying about through the years of the revolution. But we will say this for sin; it at least offered a frame of reference for personal behavior. When the frame was dismantled, guilt wasn't the only thing that fell away; we also lost the guidewire of personal responsibility.

> The revolution devalued personal responsibility because that implied unacceptable moral coercion, but it never quite produced its *magnum opus* on the proper conduct of sexual relations. Everyone was left on his or her own. It now appears that many wrecked people could have used a road map.[132]

While I do not want to sound like Oliver Stone, it seems clear that there was more than one gun. The media could not have acted alone. "Among intellectuals and commentators, judgment was long ago replaced by therapy. Ministers and priests gave way (voluntarily) to clinics and counselors. Instead of giving your kid a dressing-down, you now give him (or her) a condom," the commentary reads. A solution, however unworkable, is offered: "None of this will go away until more people in positions of responsibility are willing to come forward and explain, in frankly moral terms, that some of the things that people do nowadays are wrong."[133]

Maybe Parker, Johnson, and the *Wall Street Journal* have yet to learn that which is politically correct. "Freedom of choice" is the primary goal of mankind. It and it alone will allow us to reach nirvana, not doing what is right. If we sacrifice our children to "find ourselves," so be it.

Given the clashing viewpoints between advocates of Planned Parenthood's approach to solving problems and those endorsing opposing programs, the words of economist Sylvia Ann Hewlett are interesting to consider. Both radical feminists and conservatives disagree with her beliefs, but regardless of how Hewlett is characterized, she has views on children that should not be ignored:

> We think of ourselves as a nation that cherishes its children, but, in fact, America treats its children like excess baggage. In all other countries, childbirth is seen as an event that is vitally important to the life and future of the nation. But . . . we treat child rearing as some kind of expensive private hobby. . . .
>
> We refer to pregnancy as a "temporary disability," putting it on a par with breaking your leg. . . .[134]

In Hewlett's opinion, both liberals and conservatives have something to learn:

> The left behaves as if we do not have children. They have focused on equal opportunities, ignoring the fact that individuals who are nurturing children cannot compete on equal footing with those who are not. The left has been so concerned with the rights of people to live however they choose that they cannot decide what a family is. . . .
>
> Meanwhile, the right talks about traditional family values but does nothing to help families. They act as if we are living in the '50s, when women stayed home to raise the children. Day care was a dirty word. A hands-off government policy on families made more sense then. More families were intact, for one thing. . . .
>
> At least [then] we put the children first. These days we treat divorce as just another personal choice. Birth control has made it possible to choose when to have children, and liberalized divorce laws have made it easy to abandon them. Parents now spend 40 percent less time with their children than they did about 15 years ago.[135]

According to Hewlett, men must do their part:

> [W]e seem to expect women somehow to rear their children in their spare time. We persist in thinking of child care as a woman's issue. It's not. Fathers are more to blame for the parenting deficit in our society. . . .
>
> Too many still think that taking care of the children is women's work. And after divorce, almost half the fathers drop out of sight. . . .
>
> Twenty-four percent of the children in this country are growing up without fathers. At one time, society viewed divorced fathers as somewhat irresponsible. Now we see them as eligible males. We have forgotten that while marriages may not last, parenthood is forever.

> We are living with the appalling consequences of all this neglect. Teenage suicides have tripled since 1960. Since '71, the number of teenagers hospitalized for psychiatric care has increased from 16,000 to 263,000. More than 80 percent of them have no father at home.[136]

We need to get our priorities straight, Hewlett argues. This is true as individuals, as families, and as a society:

> In the U.S. we have confused equal rights with identical treatment, ignoring the realities of family life. After all, only women can bear children. And in this country, women must still carry most of the burden of raising them. We think that we are being fair to everyone by stressing identical opportunities, but in fact we are punishing women and children.
>
> We need access to free prenatal care. . . . We should throw sand in the machinery of divorce, force parents to think about what they are doing. We must hold parents accountable for the welfare of their children, and ourselves responsible for the care of America's youth. Otherwise we will not make it. Our standard of living will steadily decline. And the truth is, only a society that cherishes its children deserves to thrive.[137]

While neither opponents nor supporters of Planned Parenthood may be able to embrace specific details of Hewlett's ideas, they surely give one cause to consider the implications of the decisions adults are making. The one thing worse than the sexual revolution was its roots the—"me first" philosophy.

5

"STUPID" PARENTS

When speaking to adults, Planned Parenthood officials emphasize that parents are the "primary" sexuality educators of their children. This is true, of course, so long as parents are willing and able to communicate with their children. When Faye Wattleton was president of the Planned Parenthood Federation of America, she argued that, "Parents don't quite know how to approach the subject . . . ,"[1] but, of course, Planned Parenthood does know how to do so.

Planned Parenthood wants to "assist" parents in this area. Despite the assertion that parents are the primary sexuality educators, is the statement made because it is really what Planned Parenthood officials believe or is it said for political and public relations reasons? It is clear that Planned Parenthood materials often undercut the parent-child relationship.

RELATIVE RELATIONS

Planned Parenthood seems interested in giving advice to children about how parents should be regarded. This interest is evidenced in the pamphlet, *The Perils of Puberty*:

> There are certain things that you do not want to talk about to your parents. There are certain things they don't want to talk about to you.
>
> The important thing to remember is that you don't have the right to hurt *them* any more than they have the right to hurt you. The only thing you owe anyone is courtesy, and you owe everyone that. You don't owe anyone "love." You don't owe anyone "hate." You do owe courtesy, because we're humans and humans can't get along without it.
>
> If you think your parents are great, that's wonderful. If you don't get along, that's too bad but it's no lifelong tragedy. How you feel about them isn't nearly as important as how you feel about yourself, and if you start thinking and talking about them all the time, you may find yourself still doing it at age fifty with no one listening.
>
> Maybe your family is really rotten. Some families are.[2]

The pamphlet has further advice for young people:

> Don't tell your parents they don't understand you. They may not, but telling them so is only going to make them mad. . . . If you know something is going to make your family miserable, don't do it or say it unless you have to.[3]

One might wonder if the same advice applies to a pregnant teenager who is considering abortion.

Changing Bodies, Changing Lives, recommended by Planned Parenthood, tells young people, "If they [parents] seem to fear your sexuality, or if they don't want you to be sexual at all until some distant time, you may feel you have to tune out their voice entirely."[4]

Ten Heavy Facts About Sex . . . tells children in fact number ten that, "Teenagers who are afraid to get help because parents might get upset should seek counseling at a local Planned Parenthood or at a county or hospital family planning clinic."[5]

We get our best look at what Planned Parenthood thinks of the parent-child relationship in an advertisement printed in the *Dallas Observer*. The caption reads, "Since Your Parents Are Afraid to Talk to You and Your School's Hands Are Probably Tied, Here's Some Hard Facts . . . "[6] The advertisement is intended for young people and is written in a "myth/fact" format:

> Myth—I can't get birth control, I'm under 18.
>
> Fact—Wrong. If your parents are stupid enough to deny you access to birth control and you are under 18, you can get it on your own without parental consent. Call Planned Parenthood right now.[7]

HELPING PARENTS COMMUNICATE

Planned Parenthood of Central and Northern Arizona has published a workbook called *Be An Askable Parent: The Family Survival Kit.* Promoted as a tool to foster communication on sexual matters between parents and children, the workbook states that parents are the "primary sexuality educators of their children." Parents are urged, however, to keep in mind that "sexual values and behaviors differ from person to person and from generation to generation, even within a single family."[8]

Planned Parenthood states that the workbook was written for the purpose of "creating a climate for exploring personal values. Remember, whether you are a parent, child, or teen, the purpose of becoming a communicator about sexuality is not to convince others that only your views are correct or to impose your values on others."[9] In other words, the views of a 7-year-old about sex and sexual morality are just as valid as those of a 39-year-old father or mother. The workbook continues, "It is beyond the scope of this workbook to offer help in communicating sexual values based on specific philosophies, moral codes, or religious beliefs."[10]

Be An Askable Parent: The Family Survival Kit gives suggestions for what "basic sex education information" should be taught to children in each of four age groups. In reference to children between the ages of nine and twelve, it is argued that, "They are very curious about sexual behavior, and what is 'normal.' They need accurate information about both their spoken and unspoken questions, such as: 'What does sexual intercourse feel like? What do homosexuals do? What are oral and anal sex?'"[11]

These are questions of people between the ages of nine and twelve? Why? Where did these children get information that makes them wonder about such things?

This is similar to children who reportedly have nightmares about a nuclear holocaust. Adults plant such fear into the minds of children. This is often done by teachers in an effort to make children become their pawns in anti-nuclear weapons protests or projects, or by television producers who air programs on such subjects. Children should simply not have to worry about such things.

Those who claim children are naturally concerned about these weighty matters are grossly mistaken. Children are not "naturally" concerned about such issues. Any concern that does exist is exacerbated by some adults instead of dealt with in a proper manner. If a child is concerned about nuclear war or curious about "oral and anal sex," someone needs to find out why this is the case. The Planned Parenthood pamphlet titled *How to Talk to Your Teenagers About the Facts of Life*, on the other hand, recommends that parents, "Try to answer what's being asked—not what you *think* is being asked."[12]

Be An Askable Parent suggests that sixth graders learn about "sexually transmitted diseases (including AIDS), and the basics of contraception. They should understand that condoms reduce the risk of exposure to sexually transmitted diseases."[13]

Space is included in the workbook for a child to write what his or her father or mother would say about love, marriage, sex, birth control, and pregnancy. Space is provided across from this section where the child can write what he or she believes about these same issues. The child is encouraged to understand that regardless of the opinions held by his or her parents, disagreement is acceptable and even expected.[14] Once again, the implication is that children have the cognitive reasoning skills to equate their attitudes and beliefs about these important and complicated subjects with those of their parents. While a child's opinions are important and the child should be respected, such views are usually not as well-reasoned as those of their parents.

It is important to remember that children often mimic the actions of the adults in their lives. It is no secret that children will often make the same mistakes as their parents. Therefore, if parents are involved in behavior they are telling their children not to practice, parents cannot expect their children to take them seriously. Children want to look up to their parents so it is important for parents to do everything possible to enhance this respect. This is particularly true for single parents.

Be An Askable Parent includes a possible scenario which is supposed to help teenagers develop "preteen/teen refusal skills":

> John and Rachel (age 16) have been dating for 7 months. He has spent a good deal of his hard earned money on her. The initial kissing soon escalated to petting. Now John wants more—to "go all the way." Rachel is nervous. She is not in love with John and, in fact, did not want their affections to go beyond kissing. His harsh words and demands bother Rachel.[15]

The emphasis seems to be on the fact that this 16-year-old did not *feel* she loved her boyfriend. What if we changed the scenario? What if Rachel did *feel* she loved John? Would it then be acceptable to say "yes" to sex? Is a *feeling* of love by a teenager the single determining factor in answering this question? If there is not a *feeling* of love, is it being suggested that sex should absolutely not take place?

One question asked in another scenario is, "Will sex interfere with their [the teenage couple in the scenario] relationship?"[16] Is "no" a possible answer to this question? Other scenarios refer to young couples who want to "go to bed" together. The workbook was written to coincide with National Family Sexuality Education Month.

Planned Parenthood publications place young people at odds with their parents. They urge teenagers to question the teachings of their parents. Young people who choose to adhere to such teachings are made to feel "behind the times." Most parents would surely oppose any organization that works to undermine their authority and teachings on sensitive matters, particularly when those issues relate to morality and when the morality advocated by Planned Parenthood clearly endorses premarital sex.

While it is true that Planned Parenthood has created significant division between parents and children, it is just as true that some parents openly accept Planned Parenthood's brand of education and the so-called value-neutral approach. Reasons for this acceptance are most likely rooted in an approval of the Planned Parenthood premise that parents are not capable or willing to do that which Planned Parenthood leaders believe needs to be done.

How to Talk With Your Teenager About the Facts of Life seeks to assist parents in getting started talking to their children about sexual habits and sex in general. The pamphlet authors urge parents to, "Try to convey to your teenagers that you believe in them, respect their privacy, and are really more concerned with the quality of their lives and relationships than with what they did on last night's date."[17]

Planned Parenthood has published several forms of *How to Talk With Your Teenager About the Facts of Life,* often under different names, particularly as updates have become necessary. What information could change that would require an update? The definition of contraception, for one.

How to Talk to Your Teenagers About the Facts of Life, written in 1976 and revised in 1984, defines contraception generally as "any of several methods used by couples to prevent a sperm cell from uniting with an egg thereby preventing pregnancy and allowing them to plan and space the birth of children."[18] *What Teens Want to Know But Don't Know How to Ask,* written in 1987, and *How to Talk With Your Teenager About the Facts of Life,* written in late 1988, define contraception generally as "any of several methods used by couples to prevent pregnancy. Most methods prevent the sperm from uniting with an egg."[19]

The reason for the change is clear. Since many of Planned Parenthood's methods to prevent birth do not actually prevent the sperm from uniting with the egg, the previous definition did not work. Moreover, the new definition may make a young person believe there is no difference between contraception and birth control. Many organizations oppose birth control methods which do not keep the sperm and egg from uniting, at which time a unique human being is created.

For children between the ages of five and nine, *How to Talk With Your Teenager About the Facts of Life* suggests there is, "No need to get into weighty discussions of morality and behavior." While the appropriate time for such "weighty discussions" is never noted, parents are told that masturbation "is *not* harmful." The pamphlet continues by saying, "In fact, nearly all men and many women masturbate at one time or another, although many might not admit it. It is important for parents and their children to be assured that masturbation is normal behavior."[20]

How to Talk to Your Teenagers About the Facts of Life explains masturbation slightly differently. "In fact, nearly all men and women masturbate at one time or another although many perhaps don't admit it," the pamphlet states. "Masturbation is a private act and perhaps does not require lengthy discussion, but it is important that parents and their children be assured that it is not abnormal behavior."[21]

One section of *How to Talk With Your Teenager About the Facts of Life* asks, "What about premarital sex?" For Planned Parenthood, the answer is simple: "There are some people today who believe premarital sex is always wrong—and some who say it is always right. But most people stand in the middle, acknowledging that there are times when sex before marriage is appropriate behavior and times when it is not."[22]

A discussion of homosexuality, included in *What Teens Want to Know But Don't Know How to Ask*, states:

> A person's sexual needs are believed to be established before puberty, before sexual activity begins, perhaps even before birth. What determines those needs is not yet clear, but it is generally agreed that sexuality is not something that individuals can decide for themselves or for other people. Its manner of sexual expression should remain an individual and personal matter.[23]

Planned Parenthood's confidence in birth control is made clear in *What Teens Want to Know But Don't Know How to Ask*. "Without contraception, it is possible for a woman to become pregnant during sexual intercourse . . . "[24] Actually, pregnancy is possible, though statistically less likely, even with birth control and even if it is being used correctly.

How to Talk to Your Teenagers About the Facts of Life discusses God. "Love between people comes in many shapes and sizes," the pamphlet reads. "There's the love between close friends; the love between brothers and sisters; the love between parents and children, and the love in perhaps a less personal but no less real sense, for God or one's fellow-man."[25]

In *How to Talk With Your Teenager About the Facts of Life*, the question of whether abortion is dangerous receives an answer that is disputed by many:

> Abortion, safe and legal, is less risky than childbirth. (Using birth control is even safer.) Abortion is a fairly routine and simple medical procedure when done in the early months of pregnancy by a qualified medical person. Even when done later in pregnancy, when the procedure is more complicated, abortion is relatively safe. As with most surgical procedures, however, there are risks. Repeated abortions, especially if infection occurs, may increase the possibility of premature births or miscarriages in later pregnancies.
>
> Abortion should *not* be considered a substitute for effective contraception.[26]

In *How to Talk With Your Teenager About the Facts of Life*, the National Abortion Rights Action League is listed under "resource organizations" for parents who have questions about "pregnancy."[27] The pamphlet also recommends that teenagers read *Facts About Sex for Today's Youth*, by the highly controversial Sol Gordon, and *Changing Bodies, Changing Lives: A Book for Teens on Sex and Relationships*, by the controversial Ruth Bell, among others.[28]

A Man's Guide to Sexuality is recommended in *What Teens Want to Know But Don't Know How to Ask*.[29] *How to Talk to Your Teenagers About the Facts of Life* recommends *Boys and Sex* and *Girls and Sex*, both by the highly controversial

Wardell B. Pomeroy, Ph.D., as well as *A Man's Guide to Sexuality*, to teenagers. The pamphlet also lists "resource organizations" such as the Sex Information and Education Council of the United States and the Institute for the Study of Human Resources for information about homosexuality. The National Abortion Rights Action League and the pro-legal abortion American College of Obstetricians and Gynecologists are recommended for information about "pregnancy."[30]

Planned Parenthood recommends *Boys and Sex* and *Girls and Sex*, written by Wardell B. Pomeroy, Ph.D., to parents who wish to discuss sex with their children.[31] *Boys and Sex* suggests several advantages to intercourse before marriage:

> Premarital intercourse can also be a training ground, so that when people get married they already have experience in one of the most important aspects of learning to live with someone else in marriage. Of course, this means that premarital intercourse must be done with good techniques. Bad ones would no doubt be carried over into marriage, just as when one is learning to play a game and doesn't learn the fundamentals properly.[32]

Boys and Sex provides additional advice:

> If the premarital intercourse is with a girl the boy expects to marry, it will enable both of them to find out whether they are really congenial. In that sense it's like taking a car out on a test run before buying it. If that sounds too casual, remember that there are many marriages in which the two partners are well suited to each other in every other respect but sexually—something they may not discover until after they're married. Remember, too, that such intercourse with a wife-to-be would have to be done in the most relaxed circumstances to make a fair evaluation of it. If it has to be done furtively, or with strong feelings of guilt, these factors would make it so alien to the marriage state that it wouldn't be a fair test.[33]

Boys and Sex is endorsed by Mary S. Calderone, M.D., then-medical director of the Planned Parenthood Federation of America. She writes, "As I read your [Pomeroy's] manuscript, I kept saying to myself, 'At last it is being said.' . . . Congratulations."[34]

In *Girls and Sex*, Pomeroy writes that, "For those who plan on marriage eventually, early intercourse can also be a training ground." Pomeroy explains that, "There are many girls who regret after marriage that they didn't have premarital intercourse, because they've come to realize what a long, slow learning process it can often be after marriage. Sometimes, too late, they and their husbands discover that they're not suited to each other sexually."[35]

Pomeroy offers additional defense and explanation of his position, similar to that used in *Boys and Sex*. "If early intercourse is with a boy a girl expects to marry, it's a good way for her to find out if she's going to enjoy the constant intimacy of the bedroom with that particular young man. . . ."[36]

Pomeroy cites another advantage for young teenage girls to be sexually active:

> Some parents may not like to hear such things, but it's demonstratably true that girls who have orgasm when they're young—that is, up to fifteen—are those who have the least difficulty having one later on. It doesn't matter whether the orgasm comes from intercourse, petting, or masturbation. . . . Obviously, a girl who learns what orgasm is at an early point in her adolescence is going to have a more fulfilling time later on.[37]

Planned Parenthood also recommends *Sex Before Twenty: New Answers for Young People*, by Helen F. Southard (1971) and *The Sexual Adolescent*, by Dr. Sol Gordon (1973).[38]

Rachel Cressman, Planned Parenthood's national program director, suggests that parents should become more realistic regarding the use of birth control:

> Many parents are shocked to find Planned Parenthood giving their daughter birth control pills a method which became legal for minors in 1971) [sic], she [Cressman] said.
>
> Parents tend to deny the fact that their children are sexually active, she has found. "They need to overcome the immediate reaction that their teens shouldn't need or even want birth control."
>
> The ones who get caught are emotionally trapped, believes Ms. Cressman. "The message they get from their parents negates their need to engage in sexual activity and paralleling that are social pressures coupled with natural inclination."
>
> Consequently, she said, teens experiment without information. And parents aren't facing the facts because recognizing their offspring's process of maturation makes them feel older.[39]

Cressman supports school-based clinics as well.[40]

How to Talk With Your Teenager About the Facts of Life, along with other publications, reflect the basic philosophy of Planned Parenthood. This is what Planned Parenthood is teaching teens. These publications reflect values and moral indoctrination.

In her book *How to Talk With Your Child About Sexuality*, Faye Wattleton presents the negative aspects of "children raising children." Wattleton hoped to help parents talk some sense into daughters who become pregnant, give birth, and keep the child:

> Young girls commonly harbor a variety of unrealistic ideas about motherhood. When an adolescent says she wants to keep her baby, it maybe for any of the following reasons:
>
> - She thinks it will give her adult status.
> - She feels unloved and believes a baby will provide love.
> - She wants to escape from her family.
> - She hopes to stabilize the relationship with her boyfriend.
> - She is trying to change the relationship with her parents.
> - She may be morally opposed to abortion.
> - She is so guilty about having had a sexual relationship that she feels she should go through with the pregnancy as a punishment, or to take "responsibility" for the consequences of her behavior.
>
> Parents may be able to help a daughter be realistic about her reasons for continuing a pregnancy.[41]

As previously noted, Planned Parenthood leaders, at all levels, consistently use the line that parents are the primary educators of children. However, one Planned Parenthood leader includes some clarification when she says that "parents are the primary sexuality educators of their children, though not the sole educators, and social institutions such as schools, churches, family planning cents [sic] and other health professionals should supplement, not supplant, them in this role."[42] In other words, parents are given first place, but there are others who have a right to be involved. Moreover, if others are giving information that in any way conflicts with that given by the parents, it does indeed supplant the parental message. There is no way around it. The Planned Parenthood leader offers additional advice:

> The greatest gift any of us can give to our children is our value and preservation of their freedom to think, to inquire and to choose. We must also pass on to them the conviction that they too, in their turn, must either fight for these freedoms or lose them. This is why America needs sexuality education.[43]

COMPREHENSIVE SEXUALITY EDUCATION

Planned Parenthood informs parents of the importance of sex education for young people in *How to Talk With Your Teenager About the Facts of Life*:

> Fewer than 25 percent of students nationwide receive timely, comprehensive sexuality education in school.
>
> The result is reflected in our nation's high rates of sexual ignorance, sexually transmitted disease, unintended pregnancies, and out-of-wedlock births. In fact, of all industrialized countries in the world, the U.S. has the highest rates of teen pregnancy, childbearing, and abortion.
>
> Nationwide studies, for example, show that more than half of American teenagers who are 17 have had sexual intercourse. But only about a third of them always use birth control. And many rely on withdrawal or the less effective methods, such as vaginal spermicides, rather than on the more effective methods, such as the Pill.[44]

Faye Wattleton argued that those who say sex education has not worked in decreasing the rate of teen pregnancies and sexually transmitted diseases are making an inaccurate assumption. Wattleton asserts that she has yet to see "real sexuality education" in schools.[45] This is because she defines "real sexuality education" in the same way she defines "comprehensive sexuality education"—in kindergarten through grade 12 and including virtually everything. This means that instruction on issues such as abortion, contraceptive use, and several other controversial topics must be offered in schools before it can be said that sexuality education has been a failure. Therefore, the statement in *How to Talk With Your Teenager About the Facts of Life* does not mean that many schools are not offering sexuality education. It means that fewer than 25 percent are offering sexuality education written by or acceptable to Planned Parenthood.

Studies show that sexuality education does not impact the incidence of sexually transmitted diseases, unintended pregnancies, and out-of-wedlock births. It could be argued that the United States has the highest pregnancy and abortion rates because of programs which condone and even encourage teenage sexual activity.

Writing that studies "show that more than half of American teenagers who are 17 have had sexual intercourse" is misleading. Such studies are never reliable and many of these teens decided not to be sexually active for some time following the initial experience. The fact that so few use birth control is understandable. Most teens do not plan sexual activity ahead of time and many who do have sex were pressured into doing so. Moreover, people are generally irresponsible at that age, particularly when it comes to contraception. A more successful approach is necessary which means that teens are being asked to act responsibly by choosing abstinence. Interestingly, *What Teens Want to Know But Don't Know How to Ask*, written in 1987, states, "Nationwide studies . . . show that 70 percent of teenage women and 80 percent of teenage men are sexually active."[46]

Planned Parenthood states that in 1989, there were 2,572 sexuality education programs in elementary schools, 10,899 in middle schools, and 19,773 in high schools. In addition, "A total of 8,614 preschool children, 37 percent more than in 1988, participated in 450 Planned Parenthood sexuality education programs in 1989."[47] Planned Parenthood argues that "very young children need and benefit from opportunities to learn accurate vocabulary and to feel good about their bodies."[48]

Professor Jacqueline Kasun of Humboldt State University makes an important point about sexuality education. "[R]esearchers," Kasun writes, "have consistently concluded that sex education leads to increased use of contraceptives, even though this effect is offset, by the increase in sexual activity."[49]

A *Planned Parenthood Resource Guide* includes a policy statement on sexuality education. "Whether for pleasure or procreation, sexual experience can be a positive source of personal enrichment and satisfaction when it is based on informed choices and is consistent with personal values," the statement reads. It is also noted that sexuality education should include "sexual identity, sexual development and relationships across the life cycle, reproductive choices, decision-making skills, and the responsibilities of parenthood." Planned Parenthood's programs are based upon these, as well as other, objectives.[50] Planned Parenthood will almost certainly be surprised to learn that despite the widespread support it claims exists for comprehensive sexuality education, "there is little scientific evidence that sex education by itself makes any difference in the pregnancy rate."[51]

Kasun sums up the impact of comprehensive sexuality education when she writes that "the growing prevalence of sex education has been accompanied by a marked rise in adolescent pregnancy, which had been falling, as well as by an explosive increase in abortions and a cessation of the previous decline in adolescent fertility."[52] Of course, it seems Planned Parenthood leaders do not want a judgment to be made about the effectiveness of comprehensive sexuality education until every student, from kindergarten to grade 12, has been subjected to the Planned Parenthood curricula.

CONFLICTING STORIES

Parents in Missoula, Montana, told Kay Lindley, who was preparing a radio report about Planned Parenthood, that the organization's speakers bring life-size models of human genitalia to high schools when they make presentations about condoms and other birth control. Melanie Reynolds, executive director of Missoula Planned Parenthood, acknowledges that speakers from her organization do take condoms to the schools to "show students what they look like." However, she denies ever using a model of an erect penis.[53]

Lindley, whose radio special on Planned Parenthood aired on "Focus on the Family," reports that she had trouble getting cooperation from administrators at Big Sky High School. Lindley sought to get a confirmation or denial about use of the model. While school administrators would not cooperate, one student did confirm that the model was used. In fact, the student reports that it was Reynolds who used the model to demonstrate how to put on a condom:

> The model was, they told us that it was the actual size and they had a lot of detail added to it—all of the specifics. They had the testicles and the pubic hairs and it was in very much detail. . . . When we came out of the room, most of the males were making jokes about how large the model was and they were saying that they didn't have to worry any more because if they got a girl pregnant that all they'd have to do is go down to Planned Parenthood and get it all fixed up without anybody knowing.[54]

Reynolds continues to deny that a model was ever used. She also denies a report that she took various colors of condoms to class. Reynolds allegedly said that black and orange condoms are for Halloween while red and green are for Christmas. One parent decided to visit a classroom where Reynolds was speaking:

> Melanie was real light and funny. Her whole presentation was on a more humorous note and she laid colored condoms across the palm of her hand for the class to see. There was black and orange and red and green and I believe a white one, and she told the kids that condoms could be a nuisance, but if they would use them they could also be fun and she referred to how you could have your girlfriend put them on for you and then she said, "We do have the colored condoms at Planned Parenthood," and then she giggled and said, "We get a little crazy around the holidays". . . .
>
> I thought the implication was, is that sex is nothing to be taken real seriously. It's there because it's fun and everybody should take advantage of it and enjoy it and even if you're just 14-years-old you have every right to be sexually active, regardless of what your parents tell you, and Planned Parenthood is there to make sure that you have everything you need to be successful at sex.[55]

Reynolds denies the accusations:

> No, I never said that and we don't have orange and black condoms and all of that stuff. . . . I mean, I don't, I don't really know what to say. We, we do have different kinds of condoms including different colors of condoms, but we haven't done any kind of promotion along those lines.[56]

The parent discussed the presentation with Reynolds after it was over. When the same parent visited another class during a presentation made by Reynolds at a later date, the content had been modified considerably. The parent later learned that Reynolds returned to the class the following day. Reynolds allegedly told the class that she had run out of time the previous day and had returned to finish. At that time, all of the information that had been omitted while the parent was in the room was presented to the students. As the parent put it, "The essence of it is that she wants those kids to get certain information and she really doesn't care what the parents think."[57]

Reynolds says she welcomes parents to sit in when she makes presentations. "We are not embarrassed," she says. "We are very proud of the kind of information we give. We have no reason to hide any information from parents." She explains that Planned Parenthood speakers are often invited to speak to students. "We're also invited to come in and talk about responsible sexuality and in that presentation we usually talk a little bit about Planned Parenthood services and we usually do a contraceptive presentation which includes information about abstinence."[58]

Several students interviewed for the report said that abstinence played little or no part in the Planned Parenthood presentation. One female student said, "They [Planned Parenthood] made me feel like I was a nerd or I was not cool because I decided not to have sex. They made it sound like everyone, everybody's doing it and you're going to do it soon enough."[59]

A male student said that he "never heard them [Planned Parenthood] say anything about abstinence." Another male student was critical of the nature in which the presentation was made. "You know, it did bother me when they said that, you know, your parents won't understand and stuff and that you can come there and get an abortion and nobody will ever even know about it," the student says. "They just kind of made it, you know, like a statement like, like you can go get a wart removed or something."[60]

It is not surprising that Planned Parenthood speakers do not speak of abstinence as the organizations national leaders oppose such teaching. Susan Newcomer, then-director of education for the Planned Parenthood Federation of America, believes it is wrong to teach chastity. Why? Newcomer explains it is because "it's immoral and it's unethical and it's dishonest. I believe that we should respect the young people and help them learn how to think, not tell them what to think. And a program with only one answer doesn't tell kids how to think, it tells them what to think."[61]

Many school administrators and teachers will not allow parents to visit the classroom during Planned Parenthood presentations. The reason usually given is that having parents present would not allow the students to openly talk about the subjects addressed. Consequently, it is argued, parental involvement would impede the learning process. Most parents do not question such reasoning when it is offered.

6

PUBLIC RELATIONS AND THE MEDIA

Soon after the death of her daughter, Margaret Sanger, on trial for violating the Comstock Law, "decided to have a family portrait taken that would undercut all speculation about coarseness or masculinity." The photograph "was a touching depiction of a loving mother and her sons—athletic Stuart shone with health and vigor, little Grant looked boyishly cute, and Margaret was dressed in a simple blue dress and white collar, giving a tender, caring expression. The picture was printed hundreds of times over the course of the trial and was powerfully effective in winning sympathy for her side."[1]

Planned Parenthood has always understood the importance of playing and mastering the media game. The organization spends millions of dollars each year to convince the public and the media that it has the right ideas regarding sex, birth control, and abortion. Its five year plan includes a subsection called "*National Advertising Campaign —PP-WP* [Planned Parenthood-World Population]." An explanation states that the purpose of the campaign is "to design and produce a series of national advertisements on family planning which describe the Federation and its goals in a favorable fashion."[2]

CREATING MEDIA CAMPAIGNS

A 1954 Planned Parenthood Federation of America newsletter quotes Dr. William Vogt, former national director and executive vice president of the Planned Parenthood Federation of America, as arguing that Planned Parenthood must take the steps necessary to shape public opinion in the same way corporations sell a product:

> Millions have been spent determining use of and attitudes toward everything from a brand of toothpaste to a political candidate. Refined methods of measuring individual and group response, and underlying motivations have been developed. These methods can be invaluable if adapted and applied to achieving broader acceptance of Planned Parenthood.[3]

Planned Parenthood has spent a lot of money developing advertising campaigns designed to improve its public image and to get new customers. In the early 1970s, several advertisements were prepared. The advertising series was called, "Planned Parenthood: Children by Choice. Not Chance."[4]

One advertisement in the series pictures a baby cradle full of cash and is headlined "An Unexpected Child Can Really Rock the Cradle":

That's because, no matter *what* a family's income is, it costs a lot of money to raise a child to 18.

Many thousands of dollars more than most people think.

Which is why we advise every couple to plan when they want children: *when* they can be a welcome addition. Not an accidental burden.[5]

Another advertisement pictures four frames. In the first frame, a man has his arms around a woman. In the second, the pair are joined by a baby. In the third, the first child is a toddler and there is another baby. In the fourth frame, the toddler is little girl, the baby is a toddler, and there is another baby. The advertisement is headlined, "How Many Children Should a Couple Have?":

Three? Two? One? None? There's no right answer.

It depends of how many children they really want.

How many children they feel they're ready for—emotionally, and not just financially.

And *when* they feel they're ready for them.

(It could depend on their concern for the effect population growth can have on society.)

The important thing is that the question of how many children is asked.

Because asking leads to thinking.

And thinking leads to planning.

And Planning leads to us.

For further information, write Planned Parenthood . . . [6]

A third advertisement pictures a caressing young couple and is headlined, "Get to Know the Two of You Before You Become the Three of You":

Get to know what you both really like.

What you both really want out of life.

Get to enjoy your freedom together until you both decide you want to let go of a little bit of it.

But make it your choice.

Research statistics show that more than half of all the pregnancies each year are accidental. Too many of them, to couples who thought they knew all about family planning methods.

Get to know how the two of you don't have to become the three of you.

For further information, write Planned Parenthood . . . [7]

In 1979, Planned Parenthood launched a $1 million advertising campaign designed to protect legal abortion. The *Milwaukee Sentinel* explains that the organization hired a public relations firm "to come up with a program designed to have an impact on public opinion." Louise Tyrer, M.D., then a Planned Parenthood vice president, believes that more than abortion is at stake. She argues that if groups opposed to abortion succeed in making it illegal, the outlawing of contraceptives, sexuality education, and giving teenagers tests and treatments for venereal diseases will be next.[8]

In 1980, Planned Parenthood announced that "Helping Build a Strong America by Helping Build Strong American Families" would be the slogan given to a series of major nationwide advertisements:

The Planned Parenthood Federation of America will begin using the American flag and the family as a theme to fight for contraception and abortion, taking on the so-called right-to-life movement with some of its traditional weapons. . . .

The organization hopes these advertisements and others like them will counter the pro-family image of many anti-abortion groups by giving a 'pro-child, pro-family, pro-life' image to Planned Parenthood, said Fay [sic] Wattleton, the organization's president.

One advertisement opens with a shot of youngsters climbing into a 1930's-era Ford convertible and ends with a couple carrying groceries into a contemporary kitchen. The other shows clients being counseled by Planned Parenthood employees.

> Both end with a picture of the American flag and the words, "Planned Parenthood: Helping Build a Strong America by Helping Build Strong American Families."
>
> The point, said Miss Wattleton, was that the American family would be strong only if family members were free to decide how and when to have children.[9]

The advertising campaign was to be used on purchased radio time and newspaper space, but Planned Parenthood volunteers were encouraged to ask local radio and television stations to run the advertisements as public service announcements.[10]

On Inauguration Day in 1981, a full-page advertisement appeared in the *Washington Post* in the form of a letter to President Ronald Reagan. The advertisement, also part of the new campaign, is headlined, "The Strength of America is its People and Their Right to Choose." The letter begins, "Mr. President: Planned Parenthood believes in the people's right to choose." It goes on to say that Planned Parenthood is dedicated to the principle of "reproductive freedom."[11]

Frederick C. Smith, then-member of the Planned Parenthood Federation of America board of directors, writes in a letter addressed to state and federal lawmakers, "It is clear that the fundamental principles of individual privacy and justice are under the most serious attack since the days of McCarthyism." It is further written that "we will fight to overcome the clamorous attempts of a self-righteous minority to impose its own view of morality on the rest of society." The letter was written in conjunction with the Inauguration Day advertisement.[12]

Abortion opponents often accuse Planned Parenthood of being anti-child and anti-family. Without directly referring to these charges, Planned Parenthood places advertisements such as that which appeared in the *Phoenix Gazette*. The advertisement includes the names of those who paid for it:

> We believe in Planned Parenthood because we love children.
>
> We're celebrating our 50th birthday.
>
> Thanks to these supporters—and thousands more—Planned Parenthood has been a friend of the family since 1937.[13]

The advertisement also includes a coupon readers can use to request more information, volunteer, or to make a "birthday gift" to Planned Parenthood.[14]

Similar attempts to improve its public image are included in virtually all of Planned Parenthood's advertising campaigns. Along with the "Helping Build a Strong America by Helping Build Strong American Families," one advertising series is called, "For the Love of Children," but Planned Parenthood's advertising cannot change statistics regarding its rate of abortion referral.

A Planned Parenthood fund-raising letter, signed by Katharine Hepburn, espouses a strong belief in the use of advertising:

> The use of television and other media is the only way to quickly educate the public. . . .
>
> The time is now. We must buy radio, TV, and newspaper ads immediately. . . . We don't have a minute to lose.[15]

The Public Media Center produced advertisements for Planned Parenthood designed to reach new customers. The first 30 second advertisement consists of a close-up of a "father" who is speaking to the television audience:

> How do you talk to a teenage boy who thinks he invented sex? You want to say "How d'ya think you got here, the stork? You think the stork brought you? Well, I got news . . . "

I just remember how hard it was to talk to my old man about the big things . . . and how easy it was to make a big mistake. I really don't want it to be like that for my son . . . Do you?[16]

The second 30-second spot consists of a close-up of a "mother" who is speaking to the television audience:

Know what it's like to find your daughter's birth control pills . . . by mistake? You get angry. Maybe about what pills might mean. But mainly because you didn't know. And she didn't know how to tell you.

Well, one thing I can tell you is this. If you're going to find out your teenager is sexually active, I can think of worse ways. A lot worse. Can't you?[17]

The third advertisement, which pictures an "older brother," is also 30 seconds in length:

My little brother finally gets himself a girlfriend. So I say, "Bobby, you got yourself a condom?" And he says, "For what?" I say, "For protection. Condoms are strong, they're safe, they're sensitive . . . "

He looks all embarrassed. So I say, "You want to talk about this before you get your girlfriend in trouble or after?" He says, "I'm not gonna get her in trouble." I say, "You bet you're not." And I give him some condoms. Well hey, what's a big brother for?[18]

Another advertisement features a young woman. It, too, is 30 seconds long:

He said if I loved him I would prove it. So I say, "Well, I'm not ready yet." And he says, "Well then I can't love you, can I?" Right, so I say, "You're not talking about love, are you. You're not talking about love at all.

"You can't make somebody love you. All you can do is ask. And maybe the answer is no." You know what? It worked!![19]

The last 30 second advertisement in the series features a "son":

So my dad pats me on the back and calls me "son," you know. And I knew I was in trouble. He says, "Is there anything you need to know, son?" And I said, "You mean like the birds and the bees and that stuff?"

He says, "No, like how to protect your girlfriend." And I said like "Yea, sure dad, I know." And he says, "Well, that's just fine, son." Pats me on the back again. Boy, did he look relieved. And then I said, "But dad . . . What if I didn't know?"[20]

Two other advertisements were also made. All end by showing the Planned Parenthood name and logo.

Other advertisements have included television, film and music celebrities, such as Malcolm Jamal-Warner, famous for his role as "Theo" on "The Cosby Show." They often appear as public service announcements which means they are run free of charge. The advertisements appear most often on television and radio, but they have also appeared in movie theaters, magazines, and newspapers.

A 1991 full-page newspaper advertisement appearing in the *New York Times* is headlined, "What Every Teenager's Parents Need to Know. A Candid Talk With a Planned Parenthood Counselor."[21] The advertisement seeks to convince parents that Planned Parenthood counselors are interested, caring people who are serving children. Therefore, parents should not be concerned if their children go to a Planned Parenthood facility.

Part of the advertisement is correct. Most Planned Parenthood counselors are indeed interested, caring individuals. Unfortunately, they have a child-rearing philosophy which many parents find appalling.

TAKING ON THE NETWORKS

Planned Parenthood has chastised the major television networks for not allowing it and others to advertise birth control and for not including a discussion of birth control on most programs. A full-page advertisement in *USA Today* urges readers to write network officials asking them to allow the advertising of birth control and to include birth control dialogue on television programs.[22]

Another full-page advertisement appeared in *USA Today* just five days later. This advertisement focuses on the teen pregnancy rate and its alleged cost of $16 billion per year to taxpayers. Planned Parenthood said, "Instead of helping solve this problem, the TV networks have virtually banned any mention of birth control in programs and advertising. We need to turn this policy around. You can help." Readers are asked, "Does the public really want uneducated pregnant teenagers? And a tax bill for $16 billion?" Again readers are urged to contact television executives.[23] By appealing to the taxpayer, the advertisements utilize a strategy espoused by Margaret Sanger.

A high ranking Planned Parenthood official further explains the campaign on television programming in a Planned Parenthood affiliate newsletter:

> Douglas Gould, vice president for communications of the Planned Parenthood Federation of America, charges that "it is totally irresponsible for TV to offer material which unrealistically presents sex as being totally detached from consideration about pregnancy, and therefore, the practice of birth control. This, coupled with the overly romantic portrayal of sexual relationships—people being introduced to each other and then shown in bed within the span of 1 minute—teaches youngsters that this is how to be adult, popular, and beautiful."[24]

Planned Parenthood uses the controversy it created to raise money. A fund-raising letter addresses the issue:

> Television bombards our society with sexual messages of every variety. And yet the television network officials adamantly refuse to allow advertising contraceptive products on the grounds that it's too "controversial."
>
> To so openly portray sexual situations without balanced programming on the responsibility and consequences of sexual relationships exploits our children and worsens the teen pregnancy problem in our nation.[25]

Planned Parenthood knows the power of television as it relates to achieving its goals. "*Television is a most potent medium for influencing mass behavior*," the fund-raising letter reads. Faye Wattleton, who signed the letter, writes that Planned Parenthood has launched a "Campaign to Change Network Policies" which is "designed to persuade the executives of the three national TV networks to act responsibly by *balancing* their programming and *ending* their ban on contraceptive product advertising."[26]

The fund-raising letter asks Planned Parenthood supporters to take two steps:

> *FIRST*, please sign the three enclosed petitions to the heads of the three major TV networks and mail them back to Planned Parenthood today. We will deliver these petitions to the head of each network to demonstrate the public support for responsibility.
>
> *SECOND*, please make an immediate, generous contribution to help us purchase full-page newspaper space for running Planned Parenthood ads like the one I've enclosed for you. These ads will reach millions of Americans and will help to generate hundreds of thousands more petitions to the television networks.

> I'm asking for your immediate help because I believe that Planned Parenthood, as the nation's oldest and largest family planning organization, is ideally situated to carry this campaign through to victory.[27]

Wattleton writes that Planned Parenthood refuses to "stand by and wait for the TV moguls to act more responsibly." She announces full-page newspaper advertisements with a price tag in excess of $700,000, "a small price to pay for changing TV network policies and reducing the epidemic of teen pregnancy."[28]

One newspaper advertisement developed for the effort is explicit in giving Planned Parenthood's rationale and demands:

> There's a lot of sex on television. We all know that. What most people don't realize is that while the networks have been hyping sex, they've banned all mention of birth control in advertising, and censor information about it in programming. (It is permitted in the news.) Millions of dollars in sexually alluring ads are okay. Ads for vaginal sprays and hemorrhoidal products are okay. So are the ads which use nudity here and there to sell products. And characters like J.R. Ewing have been seducing women a few times an hour for eight years.
>
> In 1978, researchers counted 20,000 sexual scenes on prime-time network television (which does not even include soap operas), with nary a mention of consequences or protection. It's even higher today. The only sexual mystery left seems to be how all these people keep doing it without contraception while nobody gets pregnant.
>
> With all that worry-free hot action on television, it's no wonder American youngsters are having sex earlier and more often. *And* getting pregnant.[29]

The advertisement alleges that network executives cite "standards of public taste" as a reason for its policy. "The mention of birth control (except in the news) would somehow violate that?" Planned Parenthood responds. "Is that true? Does the public really want uneducated pregnant teens? And a tax bill for $16 billion?"[30]

While decrying the amount of sex and sexual innuendo on television, Planned Parenthood does not suggest that we work to eliminate or even decrease implicit or explicit sex from programming. Instead, its campaign is to push for advertisement of birth control and the inclusion of birth control dialogue on prime-time and other television.

Did Planned Parenthood condemn the Calvin Klein advertising campaign which consists of a supplement to *Vanity Fair*? The advertising campaign features photographs of scantily dressed, at best, young rock 'n' roll disciples, many of whom are in sexual positions.

If Planned Parenthood asked network executives to decrease the amount of sex on television, would they get anywhere? Does Planned Parenthood, with its multi-million dollar annual budget and powerful allies (see appendix G), have no influence on network executives, particularly when one considers that a Planned Parenthood fund-raiser was co-hosted by CBS entertainment head Jeff Sagansky and ABC entertainment head Robert Iger? Is Planned Parenthood really interested in the problems generated by too much sex on television or is it simply being used as a vehicle to promote the organization's agenda and business?

The Planned Parenthood campaign to change network policies seems to be working. The FOX network announced in 1991 that it would accept condom advertising. Music Television accepted such advertising long ago. Birth control has been mentioned on several prime-time television programs including "Beverly Hills 90210" (the highest rated show among teenagers for the 1991–1992 season),

"Doogie Howser, M.D.," "Roseanne," "In Living Color," along with many others. Writers of daytime television programs have also started to include birth control in scripts. Daytime talk shows seem to have discussed everything, including birth control. Phil Donahue even threw handfuls of condoms into the audience at the end of one "Donahue" program.[31]

One "Doogie Howser, M.D.," episode includes one main character, played by Max Casella, saying, "Thirty-seven girls from my senior class lost their virginity this summer. Now that puts virgins in the minority." Speaking about his girlfriend, Howser's friend says, "Now it's my honor, no, my sacred duty to put her in the in-crowd." He later says, "Tonight, we are men!" At the end of the program, Howser, played by Neil Patrick Harris, types on his word processor, "There's a difference between having sex and making love."[32] Something of a weak attempt to salvage the program—given the message that had been given during the rest of the show.

If this were not enough, an advertising agency created an advertisement picturing a "before and after" shot. The "before" shot is of Clearasil. The "after" shot is of Trojan condoms. The advertisement was killed by the advertising agency because the "promise can't be substantiated."[33] This should not be a surprise to anyone. One print condom advertisement from the 1970s is called, "A Critical Choice for Today's Eve." It shows a woman pictured with an apple pie and six packages of condoms. The advertisement reads, "Once you've decided that both the pill and IUDs [intrauterine device] are not for you, you're faced with another important decision."[34]

Encouraging network executives to accept advertisements for birth control and allowing discussion on television programs is not a new idea. The same suggestion was made by Louise Tyrer, M.D., in the 1970s when she was with Planned Parenthood.[35] Condom manufacturers had not been pushing for access to the airwaves at that time. Nevertheless, the manufacturers understand the need to take it one step at a time:

> "Using broadcast before print is like putting the cart before the horse," said [Alan] Woltz [president of Schmid Laboratories Inc.]. "The public ought to be educated first by the print media before it is ready for the broadcast media.
>
> "How do you provide information about family planning in good taste in 30 seconds of television?"[36]

An early television advertisement prepared by the makers of Trojan condoms was aired in San Jose, California, in 1975. Called "Boy and Girl," the advertisement begins with a scene of a young couple holding hands and running along the beach.[37] The person doing the voice-over adapts a passage from the Bible:

> "To everything there is a season, and a time to every purpose under heaven. . . . The makers of Trojan condoms believe there is a time for children—the right time, when they are wanted. Trojans have helped people for over half a century to practice responsible parenthood."[38]

THE BETTER WORLD SOCIETY

Planned Parenthood has teamed up with an organization called the Better World Society. In November 1987, WTBS, which is based in Atlanta, Georgia, and is carried by most cable television systems, aired a film called *Increase and Multiply?* The film was produced by the Society in conjunction with the Planned Parenthood Federation of America.

Increase and Multiply? attacks abortion foes and the Reagan Administration's policies regarding foreign aid for groups promoting abortion overseas. This includes the decision to stop American funding of the International Planned Parenthood Federation because it supports the forced abortion and sterilization policies of the People's Republic of China. The film specifically attacks the Mexico City Policy, which prohibits American funds from being used by any foreign group that promotes abortion.[39]

Based in Washington, D.C., the Better World Society lists the Alan Guttmacher Institute, the Planned Parenthood Federation of America, the International Planned Parenthood Federation, the Sierra Club, Zero Population Growth, the National Audubon Society, the Center for Population Options, and the Association for Voluntary Surgical Contraception, as organizations "concerned about population."[40]

While the Alan Guttmacher Institute is viewed and touted as an independent, reputable research organization, it is named after the man who served as president of the Planned Parenthood Federation of America from 1962 until his death in 1974. The Institute, in reality, is the research arm of Planned Parenthood. Like Margaret Sanger, Alan F. Guttmacher, M.D., is still highly regarded by Planned Parenthood leaders. Guttmacher was also vice president of the American Eugenics Society.[41]

The Alan Guttmacher Institute, with offices in New York City and Washington, D.C., professes to be "an independent [nonprofit] corporation for research, policy analysis, and public information concerning family planning and population."[42] A Planned Parenthood annual report states the relationship more clearly when it reads, "Since 1977, AGI [Alan Guttmacher Institute] has been a special affiliate of Planned Parenthood."[43] Nevertheless, the Institute's studies are often passed off as the last word in nonpartisan, unbiased research.

The purpose of the Better World Society is to make people aware of "global problems that threaten life on our planet." One of these problems is "a burgeoning world population." The Society seeks to "educate, explore solutions to our problems" and to "strive to bring together individuals, governments, corporations, foundations, and non-profit organizations to work in partnership and without regard to national boundaries."[44]

The Better World Society has a list of films that have been produced to help achieve its goals. The Society stresses the importance of television:

> We produce, acquire, commission and distribute television programming on global issues. Unlike the programs on network TV, however, our shows don't just "present" an issue. They take a stand. They . . . encourage action.[45]

The Better World Society strongly opposes the family planning policies implemented under the Reagan Administration. It notes that the United States had been the largest donor to international population control programs.[46] Such funding has been cut and tied to abortion-neutral or anti-abortion policies.

The Better World Society blames "political pressure from right-to-life groups" for the policies. It says there will be serious consequences unless the policies are reversed, but the Bush Administration is continuing them.[47]

Working with Planned Parenthood, the Better World Society could have an incredible impact on public opinion and the media. Founded by R. E. "Ted" Turner, head of Turner Broadcasting (Cable News Network, WTBS, Turner Network Television, "CNN Headline News", etc.), the Society lists the following individuals as members of its board of directors: Ambassador Zhou Boping, deputy director of the China Family Planning Association (see chapters 11 and 15); Yasushi Akashi, under secretary-general of the United Nations; Georgiy Arbatov, then-director of the Soviet Union's USA and Canada Institute; Gro Harlem Brundtland, prime minister of Norway; Jean-Michel Cousteau, executive vice president of the Cousteau Society; Jimmy Carter, former president of the United States; and Julia Henderson, formerly of the International Planned Parenthood Federation, among others. Paul Newman, John Denver, Yoko Ono, Carl Sagan, Ph.D., Joanne Woodward, Mario Cuomo, Andrew Young, Jane Alexander, Theodore Hesburgh, S.J. (former president of the University of Notre Dame), and others have "expressed an interest" in the work of the Better World Society.[48]

In December 1988, WTBS aired the 1988 Better World Society Awards. The ceremony allows the Society to present awards in numerous areas including the environment, communications, and population. Television hosts were actress Margot Kidder and actors Sam Waterston and Peter Strauss. Presenters and performers included Ben Vereen, Carl Sagan, Ph.D., Jean-Michel Cousteau, Ann Hampton Callaway, Ted Turner, Phil Donahue (who won the 1987 Communications Medal), and the Muppets (when the rights to the Muppets were owned by the late Jim Henson).[49]

In an opening speech, Turner outlines rules by which he believes all people should live. He calls his rules the Ten Voluntary Initiatives. One rule is, "I promise to have no more than two children or no more than my nation suggests."[50]

Speaking at a National Newspaper Association meeting in 1989, Turner said the Ten Commandments are out of date and not relevant to today's global problems such as overpopulation. "I bet nobody here even pays much attention to 'em, because they are too old," Turner said. "Commandments are out." Turner suggests his Ten Voluntary Initiatives as a contemporary alternative to the Ten Commandments.[51]

In October 1989, WTBS aired the Better World Society's 1989 awards program. The television host was actor Mike Farrell. The master of ceremonies was talk show host Phil Donahue. A group called City Kids Repertory Theater performed.

As part of the program, a pre-recorded report was shown during which the Society outlines three major areas of concern: the arms race, overpopulation, and environmental destruction. The announcer explains how these areas of concern are going to be addressed and why the Society is needed to do so:

> Our future, our ability to survive, depends on global action to respond to these interrelated challenges. Television is the international vehicle that will bring us together. Through television we can communicate an understanding of the issues and set an agenda for action. Through words and images we can reach out. Through television we can share a vision of a better world. The Better World Society produces and acquires Programming addressing these survival issues, and through our unique access to the Turner Broadcasting System,

distributes them worldwide. . . . The Better World Society: committed to making a difference.[52]

Phil Donahue told his audience what the Better World Society is and what it is not:

Let us understand who we are. We are not a small group of people pushing an unpopular cause up a very large incline. We are a very dedicated and informed and caring group of people who are proud to be part of a very popular ideal. The goals and the ideals advanced by this organization know no boundaries. . . . They are about common sense.[53]

Award presenters included Jimmy Carter, former president of the United States; Julia Henderson, formerly of the International Planned Parenthood Federation; and Peter Goldmark, Jr., president of the Rockefeller Foundation. Winners of 1989 awards include Time Inc. (Communications Medal), UNICEF (Humanitarian Medal), Mikhail S. Gorbachev, at the time president of what was then the Soviet Union (Peace Advocacy Medal), and Faye Wattleton, then-president of the Planned Parenthood Federation of America (Population Medal).

J. Richard Munroe, co-chairman of Time Warner Inc., accepted the Better World Society award for Time Inc. Munroe said the company "has never been afraid of having strong opinions, nor of the controversy that they often cause."[54] Time Inc. returned the favor in December 1991 when it announced its Man of the Year—Ted Turner.

During the program, Mike Farrell refers to Wattleton as "a fighter in the rights of women everywhere to decide for themselves how many children they bring into this world." In a pre-recorded report, it is said that "Planned Parenthood continues its struggle against those who threaten reproductive freedom." Wattleton said "the reason we must win the reproductive choice battle is that we have to create a world in which our children will be born wanted and loved."[55]

Wattleton gave an acceptance speech:

I know the Better World Society shares Planned Parenthood's conviction that the right to control one's childbearing is universal. The free exercise of this right must not be constrained by ignorance, by economic hardship or by political pressures. The Better World Society also understands that international family planning is not only a matter of fundamental human rights, it is a matter of planetary survival. . . . I look forward to continuing our partnership in building a better world.[56]

Viewers were shown many reports prepared by the Society. They were encouraged to join the Society by calling its toll-free telephone number.[57] (For more on the Better World Society, see chapters 11 and 15. For a list of benefactors, patrons, sponsors and staff of the Better World Society events, see Appendix A.)

CELEBRITY ASSISTANCE

Planned Parenthood has been making significant use of celebrities. Few would argue that these citizens do not have a right to voice their opinions with regard to abortion. However, it seems inappropriate for the views of these individuals to be given more weight just because they have talent in a specific area. Why, for example, should Marlo Thomas be given a stage to speak on abortion when she is not an expert in the field? Would Thomas be given the stage if she were not a well-known actress?

Whether appropriate or not, Planned Parenthood is pushing celebrities, particularly those in the entertainment industry, to speak up. Many entertainers have demonstrated support for legal abortion, Planned Parenthood, and/or the Better World Society.

One supporter of the Planned Parenthood agenda is singer Sinead O'Connor. The Associated Press reports that her single, "My Special Child," is about "the baby she would have had if she hadn't chosen to have an abortion last summer [August 1990] while on tour in the United States":

> "It was a planned pregnancy, which I was very happy about," said O'Connor. "I was completely in love with the father of the child. . . . But things didn't work out between us and we were both unhappy. . . . I made the decision that it would be better for everybody if I had the abortion."[58]

O'Connor refuses to identify the father of the child, though she was married to musician John Reynolds in 1984. They have a son who was four years old at the time of the abortion. O'Connor claims she does not "have a sense of guilt about the abortion." She explains: "If I had had the child, I wouldn't have been in any state to be the mother that child would have deserved. . . . As far as I'm concerned, that child's spirit is gone and perhaps some day it will return."[59]

The November 1991 edition of *Spin* quotes O'Connor's position on abortion from a less personal venue:

> I just believe that if a child is meant to be born it will be born. It doesn't really matter whether you have an abortion or miscarriage. The whole issue is pro-choice . . . Nobody has the right to tell anyone else what to believe. Especially the Catholic church with the amount of murdering and pillaging it has done . . .[60]

O'Connor has strong feelings about religion in general:

> I think organized religion is a crutch. 'Cause it's controlling. Organized religion tells you what to believe, tells you who to be . . . It's an abuse to tell a child that God sees everything and knows what you think and that you are going to be burnt in hell. It's a huge abuse to teach children that God is not within themselves . . . That God is bigger than them. That God is outside them. That is a lie. That's what causes the emptiness of children.[61]

Perhaps O'Connor's position on religion is the reason for her stand on abortion? The same question can be asked of actor Corbin Bernsen who says, "Religion has become an outdated mode, an outdated answer to some of our problems . . . Religion is the only reason women don't have control over their bodies."[62] Of course, there are many non-religious people who oppose abortion, so there may not be a strong correlation, but it is clear that a strong, serious religious faith generally coincides with anti-abortion beliefs.

Madonna Louise Veronica Ciccone, known to most people only by her first name, is a strong advocate of abortion. "Passion and sexuality and religion all bleed into each other for me," she says. "I think that you can be a very sexual person and also a very religious and spiritual person. I think I'm religious in the broadest sense of the word . . . "[63] A member of the National Leadership Committee to Keep Abortion Safe and Legal, a project of Planned Parenthood, Madonna is careful to pray with her dancers and others before going on stage, seemingly unconcerned about of the fact that coarse language weaves in and out of the prayer.

Another member of Planned Parenthood's National Leadership Committee, who is also known by her first name, is Cher. She discusses abortion in an interview published by *US:*

> If *Roe v. Wade* got overturned, I would do everything in my power to have women go out on a general strike and bring the country to its knees. I think that each person has to use their own conscience. We're only answerable to ourselves and to God, and it's nobody's f——— business. Rather than picketing, why not go and be a foster parent, do something for people that [sic] are here? I'm just disgusted with all of it.[64]

Norman Mailer also supports legal abortion. "If a woman decides in the depth of her soul . . . that she doesn't want to have a child," he suggests, "then I think that's her right to say no, but let's not pretend that it isn't a form of killing."[65] At least Mailer is honest.

The abortion issue has even been mentioned on a game show. One episode of "Family Feud" featured soap opera stars competing for charity. The group representing NBC, which included Charlotte Ross, John Callahan, Robin Mattson, Nicolas Coster, and Anthony Alda, chose the pro-legal abortion movement as its "charity."

"Family Feud" host Ray Combs said to NBC team captain Charlotte Ross, "You're playing for a wonderful charity and tell everyone who that is, Charlotte." Ross' response, while neither articulate nor reflective of a good understanding of the legislative process, was, "Yes, we are. We're gonna play for, ah, pro-choice, so the public can be, ah, as much aware as they can be about the state legislatures that are trying to be passed [sic]."[66]

It is ironic that one question asked of the NBC team was, "Name a place you wish people wouldn't take babies." An answer from one woman on the NBC team was your "own home."[67]

Are there any celebrities who oppose abortion? Yes, but most are unwilling to state so publicly and who can blame them? There have been reports of blacklisting against outspoken abortion foes in the entertainment industry. Nevertheless, some have spoken out.

Brooke Shields not only makes no apologies for being opposed to legal abortion, she also praises the virtues of virginity. It's "nothing to be ashamed of. It's sacred," she says. "Sex is the ultimate gift a woman can give a man, and the thought of being vulnerable and intimate with a man is very appealing to me. . . . But sex is meant for procreation, and I want to consummate a relationship with a man who's going to be the father of my children."[68]

Actor Mel Gibson has said, "God is the only one who knows how many children we should have, and we should be ready to accept them."[69] Columnist Liz Smith replies, "Mel Gibson is so divine on screen. It is awful to find out that mentally he lives in the Dark Ages."[70]

Singer Olivia Newton-John is not anti-abortion, but she has an interesting attitude about motherhood. "It's the most underestimated, exhausting and rewarding job in the world," she says. "I think women who feel being *just* a mother isn't enough shouldn't feel that way. I think women's lib, which has done wonderful things with equal pay and equal rights, has done them a disservice—if the result is that some women have been forced to feel they should be working. If you choose not to, you shouldn't feel bad about it."[71] Given that the most critical thing a person can ever do on earth is to raise a child—the chance to positively impact the life of another human being, from it's start—I could not agree more (see Appendix H).

INDOCTRINATIONAL MUSIC TELEVISION

Music Television (MTV), which targets a young audience, has aired several programs espousing a pro-legal abortion position. A wholly-owned subsidiary of Viacom, Music Television produced and aired two special programs in 1991 on sex. Titled "Sex in the '90s" and "More Sex in the '90s," the programs include sex jokes by musicians, interviews with musicians and students, countless sexual images, and other material.[72]

Planned Parenthood is listed as a "resource organization" for "Sex in the '90s" along with the Alan Guttmacher Institute, the Center for Population Options, the Gallup Organization, the Gay Men's Health Crisis, the National Gay and Lesbian Task Force, New York Women Against Rape, Rhode Island Rape Crisis Center, and the Sex Information and Education Council of the United States (SIECUS). The Feminist Majority Foundation and Playboy Enterprises are also credited.[73] Planned Parenthood of New York City, the Alan Guttmacher Institute, and the Centers for Disease Control are credited in "More Sex in the '90s."[74]

What kind of "information" is given to young people in "Sex in the '90s"? While a small effort is made to present both sides of controversial issues, the program includes rhetoric which clearly takes a stand. Program highlights include the following:

- Hugh Hefner, founder of Playboy Enterprises, gives his view about sex.[75]
- The program host, Music Television's Kurt Loder, notes that rock 'n' roll music took its name from African-American slang for "sexual frolic." He also refers to rock 'n' roll's "message of sexual liberation."[76]
- Jesse Jackson, who was once strongly opposed to legal abortion but who now supports it just as strongly, states, "Sex without love, sex without an ethic, without a purpose, can lead to vast destruction of human life."[77]
- Eric Bogosian argues that, "People don't know how to get intimate anymore. The legacy of the '70s has been that people can fall into bed so fast that they don't even know how to really say hello."[78]
- Steven Tyler, lead singer of Aerosmith, proclaims, "They say the sexual revolution is over; hogwash." Tyler also says, "Rock 'n' roll is synonymous with a lot of things, sex being one of 'em, and you can't take that away from it."[79]
- George Michael comments on surveys conducted on sexual issues. "How can you possibly listen to some survey . . . ? When you ask people about sex they say what they think you want to hear or what they think they should say. There's no such thing as an accurate sex survey."[80]

- Immediately following Michael's comment, Kurt Loder states, "Probably not, but MTV News has conducted one anyway."[81]
- University students are interviewed regarding their attitudes on sex. One woman points out that safe sex dances have been held on campus and condoms were distributed.[82]
- Regarding abortion, Loder says that "while young people can be found in both the pro-choice and anti-abortion camps on this issue, our MTV News poll [a survey of 18–35 year olds] showed that 60 percent of our respondents and 67 percent of MTV viewers favor keeping abortion legal." The poll also showed that 40 percent of the respondents said they would get an illegal abortion if abortion were outlawed. Loder summarizes the poll results by declaring, "Today's students . . . still believe strongly in abortion rights."[83]
- Students are interviewed on the abortion issue. One student who supports abortion says, "Being a male and a guy [sic] . . . I don't think I should have any say one way or another. Definitely it's a woman's issue. It should be left up to women to decide that for themselves." One female student says, "People just sort of assume that everybody's pro-choice and so I think probably the people who aren't pro-choice are afraid to say anything."[84]
- Some students argue that making abortion illegal would simply lead to back-alley abortions. Others argue that it would make young people more cautious about sex.[85]
- Loder states, as fact, that, "Making abortion illegal doesn't end the practice. There are twice as many abortions performed each year in Brazil where abortion is illegal as there are in the United States where the practice is still protected by law." He also states, as fact, that, "Every year around the world some 200,000 women die from illegal abortions—one every three minutes." This is Planned Parenthood-supported opinion and ridiculous on its face.[86]
- Regarding casual sex, one student says it "is very much alive on campus. It's part of being young, I guess."[87]
- Asked about condoms in light of acquired immunodeficiency syndrome (AIDS), some students believe people are being more careful with regard to "free love." Others argue that, in the heat of the moment, most young people neither think nor worry about condoms and acquired immunodeficiency syndrome. They apparently believe nothing will happen to them because the odds are on their side.[88]
- Loder asserts that the acquired immunodeficiency syndrome crisis has "brought with it a resurgence of homophobia . . . "[89]
- Little Richard argues that no one should criticize someone else because of a selected lifestyle.[90]
- The program highlights an erotic dancer, a man who really enjoys adult magazines, a rock music groupie who really loves having sex with hard-rock musicians, and an unmarried elderly couple who live together, among others.[91]

The somewhat more tame "More Sex in the '90s" includes the following highlights:

- Cathy Dennis believes "everyone thinks that they'll find a cure [for AIDS]. But, I mean, you know, what if they don't—ever?"[92]

- A member of the heavy-metal group Megadeth announces that he is "into kinda violent sex" but he "still likes it safe."[93]
- Sinead O'Connor, who tells a crude joke, says, "Teens are having sex and like if parents haven't noticed that by now then like they're on drugs or something."[94]
- Cyndi Lauper states that, "Condoms aren't altogether the safest thing. The safest thing is not having intercourse. Otherwise you take the chance of dying."[95]
- Kurt Loder asks whether parents have an absolute right to know if their daughter is seeking an abortion or if "young women have a right to run their own lives—even before they reach 18?" In response, MC Lyte states, "I feel that at the age 16 you really don't know what the hell is going on. I mean, everybody thinks at 16 they know what's happening, but at 16 . . . I do think a 16-year-old needs parental guidance." Queen Latifah and several others speak against requiring parental involvement.[96]
- The program features Joe, a Catholic priest, who believes "there probably is no real absolute" with regard to sex and marriage.[97]
- Lisa, a single mother, is also featured. Lisa claims that she does not believe in moral standards. "I think that is a load of baloney," she says. Lisa further states that she is very pro-choice. "I think that a man's choice comes into play when he chooses to put a condom on or not. You choose not to put a condom on, the woman that you're with gets pregnant, it's not your choice anymore."[98]
- The program also features a homosexual couple, one of whom has tested positive for the virus which leads to acquired immunodeficiency syndrome. The man who tested positive claims his sex life still exists.[99]

Even New Kids on the Block, once enjoyed by teenagers and approved by parents, have changed their tune. The group began with a wholesome image in the shadow of Bobby Sherman and Shawn Cassidy. Today, they are using profanity and grabbing their crotches while making sexual references. Is it any wonder that one album of the heavy metal group Mötley Crüe includes the statement that "those who have the youth have the future"?[100]

The National Organization for Women has condemned the "exploitation" of women in music videos. The women who appear in the videos say they want to be in them and exploitation has nothing to do with it. As bad as American music videos are, those aired in Europe are much worse.[101]

On the 1991 Music Television Video Awards program, the popular rock group R.E.M. was nominated for seven awards. The group's lead singer, Michael Stipe, planned to wear a different shirt while accepting each award. The shirts display political opinions. One shirt reads, "WEAR A CONDOM." Other shirts read, "HANDGUN CONTROL," "ALTERNATIVE ENERGY NOW," and "THE RIGHT TO VOTE," among other issues. The shirt which got the most sustained applause, however, reads, "CHOICE."[102]

You!, a magazine which targets Catholic youth, notes a "new trend" among Music Television musicians. The magazine states that "God is turning up at award ceremonies and is being acknowledged (finally) as the one responsible for all the great music, movies and TV shows that come our way." *You!* suggests that entertainers "are growing less afraid that they might trample on the toes of some industry big wigs by mentioning the fact that it was God, not the producers or directors, who really made it all possible." Several entertainers are quoted in the article including a member of In Living Colour who said, "We'd like to thank our Creator for making it possible to express our talent." A member of En Vogue claims that "God" is the reason for the group's success. Jon Bon Jovi is said to have "thanked God" and referenced prayer.[103]

Assuming these and other entertainers mean the same thing as others when they refer to the "Creator" or "God" is a mistake. Look at the work and lifestyles of many of these groups and individuals. Prince and Aerosmith's Steven Tyler have also referenced "God" or a "higher power," but their music and music videos tell a different story. While no one can judge a person's heart, it makes one wonder, considering their actions and the results of their actions. Maybe *You!* is right when it refers to thanking God as a "trend," or maybe we should simply use a small "g" when we write "god."

A "public service" announcement, featuring several popular female musicians defending legal abortion, has been produced for Music Television. The producer of the announcement, Juliet Cuming, states, "I think the women who showed up [to tape the announcement] were very brave." She also says, "We're pro-choice, not anti-children."[104] Cuming notes that she "wanted to reach 13, 14-year-old kids . . . It [the public service announcement] was geared to MTV, the kids who watch MTV." Titled "Choice: Keep Abortion Legal," the announcement endorses the National Abortion Rights Action League and, according to the *New York Guardian*, its production and promotion were funded in part by the National Endowment for the Arts.[105]

The public service announcement opens with seven musicians standing side-by-side. "The most extraordinary women in music rely on freedom of expression," a narrator states. "Motherhood is our birthright and the freedom to choose it must remain our own." The words "Keep Abortion Legal" appear on the screen, followed by a suggestion that those watching call the National Abortion Rights Action League. "Women have a right to choose," is another slogan used. A toll-free telephone number is shown.[106] While it appears Music Television will not accept the announcement, efforts to get it aired continue.

The role Music Television plays in the fight for legal abortion should not come as a surprise to anyone. Its view of religion is also negative. Music Television has featured the band Live as one of its "buzz clips." The group's album, "Mental Jewelry," includes a song of the same name which carries the recurring theme "give it up." The theme refers to religion. The band members, all of whom appear to be in their early twenties, note that Jesus lived 2,000 years ago, which means nothing to them. We must look within ourselves to solve the problems of the day, they argue, as opposed to clinging to a belief in someone or something to solve or help us solve the problems we face.

Thomas L. Jipping, J.D., director of the Center for Law and Democracy at the Free Congress Foundation, has done extensive research on the influence of music and music television on young people. "We know from experience that music dramatically affects both attitudes and behavior. Music sells coffee, it drives aerobics classes and stirs the emotions during a movie. The profession of music therapy exists because of the power of music," Jipping says. "Available research only serves to validate what experience teaches. Therefore, we are cutting our own throats if we ignore the messages being pumped into our children."[107] Jipping is author of *Heavy Metal, Rap, and America's Youth: Issues and Alternatives*.

MEDIA BIAS

Both sides in the abortion debate claim the media supports the other side. One of the best books on the subject, which deals exclusively with the print media, is *The Press and Abortion, 1838-1988*, by Marvin N. Olasky. Olasky makes a strong case in showing how the print media has been crucial in the slow change toward acceptance of abortion. His introduction includes two paragraphs that outline this influence:

> *The Press and Abortion, 1838-1988* reports the sensationalism of the 19th century abortion stories filled with specific detail concerning the depravity of abortionists, the misery of young women who sought them out, and the tragedy of unborn children victimized. It shows the triumphs of the anti-abortion campaigns—legislation tightened, abortion advertising turned down, abortionists arrested or publicly disgraced—but also points out press tendencies to back away from hard hitting exposes [sic] that could alienate some readers and advertisers. The history shows that when investigative journalism lagged, public interest decreased and laws against abortion were not enforced rigorously.
>
> The early 20th century brought both victory and defeat for anti-abortion forces. Doctors in Chicago and other cities pushed hard against newspapers that continued to accept abortion advertising. Although anti-abortionists were winning the abortion wars, they were losing the news pages. News stories emphasized the greed of abortionists but not the evil of abortion, and coverage shifted from concern for the unborn child to issues of corruption that supposedly could be dealt with through legalization of abortion. As pro-abortion public relations slowly emerged, reporting of abortion became neutral and a new set of cozy relationships developed. Newspapers from mid-century on set a pro-abortion agenda and were used by those setting agendas.[108]

Olasky explains that those involved in pro-legal abortion advocacy set out to make use of a willing media.[109] Lawrence Lader, author of *Abortion* (1966) and *Abortion II: Making the Revolution* (1973), is co-founder of the National Association for the Repeal of Abortion Laws. Lader understood the importance of using the media. "The best chance to build a movement was through public relations," Lader wrote.[110] It was Lader who decided to make an attack on the Roman Catholic Church a primary part of the crusade to make abortion legal. According to Lader, "every revolution has to have its villain."[111] A friend of Margaret Sanger, Lader became more successful in his endeavors than even he imagined possible.

One of Olasky's most poignant criticisms concerns the unwillingness of the media to verify "statistics" pro-legal abortion activists claim to be accurate. Instead of investigating these statistics, the media uses them as fact. For example, newspapers and magazines reported that state legislatures started passing laws against abortion in the early and mid-nineteenth century because of the dangers to the woman, not because of any moral reservation or concern for those not yet born. The print media reported that women faced either legal abortion that was done under sterile conditions or illegal abortion done by "back-alley butchers." This latter statement includes the printing of statistics citing anywhere between 5,000 and 10,000 maternal deaths attributed to illegal abortion each year.[112] This information, all of which is grossly false, could have been checked. It was not.

In 1974, a group called the National News Council was formed to investigate and arbitrate complaints against the news media. This was an effort by the news media to regulate itself and to assist in maintaining fairness. However, the Council had no authority, relying exclusively on publicity and peer review for its effectiveness. Not surprisingly, most in the press refused to cooperate and the Council folded.[113]

Since the April 1989 pro-legal abortion march in Washington, D.C., called the "March for Women's Equality and Women's Lives," and the United States Supreme Court decision in *Webster v. Reproductive Health Services*, some reporters are appearing to be more sensitive to accusations of bias. Some major newspapers, including the *Washington Post*, *New York Times* and *Chicago Tribune*, have reviewed their policies with regard to allowing reporters to actively participate in the abortion debate. The issue came to a head after numerous reporters from a variety of newspapers and magazines participated in the march.

Time quotes a reporter for the *Chicago Tribune* who supports legal abortion:

> To me, the struggle for abortion rights is as important to women as the struggle against slavery. This isn't about whether they're going to build some bridge downtown. This is about my body.[114]

A newspaper editor has also gone on record in support of legal abortion. She states, "As far as I'm concerned, until that thing is born, it is really no different from a kidney. It is part of the woman's body."[115]

Linda Greenhouse, who covers the United States Supreme Court for the *New York Times*, participated in the pro-legal abortion march. Several reporters from the *Washington Post* also participated.[116]

In the December 5, 1988, issue of *Time*, reporter Andrea Sachs refers to abortion as "a right that in the course of just 15 years many Americans have come to regard as no less inalienable than freedom of religion or expression." Some of Sachs' articles have been titled, "Here Come the Pregnancy Police," and "To Hell With Choice: A Cardinal Turns Excommunication Into a Political Weapon."[117]

According to a University of Michigan Law School newspaper article, Sachs, who admits to participating in the pro-legal abortion march, has decided to refrain from doing so in future events since she often writes about the abortion issue. Sachs was asked "whether her decision was based on a need to remain objective or to be perceived as objective." Sachs says it is for "the latter" reason.[118]

Barbara Reynolds, editor of *USA Today*'s "Inquiry" section, makes her view of abortion clear:

> How can you who protest abortion be so certain that we aren't swimming toward a fate worse than death? Is homicide in the womb, swift and merciful, not better than the slow death that lies ahead for some of us once our lives begin? . . . Better to die now, before we can feel real pain, than to enter a world where life is so painful it's criminal to be born.[119]

ABC's David Brinkley ends one of his television programs with these words:

> What was astonishing here was not that the [United States Supreme] Court opposes abortion. What was astonishing was its absurd view that medical personnel paid with government money lose their right to free speech. The Constitution says no law shall abridge freedom of speech, no law. Could it be that the Court hasn't read that part? . . . Was (David Souter) able and willing to read the Constitution as a member of the Court? Would he abide by it? Well, now we know the answer. It's no.[120]

Bert Quint, a correspondent for CBS News, reports that most citizens of Poland "do not share [Pope] John Paul's concept of morality . . . Many here expect John Paul to use his authority to support Church efforts to ban abortion, perhaps the country's principal means of birth control. And this, they say, could deprive them of a freedom of choice the communists never tried to take away from them."[121]

Just six months after Quint made this comment, Poland's Congress of Physicians, by a vote of 449-75, adopted a medical code of ethics which states that doctors who perform abortions could be stripped of their medical licenses. Exceptions are made only if the pregnancy is a threat to the mother's life or if a result of rape. The Congress of Physicians also pledged to lobby the Polish government for laws consistent with the code. Senator Zofia Kuratowska, M.D., calls the law "simply unethical" and argues that, "Abortion is evil from every point of view, but I think it is the woman who should always make the final decision."[122]

Lynn Sherr, a correspondent for the ABC News program "20/20," prepared a report on the abortion pill RU 486 which aired on April 7, 1989. While reporters are expected to present material in an impartial way, Sherr makes her position clear:

> The movement to ban the new drug and all abortions in the United States is being led by a minority. According to polls, a majority of Americans support legal abortion, but the protesters have support in the White House. President Bush is opposed to abortion.[123]

Ken Auletta of the *New York Daily News* has written of the "incalculable costs" of limiting access to abortion. "More future city criminals will be incubated, unwanted kids, entering the world without nurturing and self-esteem."[124]

Such statements have led some journalists to question their colleagues. Auletta's comments prompted Nat Hentoff of the *Village Voice* to respond:

> So the battle for abortion rights is not—as we've been told all along—solely a matter of preserving an individual woman's right to decide how she shall manage her life. There is an added dimension—the equation of abortion with a public service responsibility to keep the population down. Especially to keep the population in the ghetto down.[125]

Ethan Bronner, legal affairs reporter for the *Boston Globe*, acknowledges that bias exists:

> Journalists tend to regard opponents of abortion as "religious fanatics" and "bug eyed zealots." Opposing abortion, in the eyes of most journalists, is not a legitimate, civilized position in our society. I think that when abortion opponents complain about a bias in newsrooms against their cause, they're absolutely right.[126]

Many reporters and columnists are actively involved in Planned Parenthood. For example, Eleanor Clift of *Newsweek* and "The McLaughlin Group" presented Maggie Awards at Planned Parenthood's 75th anniversary gala.[127]

Most news organizations do not limit a reporter's political activity so long as it does not directly relate to the reporter's regular field of writing.[128] Given the turbulent situation with abortion, however, it appears that news organizations may impose more restrictions which may apply to all reporters. For example, some who regularly write movie reviews could be prohibited from active participation in either the pro-legal abortion or anti-legal abortion movements.

Marvin Olasky writes, "If one thing is clear from the history of press coverage of abortion, it is that journalists' beliefs, whether for or against abortion, do heavily influence coverage."[129] Even *Time* agrees:

> All reporters have personal opinions on a wide range of issues, just like everyone else, even if they do not choose to proclaim them publicly. The best solution for journalists with strong political beliefs is to disqualify themselves from covering stories on which they feel their reporting cannot be fair. Deni Elliot of Dartmouth's Institute for the Study of Applied and Professional Ethics believes every reporter has at least one such issue.[130]

While most abortion opponents would surely approve of restrictions on reporters when it comes to participation in pro-legal abortion activities, it could be argued that such restrictions are useless. Do the restrictions really help to balance news reporting? Does anyone believe the stories would change one way or the other? Could reporters excluded from such activities against their will believe they have more reason to be unfair? Are reporters likely to ask to be excused from stories because they feel strongly about the issue being covered? Is a reporter likely to say that he or she cannot be objective when writing about any subject? Don't reporters believe they can always put their personal opinions aside?

It seems that allowing reporters to become openly vocal on such issues would have the desired effect of creating more objectivity. After all, if everyone knows a reporter has a strong interest in supporting one particular side of the abortion debate, this could force the reporter to take extra steps to at least *appear* fair. As it now stands, reporters make their positions known in their reporting as opposed to in their private activities. At least people would know the reporter's position on abortion and this kind of information would be helpful to leaders of both sides in the abortion debate.

It surely is no secret that most national journalists and most of America's largest news organizations support legal abortion (90 percent, according to a survey[131]). It could be argued that much of the resulting coverage has been part of a conspiracy. Cal Thomas, a nationally syndicated columnist, writes that such a conspiracy exists among the editors of many national women's magazines:

> Editors from *Women's Day*, *Family Circle*, *Good Housekeeping* and *Ladies' Home Journal* met with editors from more politically and socially trendy publications such as *Redbook*, *Harper's Bazaar*, *Savvy*, *Lear's*, Ms., *Cosmopolitan* and *Mirabella* to discuss whether their magazines should be used to support and maintain abortion on demand.[132]

The meeting of the magazine editors was organized by Helen Gurley Brown, editor of *Cosmopolitan*. Brown has been quoted as saying that the editors discussed what they can do to protect *Roe v. Wade*. Attending the meeting with the editors was Kate Michelman, executive director of the National Abortion Rights Action League. Michelman offered to assist the editors by making available a letter for their magazines that "readers could send to state and federal legislators." *Mademoiselle* published such a letter in June 1989. The former editor of Ms., Suzanne Levine, also attended the meeting. Levine left Ms. to become editor of the *Columbia Journalism Review*.[133]

The Thomas column, which appeared in the *Washington Times*, quotes the National Abortion Rights Action League letter in part:

> I strongly believe that each woman must be able to decide when and whether to bear a child, and that government must not intrude on this most personal decision. Religious

extremists must not be allowed to impose their narrow beliefs on society as a whole rather, each of us must be permitted to heed our own conscience and faith.[134]

Thomas reports that *Spy*, not represented at the meeting, printed a full-page National Abortion Rights Action League advertisement in its April 1989 issue at no charge. The printing of this advertisement, along with the meeting, brings Thomas to ask an important question—a question he answers:

> Will there be an outcry from the journalistic establishment over the conspiracy and scheming by the women's and other magazines . . . to promote a political agenda and objective for a single issue? Not likely.
>
> Gone, apparently, are all pretenses to objectivity, balance and truth. Some of these magazines are saying to women, we want you to think the way we do.[135]

Thomas ends his column by urging women who oppose abortion to "send a message by refusing to pick up their magazines in the market and canceling their subscriptions."[136]

Another Cal Thomas commentary blasts a *Washington Post* article by Richard Harwood:

> Mr. Harwood wrote, "The anti-abortion forces . . . believe that *The Post*, institutionally, is 'pro-choice.' Of course it is. Any reader of the paper's editorials and home-grown columnists is aware of that. Moreover, while the shadings are more subtle, close textual analysis probably would reveal that, all things considered, our news coverage has favored the 'pro-choice' side."
>
> What a startling admission. And written with a defiant, "What are you going to do about it" attitude.
>
> This is frightening stuff, but there's more.
>
> Because of *The Post*'s pro-abortion bias, he writes, "it is argued . . . that *The Post* is obliged in the interest of 'fairness' [why does he put the word is quotes?] to now devote more space to anti-abortion activities and to anti-abortion letters to the editor. I do not agree. The news value of pro- and anti-abortion demonstrations was exhausted long ago. The intellectual enlightenment derived from letters to the editor or Op-Ed pieces of this subject also has been exhausted. The arguments are known to all, and they are stale . . .[137]

Media bias goes beyond general support for legal abortion by reporters. Could it be that Planned Parenthood is "buying" good coverage? If not, it is certainly rewarding it. The Planned Parenthood Federation of America presents annual Maggie Awards (named after Margaret Sanger) to recognize news writing that "covers issues of concern" to Planned Parenthood.

In 1985, Maggie Awards were given to: ABC's "20/20" and "World News Tonight," NBC's "Today," WJLA-TV (Washington, D.C.), NBC Radio, Dr. Lonnie Carton for "The Learning Center" (a syndicated radio program), Youth News Radio (Oakland, California), *Ms.*, *Time*, *Boston Globe*, *Glamour*, *Image* (Texas Christian University), and Mike Peters (editorial cartoonist.)[138] The announcement did not include specifics about the awards.

In 1989, awards were given to the *Arkansas Gazette* for its series, "Children Having Children," to ABC for "American Agenda: Abortion," and a "20/20" segment which focused on efforts to contain the spread of RU 486, to NBC for an episode of "A Different World" that focused on date rape and for its production of the television movie *Roe vs. Wade* which dramatized the events leading to the 1973 Supreme Court decision. *New Woman* also received a Maggie Award for an article about a woman who chose to abort a baby which tests showed may have been born handicapped. The article was titled, "A Matter of Life and Love."[139]

Maggie Awards for 1990 were presented to: "L. A. Law" (NBC-TV), WPLG-TV (Miami), "Geraldo" (Tribune Entertainment), Lifetime Television, *Newsweek*, and the *San Francisco Examiner*.[140] The announcement did not include specifics about the 1990 awards.

In 1991, Maggie Awards were presented to the *Dallas Morning News* for its six-part series titled, "Sex, Lies and Big Brother: Sexual Tyranny in Romania," *Glamour* for "Teenage and Pregnant" and for "The Politics of Birth Control," the *Washington Post* for a series of cartoons by Herb Block which addressed family planning and legislation, NBC/Carsey-Werner Company for an episode of "A Different World" titled, "If I Should Die Before I Wake," World Monitor Television for "Women with AIDS," and to Capital Cities/ABC for "Peter Jennings Reporting: The New Civil War." In her acceptance speech, "A Different World" writer Susan Fales warned that "the same forces that are blocking abortion clinics around the country are exerting tremendous pressure both on the networks and on the corporations that advertise through them."[141]

Planned Parenthood affiliates present Maggie Awards at the local level. One affiliate gave awards to three *Arizona Republic* reporters. One writer received a Maggie for an article titled "Too Soon Parents," a piece that discusses the "emotional, financial and physical costs of teenagers' having babies." Another writer received a Maggie for a story "detailing the struggles of an unmarried 16-year-old after she gave birth to twins." Maggies are presented in the categories of newspaper feature, magazine feature, editorials, broadcast, and columns.[142]

There is little doubt that had an anti-abortion group given an award to a reporter, Planned Parenthood would have attacked not only the group, but also the newspaper and the reporter for accepting the award. The charge would have been that one cannot expect fair reporting when accepting awards from an anti-abortion organization.

Writing for the *Los Angeles Times*, David Shaw examines the abortion bias among reporters, editors, and producers. He writes that the news media "consistently use language and images that frame the entire abortion debate in terms that implicitly favor abortion-rights advocates."[143]

Shaw notes that the media quotes supporters of legal abortion more frequently than those opposed and characterize supporters of abortion in a more favorable manner. In addition, "Events and issues favorable to abortion opponents are sometimes ignored or given minimal attention by the media." The reverse is also true. "Many news organizations have given more prominent play to stories on rallies and electoral and legislative victories by abortion rights advocates than to stories on rallies and electoral and legislative victories by abortion-rights opponents." Shaw believes the electronic media is more guilty of bias than the print media but they both are clearly prejudiced.[144]

Even leaders in the movement to protect and expand legal abortion admit that the vast majority of those in the media support their cause. Susanne Millsaps, executive director of the Utah affiliate of the National Abortion Rights Action League, received a call from a reporter who, at the end of the interview, asked how Millsaps could be reached in the event the reporter had additional questions. After getting the information, the reporter thanked Millsaps who immediately expressed an eager willingness to be of assistance. "The media has been our best friends in this fight," Millsaps told the reporter. "They claim objectivity, but I know they're all pro-choice."[145]

While most in the media are clearly supportive of legal abortion, some are making an effort to, as Millsaps notes, be able to *claim* objectivity. A *Wall Street Journal* internal bulletin notes that the newspaper will no longer use the term "pro-choice" when referring to advocates of legal abortion:

> A year ago S&S [Style and Substance—the name of the bulletin] discussed terminology to refer to the adversaries in the abortion debate. We opined that *pro-life* is a euphemism for *anti-abortion* and should be avoided except in formal names of groups, while *pro-choice* accurately reflects the attitude of those given the label.
>
> Some second thoughts on pro-choice: The term by itself isn't specific to the abortion issue, and it also is perceived by some as putting an unfairly positive spin on the ball. So let's use abortion rights to describe the philosophy of those who aren't opposed to induced abortions per se [sic].
>
> As for anti-abortion, the term still strikes us as appropriate, though groups may of course call themselves right-to-life groups.[146]

It may be a slow start, but it is a start nevertheless.

It is no wonder that Faye Wattleton, after taking the Planned Parenthood leadership, hired media consultants. They have obviously been worth the money. Such efforts have paid off with statements that refer to Planned Parenthood in positive terms. One newspaper, criticizing a bill before a state legislature, refered to Planned Parenthood as a "reliable" group.[147] Another newspaper refered to "the good work of Planned Parenthood."[148] A third newspaper suggested that support be given to Planned Parenthood because it is a choice "between Planned Parenthood and the back-alley quacks of old."[149]

One of the most blatantly biased pieces of "journalism" is the May 4, 1992, edition of *Time*. The featured article, titled "Abortion: The Future is Already Here," is authored by Richard LaCayo. The piece begins by citing the difficulty some women have in finding an abortionist and how a Texas abortionist has been "under siege for weeks by antiabortion demonstrators." The alleged activities of some abortion foes, those which would be condemned by the vast majority of anti-abortion leaders (firebombing, threats against abortionists and their families, and so forth), are described.[150]

The author of the *Time* article refers to the "last days for a woman's constitutionally protected right to abortion in America."[151] Referring to pictures of aborted preborn human beings, he goes on to say that, "The predicament of women trying to get abortions is harder to distill into a single wrenching image."[152]

Time attacks the Pennsylvania law requiring a 24-hour waiting period before an abortion is performed. "Though it sounds benign enough," the author writes, "it can confound poor women who already have to travel long distances to find a clinic, only to discover they must also scrape together the price of overnight accommodations. Often by the time they get the money together, they have advanced into the second trimester, when the cost is higher."[153]

The *Time* article frames the debate in the same way supporters of legal abortion do so. "Who decides whether a woman can have an abortion?," is said to be "the most fundamental question."[154]

Planned Parenthood is given a plug as a champion for the poor:

> Partly from a desire to keep abortion within reach of poor women, Planned Parenthood, which operates 900 clinics around the country, has succeeded in keeping prices low at their facilities. That in turn has put competitive pressure on everyone else, keeping the average cost for a first-trimester abortion at just $251, not much of an increase over the $196 price of 20 years ago. At a Planned Parenthood clinic in New York City, a physician earns up to $125,000 annually for a four-day week, perhaps half of what he or she might make in private practice.[155]

David Grimes, M.D., identified in the *Time* article only as part of the University of Southern California School of Medicine, is quoted as saying he has "personally" cared for women who have attempted to self-abort. Grimes has served on the board of directors of the Planned Parenthood Federation of America and is one of the world's most out-spoken proponents of unrestricted abortion.[156] Other "experts" from the National Abortion Federation and abortion providers are quoted to support other arguments.

It is noted by the article's author that "past experience suggests that when women are sufficiently desperate, they will terminate their pregnancies by any means necessary." A figure of "as many as 1.2 million illegal abortions annually" prior to *Roe v. Wade* is given as fact-without citation. We are warned that if abortion becomes illegal in some states, the price could skyrocket and "hustlers" could become involved. In order to prevent such activity, it is reported that, "Pro-choice groups are preparing for the day when they will have to provide an abortion underground, with networks to help women get to states where abortion is available." However, home abortion kits are also mentioned in the article.[157]

The author of the article notes that, "A generation [of doctors] raised in the era of safe and legal abortion is less likely to produce doctors ready to go to the barricades at the first sign of women being forced to undergo illegal—and dangerous—abortions. He also writes that restrictions states may place on abortion after the fall of *Roe v. Wade* "are hardly insurmountable." However, they will likely "make it take longer for women to afford and arrange an abortion, which makes the procedure more dangerous."[158]

The *Time* article takes on laws which require spousal notification. It is argued that the vast majority of women talk to their husbands, and those who do not "may have good reason not to" do so. In support of this statement, the head of the Elizabeth Blackwell Health Center for Women, a Philadelphia, Pennsylvania, abortion facility, is quoted. The argument used by supporters of legal abortion against parental notification is also mentioned.[159]

Consider the conclusion to the article:

> . . . America is bracing itself for a partial return to the past. In the two decades since *Roe* was handed down, a generation has grown up that knows nothing of the days of illicit abortions conducted on kitchen tables, or in doctor's offices at night with the blinds drawn.
>
> For the same two decades, while pro-lifers have waved pictures of the developing fetus, there were no more new images of women victimized by illegal abortion. In the year to come, those pictures, and the desolate realities they represent, are sure to reappear. It was harsh experience that led to the climate of opinion that welcomed *Roe*. Will it take harsh experience again to sort out the national will on abortion once and for all?[160]

Time should be ashamed to refer to the content of its magazine as "journalism." As for supporters of unrestricted abortion, one could not buy better coverage.

7

THE ABORTION CONNECTION

For many years, Planned Parenthood went to great lengths to claim it was not involved in abortion advocacy. Officials either stated that Planned Parenthood did not take a stand on abortion or that it was simply "pro-choice." However, Planned Parenthood leaders have become bold about their advocacy of unrestricted legal abortion.

Mimi Grinker of Planned Parenthood's Margaret Sanger Clinic in New York City said, "We believe that women have the right to choose when and how many children they wish to bear and that children who are wanted are loved and we believe that that is very, very pro-child and pro-family."[1]

The *Detroit News* reports that Planned Parenthood is "the premier institution providing abortions around the country . . . "[2] In fact, the organization does more abortions than any other single entity in the United States and no group works harder to protect legal abortion worldwide.

ABORTION LAW REFORM

At the start of the 1960s, Planned Parenthood was generally known as a private organization that advocated and provided birth control and sterilization. Throughout that decade, Planned Parenthood avoided the subject of abortion, although Alan F. Guttmacher, M.D., then-president of the Planned Parenthood Federation of America, vocally supported legal abortion during the early part of his medical career:

> We have accepted the baton of leadership and we cannot now refuse to run the race. Indeed we have to run faster to win it. The prize is nothing less than . . . "the perfect contracepting society." To achieve this society we in Planned Parenthood must establish a multi-faceted program which would include . . . abortion and sterilization.[3]

Other Planned Parenthood officials of the time, including the late Harriet Fleischl Pilpel, J.D., general counsel, who also served as counsel to the Rev. Billy Graham, and George Langmyhr, M.D., medical director, also supported abortion law reform. By 1970, Planned Parenthood had become a powerful and, in part, publicly funded organization. It gained the support of key elected and appointed government officials. Today, many people see Planned Parenthood as a respectable charity.

In its five year plan, Planned Parenthood states that one of its foremost "truths" is that "'universal reproductive freedom' is a most essential, if not *the* most essential step in providing our civilization with the opportunity to solve the most critical problems of hunger, deprivation, and the hopelessness of poverty . . ." Planned Parenthood pledges to abolish "the arbitrary and outmoded restrictions—legal, regulatory and cultural—which continue to limit the individual's freedom of choice in fertility matters."[4]

Since Planned Parenthood has targeted cultural as well as legal restrictions to "freedom of choice," it took aim at every institution perceived as a menace. At the top of the list was the Roman Catholic Church which had repeatedly expressed opposition to abortion. Planned Parenthood's response to such opposition was most often to ridicule the Roman Catholic Church and its leaders.

Planned Parenthood had viewed the judicial system as the best avenue for change. It has been part of almost every case involving abortion since the 1960s. Even before the Supreme Court's 1973 *Roe v. Wade* decision, Planned Parenthood worked in many states to establish a constitutional right to abortion. It had been active in providing testimony and research to aid those working toward legalized abortion.

Before *Roe v. Wade*, several Planned Parenthood affiliates aided women seeking an abortion by taking them to states where it was legal, such as California, Washington, and New York. Planned Parenthood of Central and Northern Arizona was one affiliate doing so:

> After California liberalized its abortion laws in 1971, many Arizona women chose to travel to California to obtain services. Planned Parenthood's Clergy Counseling Committee helped relieve some of the hardship, providing pregnancy counseling, emotional support, referral to reputable clinics in California—and reserved airline seats.
>
> "We obtained a discount on the flights through a sympathetic travel agent," volunteer Sally Boyd recalls. "Lots of people helped the agency in so many ways." A minister accompanied the women—sometimes as many as 20 at once—on the flight.[5]

On January 22, 1973, in the case known as *Roe v. Wade*, the United States Supreme Court ruled that abortion is a constitutional right. All abortion laws were effectively struck down. The *Roe* companion case, *Doe v. Bolton*, essentially made abortion on demand the law throughout the United States. A woman may get an abortion for any reason at any time during her pregnancy. The Supreme Court ruled in *Roe* that a woman may get an abortion if her life or health are in danger. In defining "health" in *Doe*, the Court said it involves "all of the attending circumstances" including "physical, emotional, psychological, familial and the woman's age."[6]

The Supreme Court relied heavily on the right to privacy in deciding *Roe v. Wade*. While the Constitution does not state that such a right exists, the Court interpreted the document in a way which created one. More precisely, the Court held that a right to privacy exists but it was not specifically spelled out in the Constitution. This interpretation was used and extended to create what has amounted to a constitutional right to abortion.

As noted it is the *Doe v. Bolton* decision, with its broad definition of "health," which effectively makes abortion legal throughout nine months of pregnancy—a fact often ignored, incorrectly explained, or denied by supporters of legal abortion. While *Roe* allows states to regulate and, in the last trimester of pregnancy, outlaw abortion, it cannot be done when the woman's "health," as defined in *Doe*, is at risk. The effect is that no laws restricting abortion may be passed. Even many supporters of legal abortion find no constitutional basis for the decision.

On the same day *Roe* and *Doe* were handed down, a constitutional amendment was proposed in Congress which would have nullified decisions. The Human Life Amendment would declare personhood from the moment of conception. As part of *Roe,* it was decided that preborn human beings are not legal persons and, since the Constitution refers to "persons," those not yet born are unprotected.

Shortly after the Supreme Court acted, Planned Parenthood published a pamphlet titled *Facts and Figures on Legal Abortion of Importance to All Americans*. The pamphlet cites public opinion polls which, according to Planned Parenthood, support the Supreme Court's decisions.[7]

The first section of the pamphlet, headlined, "Majority of Americans Favor Abortion Decision," summarizes one poll by saying that most Americans believe the abortion decision, "in the early months of pregnancy," should be left to "the woman (couple) and her (their) doctor." The actual question asked in the Gallup poll is, "Do you favor a law which would permit a woman to go to a doctor to end a pregnancy at any time during the first three months?" A Harris poll asks, "Do you favor the Supreme Court decision making abortions legal up to three months of pregnancy?"[8] Of course, the questions and answers have little to do with the decisions in *Roe* and *Doe* as abortion was not limited to three months.

The Planned Parenthood pamphlet argues that since the Supreme Court decisions, "declines have been reported in the numbers of women admitted to hospitals for aftercare following abortions begun elsewhere, suggesting a sharp reduction in unsafe illegal abortions." Most legal abortions, it is stated, are "replacements of illegal ones." It is also argued that legal abortion has prevented "unwanted births which otherwise would have occurred" and that abortion has led to declines in maternal and infant mortality rates.[9]

The pamphlet concludes by stating that, "Despite the record of medical, social and economic improvements cited, legal abortion is under attack." It is suggested that if the many attempts to restrict abortion should succeed, the United States could face a situation similar to that in Romania.[10]

Planned Parenthood opened its first abortion facility in Syracuse, New York, when abortion was legalized in that state in 1970. At least 75 affiliates are doing abortions or have agreed to do so in the near future.[11]

PRINT MEDIA CAMPAIGNS

Planned Parenthood has placed full-page advertisements in many major magazines and newspapers including *Time, Newsweek,* the *Washington Post* and the *New York Times*. Designed to convince the public that abortion should remain unrestricted and unregulated, the advertisements have proved successful in getting Planned Parenthood's point of view in front of the public, as well as in raising money for its efforts.

Opponents of legal abortion have a difficult time competing with such advertising. There is simply no way they can compete—advertisement for advertisement, dollar for dollar. Nevertheless, foes of legal abortion believe that money will not determine the outcome of the abortion debate.

One advertisement, which appeared in the *New York Times*, is headlined, "Nine Reasons Why Abortions Are Legal." The text includes language strongly supportive of legal abortion:

> Whenever a society has sought to outlaw abortions, it has only driven them into back alleys where they became dangerous, expensive and humiliating. Amazingly, this was the case in the United States until 15 years ago when abortion was legalized. Thousands of American women died. Thousands more were maimed. For this reason and others, women and men fought for and achieved women's legal right to make their own decisions about abortion.
>
> No nation committed to individual liberty could seriously consider returning to the days of back-alley abortions to the revolting specter of a government forcing women to bear children against their will.[12]

After nine arguments are given for keeping abortion legal, all of which include unsubstantiated information, the advertisement notes that "the abortion issue is not really about abortion. It is about the value of women in society." Of course, it is common for Planned Parenthood to claim that abortion is not the real issue regardless of the point being discussed. The advertisement concludes by saying, "If you agree with this, you can help." Readers are urged to write their elected officials and to send money to Planned Parenthood.[13]

It should be noted that constant references to "back-alley abortions" and the danger they involved lack substance, and Planned Parenthood officials know the argument is erroneous. Mary S. Calderone, former medical director of the Planned Parenthood Federation of America and founder of the Sex Information and Education Council of the United States, said in 1960 that "98 percent of all illegal abortions are presently done by physicians."[14] Similarly, a study conducted by the Kinsey Institute in the 1950s shows that 85 percent of illegal abortions were done by "regular doctors under clean conditions."[15] Nevertheless, the argument continues to prove profitable, so it is still used.

A second full-page advertisement appeared in the same newspaper one day later. This advertisement is headlined, "Five Ways to Prevent Abortion (And One Way That Won't)." An explanation is offered. "The way to prevent abortion is *not* to make it illegal. That won't work. It never has," Planned Parenthood argues. Without citing a source for its claim, Planned Parenthood asserts that "nearly one million American women went 'underground' each year for illegal operations. Thousands died for lack of medical care. Tens of thousands were maimed. *All* were forced to behave as if they were criminals in order to do what they felt was right for themselves."[16]

Planned Parenthood uses most of the remaining advertising space to offer ways it claims will prevent the "need" for abortion. This includes making contraception more easily accessible, providing young people with sex education, increasing the involvement of men, creating new birth control methods, and making America "friendlier to children." The advertisement concludes by urging readers to contact elected officials, send money to Planned Parenthood, and post the advertisement in a public place.[17]

One of Planned Parenthood's most common arguments has been that men have little or nothing to say about abortion since it is the woman who must carry the preborn human being. However, as part of its "The decision is yours" series, one advertisement is headlined, "What Every Man Should Know About Abortion." The advertisement points out that women must face the abortion decision, but "that doesn't make abortion a 'women's issue' any more than birth control is. Because no woman ever made herself pregnant. Men are responsible too."[18]

The advertisement attempts to draw men into the abortion battle:

> So the public controversy over keeping abortion safe and legal concerns your freedom as well. To marry when and if you want. To decide with your partner to have children when you want them. If you want them. Yet an increasingly vocal and violent minority wants to outlaw abortion. For all women. Regardless of circumstances. Even if her life or health is endangered by a pregnancy. Even if she's a victim of rape or incest. Even if she's too young to be a mother.
>
> But outlawing abortion won't stop it. Women have always had abortions when they've felt there's no other way. Even at the risk of being maimed or killed with a back-alley abortion.
>
> Ironically, it's mostly men who want to outlaw abortion—men in the White House, in Congress, in the Courts. Many of them even want to ban contraceptives and sex education.
>
> These people must know there's a man intimately involved in every unwanted pregnancy. Why don't they ever mention it?
>
> Maybe they're hoping to buy your silence until it's too late. And they think you're too selfish to care. If you'd like to prove them wrong, start by returning the coupon.[19]

Men are urged to write members of Congress to express support for legal abortion and family planning programs. Planned Parenthood also requests a tax-deductible contribution.[20]

Another advertisement in the series shows a professional woman with the headline, "The Right to Choose Abortion Makes All My Other Rights Possible":

> The right to choose abortion gives you the right to protect your health, your education, your career, and your future. It gives you the right to defend yourself against contraceptive failure and unwanted pregnancy.
>
> The right to decide when and whether to bear children gives women genuine control over their own lives. Not in the abstract. But in real, practical terms. Anatomy is no longer destiny.[21]

The advertising series includes much of the same language when referring to the "increasingly vocal and violent minority":

> Many are fanatics who even object to birth control and sex education. They believe there's only one place for women. At home, in the kitchen and nursery.
>
> Even if you've never had to make a personal decision about abortion, your right to decide for yourself is one of your most precious and fragile freedoms. Speak out *now.* Use the coupon below.
>
> Because if you're not free to decide the important things for yourself, you're not free at all.[22]

PRONOUNCEMENTS

Planned Parenthood has published countless documents which make its position clear. The best evidence comes from its five year plan:

> The Purpose of the Federation shall be:
>
> a) to provide leadership:

> in making effective means of voluntary fertility control, including contraception, abortion and sterilization, available and fully accessible to all.[23]

The document "'Til Victory is Won . . . An Action Agenda for 1982-84" outlines the goals of the Planned Parenthood Federation of America which include addressing "the unmet need for fertility regulation services in the United States, regardless of age or ability to pay," and to "preserve the legality of and assure equal access to safe abortion services and pregnancy-options counseling for all women, regardless of age or ability to pay."[24]

Faye Wattleton, former president of the Planned Parenthood Federation of America, said, "We committed ourselves to restoring access to abortion to the poor and to preserving it as a matter of choice to individuals throughout the economic spectrum . . . "[25]

In the pamphlet *Ten Heavy Facts About Sex . . .*, number ten tells teens that Planned Parenthood or a county or hospital family planning clinic can help them "arrange an abortion . . . "[26]

They Learn History at Yale . . . Economics at Harvard . . . Sex Education at State Street and Main, continues with, "But, where do they learn sexual responsibility?" Planned Parenthood writes that, "Those who wished an abortion were guided to high quality medical services. . . . [Some of Planned Parenthood's] community based clinics provided abortion services and follow-up contraceptive guidance in their own facilities." Its slogan for this publication is "Planned Parenthood: The Sane Way."[27]

One section of "'Til Victory is Won . . . An Action Agenda for 1982-84," is called, "Planned Parenthood Advocates Freedom of Choice":

> We are deeply committed to an individual's right of choice in regard to human reproduction, and we affirm the dignity and worth of each individual. We believe that the benefits of medical science and contraceptive technology are not luxuries afforded the affluent, but are necessities that are fundamental to the strength and stability of the family. Without the right of reproductive choice, other freedoms become academic . . . and opportunities become severely limited.[28]

Another section of the document is titled, "Planned Parenthood Advocates Moral Decision-Making."

> Moral concepts are central to our principles and our programs. We believe in, and will fight for, the continued right of individuals to exercise their own moral principles with regard to reproductive choices. Rarely does a human being make a more profoundly moral decision than when he or she contemplates creating a new life. Choosing to become a parent is to accept a long-lasting and often enriching moral obligation which should be approached with the most careful deliberation. Though we may wish otherwise many who are forced to become parents cannot accept the responsibilities of parenthood. Bringing children into the world who, from the day they are born are unwanted and unloved, is profoundly immoral.[29]

In *Implementation of Legal Abortion: A National Problem*, George Langmyhr, M.D., writes a section called, "The Role of Planned Parenthood-World Population in Abortion." He acknowledges that "most professionals and volunteers associated with Planned Parenthood have accepted, for a long time, the necessity of abortion as an integral part of any complete or total family planning program."[30]

In the pamphlet, *Planned Parenthood: A Strong Voice for the Most Personal of Human Rights*, the authors write that unless the "right to choose" is retained, "in a few years, compulsory childbirth could be the law of the land for every woman who becomes pregnant unintentionally." It is also written that the freedom to choose abortion is "the most personal of rights . . ." The pamphlet informs us that overturning *Roe v. Wade* "would bring back the horrors of back-alley abortions. Horrors most of us thought were gone forever." Near the end of the pamphlet the reader is told that, "Planned Parenthood leads in advancing and defending these rights."[31]

Pro-Child, Pro-Family, Pro-Choice, lists the services offered by Planned Parenthood of Orange and San Bernadino Counties (California). The number 10 service is called, "Pregnancy options counseling—for persons dealing with unintended pregnancies who wish to explore all their choices."[32] Service number 20 is public affairs support:

> Advocacy—promoting the right to choose, our public affairs department works to build a broad-based constituency to speak out on family planning and reproductive rights issues. You are invited to join our Alert Network of persons who support freedom of choice.[33]

So You Don't Want to Be a Sex Object, a Planned Parenthood publication, describes the real relationship that is suggested to exist between a woman and her doctor. "You should expect the doctor to take *your* choices into consideration in the matter of contraception, [and] abortion . . . ," the pamphlet reads. If, in any way, a doctor urges a woman not to have an abortion, Planned Parenthood says she might want to say, "Doctor, unless you're proposing marriage, my personal life shouldn't concern you," or, "Doctor, I'll have a baby when I choose to do so."[34]

One Planned Parenthood affiliate released a general statement in defense of abortion:

> Before 1973, up to one million women each year sought out dangerous, illegal abortions. [One Margaret Sanger biographer writes, "In the United States the number of illegal abortions is estimated at an annual figure of between 200,000 and 1,200,000."[35]] Many died. Countless thousands more survived life-threatening and painful infections, gangrene, or other complications related to unsafe methods. The abortion rate is approximately the same today as before legalization, however legalized abortion has dramatically reduced the number of abortion related deaths in this country. Today, legal abortion is considered at least 5 times safer than childbearing.[36]

These statements are presented without documentation. Common sense says there were not "up to one million" illegal abortions done prior to 1973 as most people obey the law. Moreover, illegal abortions were not reported so there is no way to estimate the number performed. To say the abortion rate is "approximately the same today as before legalization" is simply ludicrous. It is interesting to note there is no requirement to report today's legal abortions so the reported statistics are surely low.

The argument that abortion is "considered at least five times safer than childbearing" is a fallacy. Statistics on childbirth mortality rates include all maternal deaths of any nature, including those not relating to pregnancy or childbirth (such as automobile accidents) when death occurs during pregnancy, during childbirth, or up to 189 days following childbirth. Methods of statistical gathering in this area vary from state-to-state. Abortion-related deaths, on the other hand, are recorded only if they are directly related to abortion and if the death is reported at the time the abortion report is completed. Furthermore, late-term abortion-related deaths may be reported as a maternal death.

The fact is that doctors, particularly abortionists, have nothing to gain by attributing complications and deaths to an abortion procedure. The Centers for Disease Control no longer tracks the number of deaths attributed to legal abortion (see chapter 15).

Despite these facts, Louis B. Tyrer, M.D., and Julie E. Salas write:

> In all fairness, the inherent risks of contraceptive options must not be weighed only against the health risks to a woman who is not pregnant but most specifically against the infrequently acknowledged danger to a woman's life from becoming pregnant.
>
> The US public and government must recognize the grave social and health consequences of unintended pregnancies in the United States and in the rest of the world. It is estimated that approximately 500,000 women die annually from pregnancy complications. Approximately 200,000 of these result from complications of illegal abortions. The widespread use of birth control can substantially reduce this unacceptable high toll.[37]

FUND-RAISING LETTERS

One fund-raising letter, signed by Katharine Hepburn, refers to Planned Parenthood efforts to inform "millions of Americans" that passage of a Human Life Amendment would have several disastrous consequences:

> [The Human Life Amendment would] Prevent an abortion for a woman who has been exposed to X-ray treatments or proven dangerous drugs and whose doctor expects brain damage or deformity to the fetus. . . .
>
> Prevent an abortion for a 14-year-old girl impregnated by her father.
>
> Prevent an abortion for a woman who already has several children and whose husband is guilty of family brutality, causing the woman serious emotional problems.
>
> Prevent an abortion for a 16-year-old high school student who has no prospect for a stable home and whose pregnancy will end her chance for an education.
>
> Cause medically safe abortions to be replaced by back-alley butchery, and by self-induced procedures of desperate women, many on the verge of nervous breakdown, or even suicide.
>
> Substitute cold constitutional prohibitions for individual choice based on sound advice from a woman's personal physician.
>
> Like the Prohibition Amendment, a constitutional amendment banning abortion would give crime another lucrative market in illegal abortions and black market adoptions.
>
> Most reasonable people, learning these *uncontested facts*, would agree that abortions certainly should be available to women like these, and those in many more similar situations.
>
> Most reasonable people agree that the decision for an abortion should be left to the woman and her physician . . . as are other medical procedures.[38]

A chief component of the *Roe v. Wade* decision is that abortion should be a matter between a woman and her doctor. The point is raised in the Hepburn fund-raising letter,[39] and Faye Wattleton often referred to this part of the United States Supreme Court decision in public when she was president of the Planned Parenthood Federation of America.

In a fund-raising letter, Faye Wattleton writes that "when you support Planned Parenthood you support a . . . campaign to . . . work against the enactment of laws that restrict the availability of abortions."[40]

A Wattleton fund-raising letter also states, "For over sixty years we have been the acknowledged preeminent force *in advancing the right of all Americans to know the facts about their bodies and in defending our right to determine our own fertility*."[41]

CRITIQUE OF
THE SILENT SCREAM

Planned Parenthood was seriously concerned about the impact of the anti-abortion film produced by former abortionist and co-founder of the pro-legal abortion movement, Bernard N. Nathanson, M.D. *The Silent Scream* shows the abortion of a preborn human being at between 12 and 14 weeks gestation.

In "The Facts Speak Louder: Planned Parenthood's Critique of *The Silent Scream*," we are told an attempt is made to shift the focus of the film to more comfortable and slightly more defensible territory, a tactic Planned Parenthood leaders know well:

> The film represents an attempt to shift the focus in the abortion debate to the fetus and away from any concern or compassion for women in need of abortion services. It is an attempt to deny the desperation that once forced American women into the life threatening, humiliating experiences of unsafe and often lethal abortions.[42]

Planned Parenthood argues that the film is filled with errors:

> *The Silent Scream* . . . has been treated as factual, when the opposite is true.
>
> From its title, to the description of a fetus as a "person," . . . the documentary aspects of this film are flawed and biased. The film is riddled with scientific, medical, and legal inaccuracies, misleading statements, and exaggerations. And through innuendo, the film attempts to denigrate the efforts of Planned Parenthood and other reproductive health and rights organizations to provide safe, legal, inexpensive reproductive health care services, including abortion, for women who want and need these services.[43]

The writers of the publication explain the purpose of Planned Parenthood:

> Planned Parenthood Federation of America is committed to assuring that all individuals have the freedom to make their own decisions about whether or when to have a child. To help individuals make and implement those decisions, Planned Parenthood is committed to expanding access to all of the information and services needed to prevent unintended pregnancies. Likewise, for all women who are faced with unintended pregnancies, Planned Parenthood is committed to preserving the constitutionally protected right to obtain medically safe, legal abortions.[44]

According to Planned Parenthood, "The abolition of legal abortion would have a serious negative impact on the health of women and children in the United States." Additionally, it is argued that, "Pregnancy and childbearing in young teenagers are associated with both maternal and fetal problems."[45]

On the concluding page, the authors look to the future. Reasons why abortion should remain legal are offered:

> In the absence of legal abortion, even more illegal abortions might be performed in the 1980s than in the 1960s for two reasons: 1) a generation of American women has come to expect the right to choose legal abortion as part of their reproductive health care; 2) a cohort of abortion providers throughout the country has been trained to deliver abortion services.[46]

KIRO television, the Seattle area CBS affiliate, decided to air *The Silent Scream*, but they wanted to give Planned Parenthood a chance to respond. Planned Parenthood of Seattle-King County, using the facilities of KIRO, prepared a video responding to the film. When first aired, Nathanson's film was shown, followed by the Planned Parenthood video. The results were positive for

Planned Parenthood. The Planned Parenthood video served as an effective rebuttal and was eventually used intermantionally.

There are several things wrong with the process. First, KIRO did not supply funds or facilities for the making of *The Silent Scream*. Why should it give Planned Parenthood the chance to respond unless the organization was willing to fully pay for production of the video? Second, Planned Parenthood was able to use *The Silent Scream* as a resource in making its response. It would be similar to President Bush sending a copy of his debate arguments to his opponent before the debate, without getting the same favor in return. Planned Parenthood could specifically address the arguments made in the film. Third, Planned Parenthood had the last word. With both pieces aired, inaccuracies in the Planned Parenthood production could not be addressed.

The media was quick to join Planned Parenthood in spreading the word that the Nathanson film could not be taken seriously. In one article which appeared in the *New York Times*, Hart Peterson, M.D., acting chairman of pediatric neurology at New York Hospital at Cornell Medical Center in New York, said, "The notion that a 12-week fetus screams in discomfort is erroneous." Peterson argues that if you poke an earthworm with a stick, "it responds, too." In response, Nathanson argues that pain is a "reflex," not an "intellectual exercise."[47]

A Planned Parenthood ally, the American Humanist Association, released a publication attacking the film. *The Abortion of* The Silent Scream: *A False and Wrongful Cry for Human Pain, Suffering and Violence*, authored by James W. Prescott, was originally printed as an article in *The Humanist*, the association's newsletter.

The publication begins by quoting Proverbs 23:13–14 which reads, "Withhold not correction from a child; for if thou strike him with the rod, he shall not die. Thou shalt beat him with the rod, and deliver his soul from hell." Matthew 26:24 is also quoted: "It would be better for that man if he had never been born"[48]:

> Is it appropriate to compare from a *moral perspective* the production of *The Silent Scream* and the production of "snuff" films in which women are enticed into a sexual encounter and, unbeknownst to them, are scheduled for sexual torture, mutilation, and murder? Assuming that abortion is murder and "snuff" is murder, do the producers and supporters of these two kinds of films share a *certain common morality?* If so, what would be the nature of that common morality?[49]

Prescott has served on the board of directors of the American Humanist Association and is a signer of Humanist Manifesto II.[50]

CRITIQUE OF ECLIPSE OF REASON

Planned Parenthood has had help attacking the follow-up to *The Silent Scream*. In *Eclipse of Reason*, a second-trimester abortion is shown in vivid detail. The most shocking aspect of the film is that the abortion is shown *in utero*, not by using ultrasound. Instead, a camera is inserted into the uterus capturing the death of the preborn human being as it happens.

Eclipse of Reason is attacked in the September 1987 edition of *Self*. The article, authored by Sue Woodman, asserts that "instead of exploring" late abortions,

Eclipse of Reason "exploits them." Comparing *Eclipse of Reason* to *The Silent Scream*, Woodman writes that "once again, according to several doctors, it's an overall misleading portrait, gorily graphic and often inaccurate . . ." She also calls *The Silent Scream* an admitted piece of anti-abortion propaganda that was widely denounced for presenting sensationalist, misleading and often false information about early abortions.[51]

"The last thing any woman trying to sort out her own ethics and feelings about abortion needs is to be lied to," Woodman writes.[52] Few if any people would disagree. What does she allege to be distortions in *Eclipse of Reason?* The author cites the following problems:

- The film was made by photographing several abortions and "using the most gory and distressing parts." It is argued that all surgery is bloody, including heart transplants. It is noted that even childbirth can be bloody.[53] A comment is not made about the fact that what seems to make the viewing of an abortion much more heart-wrenching is that in a heart transplant or childbirth, life is being revered. In an abortion, life is being taken, and the victim is clearly not happy about it.
- Nathanson lumps second and third trimester abortion statistics which he classifies as "late abortions." According to the author, Nathanson "implies that one in ten takes place after 20 weeks."[54] I have seen the film and did not come to this conclusion. The author writes that, "According to the Centers for Disease Control, about 10 percent of abortions are performed in the second trimester and less than 1 percent after 21 weeks, or late in the second and into the third trimester." To further attack Nathanson's use of statistics, the author quotes Douglas Gould, vice president for communications of the Planned Parenthood Federation of America who, in turn, cites "'the respected Alan Guttmacher Institute' which states that there are 'no more than 120 third-trimester abortions each year, and these are done because of extreme need.'"
- The "needs of the pregnant woman are never addressed in its emotional, melodramatic commentary. In its near-exclusive concern for fetuses, the women who bear them are mentioned only once . . ." To support this claim, the author quotes Kate Michelman, executive director of the National Abortion Rights Action League.[55] Woodman must have missed the section of the film where several women discuss their abortions and how damaging they have been.

The fact is that both *The Silent Scream* and *Eclipse of Reason* show the world exactly what its makers claim. The films begin with living preborn human beings and end with dead human beings. Advocates of legal abortion cannot dispute this fact, so they prefer to discuss other issues.

ABORTION ENTERPRISE

In 1991, as part of its 75th anniversary celebration, the Planned Parenthood Federation of America launched a campaign to convince at least 75 of its affiliates to do abortions or to plan on doing them in the near future. The slogan for the campaign was "75 in 75."[56]

The specific nature of the project is described in the newsletter of the Consortium of Abortion Providers (CAPS), a coalition of Planned Parenthood affiliates which do abortions. The "major goal" was to "encourage and assist affiliates in the initiation of abortion services, but support of all CAPS activities and current abortion providers is also an important focus of the Project." It is also reported that Consortium officials visited many affiliates where abortions were not being done in order to urge that abortions be performed. "With luck and commitment," the newsletter reads, "the members of CAPS could soon number more than 70."[57]

The Consortium newsletter states that the "'magic ingredients' which can motivate a board to move forward and approve abortion services" include "giving [the] board (and staff) the opportunity to learn basic facts about abortion as a medical procedure and service . . ." Three other "ingredients" are mentioned: "putting client need first, valuing abortion as an integral part of reproductive health care, and having board and staff members willing and determined to lead on this issue." The article notes that abortion "fits within the Planned Parenthood mission" and it involves "the traditions of Planned Parenthood."[58]

The goal to establish "75 in 75" was achieved and announced in *INsider*, the newspaper of the Planned Parenthood Federation of America:

> In August, the CAPS Project to Expand Abortion Services will begin its third year of operation. Created by the Consortium of Abortion Providers (the abortion-providing affiliates of PPFA [Planned Parenthood Federation of America]), the project is based at Planned Parenthood of Houston and Southeast Texas. It recently attained a special goal in time for PPFA's 75th anniversary—an increase in the number of current and future affiliate abortion providers that brought the total to 75.
>
> Planned Parenthood of West Texas (Odessa, Texas) in PPFA's Southern Region became "the official number 75" this spring. Pam Feist, board president, said her board approved abortion services unanimously because of the tremendous need in the affiliate's 30-county area. "This board felt that by offering abortion services we had a real opportunity to provide complete reproductive health care to our clients," she said.[59]

Julie Bloom, chairman of the Patient Services Committee of Planned Parenthood of Southern Indiana (Bloomington, Indiana), claims her affiliate decided to do abortions in order to be "true" to the organization's "mission." Beth Calleton, executive director of the Pasadena Planned Parenthood Committee (Pasadena, California), wrote to her board about its decision to allow the affiliate to do abortions as part of a "special goal."[60]

> I was very touched that the first patient we were able to help was a 16-year-old who came with her 17-year-old boyfriend. As the mother of two daughters who were once 16-trying-to-act-26, I was sure, emotionally as well as philosophically and intellectually, that one of the best decisions our board has ever made was to offer first-trimester abortion services.[61]

The Project to Expand Abortion Services, which is funded by a major foundation,[62] began following the decision of the United States Supreme Court in *Webster v. Reproductive Health Services*.[63]

The October 1990 newsletter of the Consortium of Abortion Providers is headlined, "'Hats Off' to the Newest Members of CAPS." Along with congratulating the newest Planned Parenthood affiliates that have started doing abortions, the newsletter includes a notice regarding a workshop titled "On the Verge: Initiating Abortion Services."[64]

In 1986, Planned Parenthood did at least 98,638 abortions. In 1987 the number increased to 104,411. Planned Parenthood reports having done 111,189 abortions in 1988 and 122,191 in 1989. The number of abortions done at Planned Parenthood increased to 129,155 in 1990.[65] Planned Parenthood reports referring 100,248 women to other abortion facilities in 1988 and 83,835 in 1989.[66] All affiliates are required to refer for abortions if they do not do them.

Former abortion clinic operator Carol Everett charges that "kickbacks" are involved in the abortion business. She answers statements made by a woman who claims Planned Parenthood does not receive kickbacks for making abortion referrals. "I found . . . [the] letter stating that Planned Parenthood did not receive kickbacks very interesting," Everett writes, "as the Texas corporation DOCTA furnished a Fort Worth [Texas] Planned Parenthood director a new Cadillac—until she retired! What is your definition of a kickback?"[67]

The defender of Planned Parenthood alleges that the organization is not in the business to make a profit. Everett responds:

> . . . I worked on a straight commission basis in the abortion clinics. My commission was $25.00 for each abortion, and the last month in the industry, we did 545 abortions which made my income $13,625.00 for that month. Our doctors worked on a straight commission also, usually making 1/3 to 1/2 of the total abortion fee. An average abortionist can do 10 to 12 first trimester abortions per hour. About the lowest fee an abortionist can make now is $75.00 per case, which means 10 times $75.00 equals $750.00 per hour and 12 times $75.00 equals $900.00 per hour.
>
> As an ex-abortion provider, I saw one out of 500 women die or have major surgery the last 18 months I was involved in the abortion industry. Not one of those complications made the newspapers because of the built-in cover-up. The women and their families do not come forward to share with the public the truth about abortion—so the cover-up and the big money goes on!
>
> . . . Abortion is about money! Abortion is a skillfully marketed product sold to . . . women in a crisis pregnancy. She buys the product; finds it defective, but cannot return it for a refund.[68]

In 1990, the Alan Guttmacher Institute issued a report detailing the average cost of an abortion. Up to eight weeks after the last missed menstrual period, the average cost was listed at $231. The average cost was $247 for up to 12 weeks gestation. Abortions done up to 16 weeks cost an average of $400. Those done up to 20 weeks cost an average of $697. No averages are provided for abortions done after five months gestation.[69]

Figuring an average cost of $251 for a first trimester abortion,[70] it is estimated that Planned Parenthood generated more than $32.4 million in 1990 alone. This does not take into account increased profits from second trimester abortions.

It is interesting to note that Planned Parenthood affiliates may run an abortion facility under a different name. For example, a name such as "Yellow Valley Women's Clinic" might seem as though it is independent from Planned Parenthood when, in effect, the facility is controlled by a board of directors which is remarkably similar to that of the Planned Parenthood affiliate. In a memorandum to an affiliate from Eve W. Paul of the Planned Parenthood Federation of America, it is suggested that "the concept of a separate corporation for the performance of abortion or any other service does not seem to me to present any insuperable obstacles and may indeed be a valuable tool . . . This has been done with great success by our Columbus, Ohio, affiliate. However, it seems to me essential that the separate corporation be so structured that the affiliate retains control . . ." The memorandum also states that the abortion service must be treated "as a chapter" and suggests that the affiliate retain the power to appoint members of the board of directors who would oversee the "chapter."[71]

While some Planned Parenthood affiliates have shied away from doing abortions, Faye Wattleton argued that all affiliates should do them. "Abortion invites controversy," she explained. "The problem is, whether affiliates do abortions or not, they are still labeled as being part of abortion services, so you may as well provide them."[72]

Affiliates seem to be listening. In 1980, Planned Parenthood performed 77,880 abortions at 36 clinics. In 1990, Planned Parenthood's 129,155 abortions were done at 57 sites.[73] The statistics are likely to change dramatically when Planned Parenthood releases its report covering 1991. Subsequent reports should prove even more interesting considering the Consortium of Abortion Providers project previously described:

> Although only two affiliates added the service [abortion] in 1989, bringing the total number to 53, the boards of an additional 13 affiliates have approved plans to offer abortion services, and many of those plans will be implemented in 1990. The loss of abortion providers in affiliate communities is one of the most compelling reasons for offering the service.[74]

The number of Planned Parenthood affiliates providing abortions increased by 10 percent between 1982 and 1989.[75] These facts, along with the Consortium of Abortion Providers project, are the most concrete evidence of Planned Parenthood's determination to increase its share of the abortion market.

The Consortium of Abortion Providers "Confidential—In-House Use Only" report, titled "CAPS Survey '90," offers an interesting look into Planned Parenthood's abortion business. All but one of the Consortium's members responded to the survey. Consider these 1990 statistics:

- 25 affiliates did abortions through three months since the last missed menstrual period; 21 affiliates through three and one-half months; six affiliates through four months; three through four and one-half months; and one affiliate did abortions through five and one-half weeks since the last missed period.[76]
- 15 affiliates did fewer than 1,000 abortions; 15 affiliates did between 1,000 and 2,000 abortions; nine affiliates did between 2,000 and 3,000 abortions; nine affiliates did between 3,000 and 4,000 abortions; three affiliates did between 4,000 and 5,000 abortions, three affiliates did between 5,000 and 10,000 abortions; and one affiliate did more than 10,000 abortions.[77]
- 33 affiliates reported an increase in the number of abortions done over the previous year; 14 reported little or no change; and seven affiliates reported a decrease in the number of abortions done. The most frequently cited reasons for an increase in the number of abortions were quality of service, more physician accountability, low cost, and good word of mouth. The most frequently cited reason for a decrease in the number of abortions done was a shortage of physicians.[78]
- 45 affiliates reported using Obstetrician/Gynecologists for abortions; 10 affiliates used family practitioners; two affiliates used doctors of osteopathy; two affiliates used surgeons; two affiliates used emergency room doctors, and one affiliate used a pediatrician.[79]

- Recommendations were made regarding the recruitment of physicians. Affiliates were urged to: target older doctors reducing their practices and doctors doing research at medical schools, put university medical school faculty (Obstetrician/Gynecologists) on the affiliate's medical committee because it will serve as a pipeline to medical residents, have the affiliate medical director contact potential abortionists because of the advantage of peer-to-peer contact, subscribe to local medical bulletins to learn about physicians new to the area, join with or establish a national and regional recruitment network/mechanism, try getting approval to allow physician assistants to perform abortions, urge licensure of mid-level practitioners, and "Prayer X 2."[80]
- 37 affiliates reported that physician recruitment and training was the biggest problem with doing abortions; 11 reported the biggest problem was staff retention, training, and stress; seven affiliates reported cost containment; four reported that picketers were the biggest problem; and four reported that the biggest problem was finding registered nurses. Sixteen affiliates suggested that the Planned Parenthood Federation of America develop a national/regional system for finding, recruiting, and training physicians to do abortions.[81]
- 28 affiliates reported that salaries had been the biggest cost increase; 10 affiliates reported lab expenses; seven reported security; and four reported that "P.O.C. [product of conception] Disposal" represented the biggest cost increase.[82]
- All members of the Consortium of Abortion Providers are listed, including the names of executive directors and their telephone numbers.[83]
- A breakdown for all Consortium members is also included listing the following information for each: total budget, number of abortion sites, whether Title X (pronounced "title ten") funds are received, the number of abortions performed, the gestational age limit for performing abortions, future plans of the affiliate regarding abortion (most are adding weeks to the gestational age limit for their performing abortions or adding equipment), biggest problems faced by each affiliate, types of anesthesia/analgesia used, routine regarding the use of ultrasound (if any), the length of stay for the client (none exceed two days), the cost to the affiliate for performing abortions, the amount of money paid to the abortionist (per abortion), the fee range charged clients for doing an abortion, staffing at the abortion site, and tips for cutting costs.[84]

An interesting interview was conducted with the director of public relations of the Upper Hudson Planned Parenthood regarding a lawsuit it had filed. Referring to abortion foes, the Planned Parenthood employee said, "They're small in number but they continue. And when it affects our business, uh, not our business, our patients, we have to do something."[85]

Some Planned Parenthood affiliates have started a loan fund to "assist" women who "need" an abortion but who do not have money to pay for them.[86] Women may borrow from the fund interest free, in most cases. It is not known whether Planned Parenthood would make such a loan if a woman wanted to get her abortion at a non-Planned Parenthood facility. No such fund exists for poor women who wish to give birth.

Every Planned Parenthood affiliate pays dues to the national headquarters. This money, along with other contributions, fund a pro-legal abortion advertising and lobbying campaign.

MORE PLANS

A June 1977 document titled "Planned Birth, the Future of the Family and the Quality of American Life" was written with the involvement of several organizations including the National Family Planning Forum, the Metropolitan Executive Directors Council of Planned Parenthood, the National Executive Directors Council of Planned Parenthood, the Great Lakes Family Planning Coalition, and Zero Population Growth. Conclusions and recommendations are endorsed in principle by the Planned Parenthood Federation of America, the National Council of the Alan Guttmacher Institute, the Population Institute, and the Population Section of the American Public Health Association. The document sets goals for the family planning movement:

> The goals of government should be to press for the extension, on a universal basis, of services to prevent unwanted conceptions and the development of contraceptive technologies necessary to that end; to insure that all pregnant women have full freedom to choose any of the legal means of resolving their pregnancies; and to improve equality of access to abortion services for American women in all walks of life who might choose to terminate unwanted pregnancies.[87]

The document suggests other goals:

> Continuing reimbursement for pregnancy detection, referral and abortion services for women on welfare and/or Medicaid.
>
> Assessing the financial obstacles to obtaining abortion services encountered by low- and marginal-income women and adolescents not eligible for Medicaid and exploring the consequences for the women, their families and society.
>
> Requiring Health Systems Agencies to assess the adequacy of abortion services in their areas and to develop plans for remedying service deficits.
>
> Encouraging greater participation by hospitals in provision of abortions, or development of alternative facilities, in order to equalize geographical access to abortion in all areas of the country.
>
> Developing suitable "catchment areas" and regional facilities to specialize in second trimester abortions and prenatal diagnosis of fetal defects.
>
> Encouraging greater attention to abortion in professional education by medical, nursing, hospital and public health schools and organizations.
>
> Conducting on an on going basis, a nationwide education program to inform American women on their options in coping with pregnancy, including their right to legal abortion, the importance of early pregnancy detection, and the differential and adverse risks involved in late versus early abortion.[88]

Elizabeth Hrenda-Roberts, executive director of a Pennsylvania affiliate of the Planned Parenthood Federation of America, clearly summarizes the organization's position. "The alternative to aborting a fetus that is unwanted because of its sex is giving birth to a child that is unwanted because of its sex," she writes. "When we acknowledge the importance of motherhood, the significance of pregnancy, and the moral competence of each individual, we accept that each woman has the right to continue or to terminate a pregnancy for her own reasons—even reasons that seem frivolous or unwise to others."[89]

Such militant abortion advocacy seems a rather large shift from the ideal written in a 1965 book, *Planned Parenthood: A Practical Handbook of Birth-Control Methods*, which says that contraception "is of course not abortion." The authors correctly write that contraception "is the prevention of conception, whereas abortion destroys an already fertilized ovum. Abortion destroys a life already begun;

birth control prevents its beginning by keeping the sperm and egg cell separated." It is noted that contraception prevents the beginning of human life.[90]

Likewise, a 1963 Planned Parenthood pamphlet answers the question of whether abortion is a form of birth control. The answer is clear:

> Definitely not. An abortion kills the life of a baby after it has begun. It is dangerous to your life and health. It may make you sterile so that when you want a child you cannot have it. Birth control merely postpones the beginning of life.[91]

Has Planned Parenthood changed or has the preborn human changed?

8

"WHAT WOMEN DON'T KNOW . . ."

Not all women who have been to Planned Parenthood have been pleased with its services. Reports range from not being given full and accurate information to physical, sexual, and psychological abuse.

Planned Parenthood's unwillingness to discuss abortion in detail, including possible complications (emotional and physical), the nature of the preborn human being, and alternatives to abortion, have brought the organization under fire from women. Nevertheless, Planned Parenthood shows no sign of changing its procedures.

COUNSELING

In a Planned Parenthood publication called "Pregnancy Counseling Standards for Planned Parenthood Federation of America," the second standard addresses the counseling interview process:

> Pregnancy counseling interviews should be scheduled to allow adequate time to review the medical diagnosis and to explore the options available to the woman. As a minimum, a woman should be given the opportunity to consider . . . options available for continuing or terminating the pregnancy . . . [and the] potential effect each option suggests for the future.[1]

Some observers charge that counseling on the "potential effect each option suggests for the future" is often a slanted discussion intended to lead patients down the abortion path. A counselor can easily give a bad potential outlook by emphasizing those things the woman would not be able to do while pregnant and if she has to raise the child alone.

Planned Parenthood counselors are required to pressure customers into using contraceptives. The third standard listed in this publication states, "Patients shall be advised of the availability and advisability of contraceptives following the termination of pregnancy."[2] Planned Parenthood counselors are trained in-house by fellow employees.

A study of women who received counseling and, in many cases, abortions at Planned Parenthood, shows that 89 percent believe their counselor was strongly biased in favor of abortion. Eighty percent claim Planned Parenthood gave little or no information about possible abortion complications. Ninety-five percent say their counselors gave little or no information about fetal development. Most surprisingly, 90 percent say there was a strong chance abortion would not be chosen had it not been so forcefully advocated by the Planned Parenthood counselor.[3]

When deemed necessary, Planned Parenthood uses the "automobile sales technique" in its abortion counseling. This is especially true when religious concerns need to be overcome. This means that many people become involved in the "sale." The initial Planned Parenthood counselor may refer the pregnant client to another "specialist," a Planned Parenthood-approved psychiatrist, or a Planned Parenthood-approved minister.[4]

Is it really fair to say Planned Parenthood sees its services like an automobile dealer? An article in Planned Parenthood's *Papers 1975* argues it is necessary to "take into account the customer motivation necessary, [and] its strength related to the immediacy of the reward or benefit." The article suggests "that the promotion of a concept, such as 'every child a wanted child' or 'adopt family planning' is not specific enough nor implies immediate benefit." Instead, "family planning should concentrate on selling different brands of contraceptives, clinic services, techniques, in other words create a 'Brand X situation', selling a product which 'makes a specific product related promise—infertile sex.'" The article endorses and quotes the ideas of Dr. Timothy Black.[5]

The Planned Parenthood Federation of America has initiated a national recruitment program to augment its staff. The organization is seeking nurse practitioners, physicians, physicians' assistants, clinic managers, and certified nurse midwives. Planned Parenthood is having trouble recruiting qualified staff.[6] Its recruitment brochure is called *Planned Parenthood . . . The Career of Choice! . . . It's More than a Living . . . It's Living Your Ideals*. It is noted that Planned Parenthood employees "find fulfillment—knowing they are doing something about their deeply felt convictions regarding the rights of individuals to make their own child-bearing decisions." The brochure emphasizes a "commitment to reproductive freedom."[7]

Planned Parenthood's counseling has a direct impact on the number of women who choose abortion. In 1982, Planned Parenthood of Seattle-King County (Washington state), where abortions were referred out after Planned Parenthood did the "counseling," almost 21.4 percent of its pregnant customers were referred for prenatal care and fewer than 1 percent were referred for adoption. Almost 77.7 percent were referred for abortions.[8] One year later, the Planned Parenthood affiliate referred nearly 22.6 percent of its pregnant customers for prenatal care. Fewer than one-half of 1 percent were referred for adoption. Nearly 77 percent were referred for abortion. This means that in 1983 a total of only 23 percent of Planned Parenthood's pregnant customers were referred for something other than abortion.[9] The national average of women who abort is about one-third.

At one time, the Seattle-King County Planned Parenthood affiliate made a point of telling people it did not perform abortions in order to secure funding from groups like the United Way. The Seattle-King County affiliate is now performing abortions (see chapters 9 and 16).

Jo Ann Gasper, former deputy assistant secretary for population affairs with the Department of Health and Human Services, reports that an audit of some federally funded family planning clinics, conducted by the United States General Accounting Office, found that Planned Parenthood has the highest average abortion referral rate. The nationwide survey does, however, show a significant improvement over the results reported by Seattle-King County. The audit revealed that Planned Parenthood's average rate for abortion referral is 35.2 percent compared to an average of 5.7 percent for all family planning clinics. The audit found that one Planned Parenthood clinic referred 86.4 percent of women with positive pregnancy tests for abortion.[10] Of course, the high Planned Parenthood figure significantly increases the overall abortion referral rate.

These statistics could help account for the fact that there are approximately 319 abortions per 1,000 live births and only seven adoptions per 1,000 live births in the United States. Furthermore, since the legalization of abortion, the number of adoptions have dropped at an astounding rate.[11] Abortion is surely the primary reason for this statistic. However, another reason is that many teenagers who give birth are now choosing to raise their children, a fact Faye Wattleton found disturbing. "Many professionals believe this trend of teenage parenting is as great a concern as teenage pregnancy," she wrote.[12]

Simply put, according to Planned Parenthood, abortion is better for teenagers than is childbirth, even if adoption is chosen. Nevertheless, while adoption is truly a hard choice, it is a loving, life-affirming, and selfless one. One teenager who chose the option explains:

> Giving my baby up for adoption was something I did out of love. I've made two people who weren't able to have children the happiest people in the world. I get letters and pictures from them, and they call me every couple of weeks. I never worry about the baby's well-being.[13]

In an effort to diffuse arguments that it pushes abortion over childbirth, an allegation which is based on statistics, Planned Parenthood is now urging its affiliates to implement more popular programs. Speakers are urged to shift arguments about abortion to these new programs. For example, local Planned Parenthood clinics are being urged to offer prenatal care:

> Several administrators note that a prenatal program can enhance the public image of a clinic and, if the clinic also offers abortion services, help deflate charges leveled by right-to-life groups that the clinic encourages pregnant women to have abortions. "When you have prenatal services, the community sees you differently, more sympathetically," according to [Shirley] Mirow [executive director, Planned Parenthood of South Palm Beach and Broward Counties, Florida]. [Nancy] Mosher [regional director of Planned Parenthood of Northern New England], whose clinic in Barre, Vermont, initiated abortion services in 1987, agrees, noting that "it is definitely helpful to be able to say we offer women the options they need."[14]

The article also notes that prenatal care can be effective in "reaching certain groups (Hispanic women, for example) who may be reluctant to come to the clinic for contraceptives."[15]

Planned Parenthood leaders are increasing references to its prenatal care and other services. As noted in one *Detroit News* article, Planned Parenthood offers "everything from infertility counseling to prenatal care."[16] This is not a surprise. As one writer notes, "Planned Parenthood has supported abortion rights for two decades, but its preferred image was as a provider of general reproductive health services to young or poor women."[17]

Planned Parenthood affiliates added many services to their menus in 1990, including testing for the human immunodeficiency virus, which causes acquired immunodeficiency syndrome, and counseling for those tested or interested in being tested for the virus. Once again, services have been added primarily to diffuse arguments that Planned Parenthood is only interested in abortion.[18]

Planned Parenthood boasts of its 10 percent increase in the number of abortions done in 1989 over the previous year, as well as an increase in the number of affiliates doing abortions, but it notes that "only one affiliate added prenatal services" in the same year. A prediction is not made concerning an increase in the number of affiliates offering prenatal services, but the number in 1990 totalled 26.[19] Some affiliates which do not offer prenatal care provide "prenatal counseling."[20]

While it is suggested that prenatal care be offered, it is not suggested that equal weight be given to the option during counseling sessions. It is merely the most recent tactic designed to improve Planned Parenthood's public image, in the same way that its advertising campaigns are designed to do so.

16-YEAR-OLD CLIENT

The *Mogollan Advisor*, an Arizona newspaper, interviewed a former Planned Parenthood client. The 16-year-old being interviewed said that when she was in school "we were even told by one teacher that if we did not have intercourse by the time we were 11 years old, we were probably homosexual. The teacher would show films and they referred us to Planned Parenthood."[21] The student continues:

> "In 9th grade, I had a friend who had already had four abortions and was getting ready for her fifth one. By the time I was 12, I was sexually active and had a number of partners . . . and the schools were telling us it's okay before marriage."
>
> She blames her situation on the kind of sex education she received in school. "Nowadays, the schools have gotten away from moral standings. There is little support at home in this area. Most parents don't even know what the kids are learning. And Planned Parenthood furnishes the educational materials for the schools. Some of the schools are teaching its okay to . . . practice bestiality. When I read about Planned Parenthood coming here [to Payson, Arizona], inside I got mad. . . . I have no use for them at all. They tell you to come in and get an abortion. They don't tell you the dangers down the road, the emotional price."[22]

This former client contracted numerous venereal diseases and was diagnosed with cancer of the cervix. She was not expected to live past 21 years of age.

KATHY'S STORY

Kathy, a woman from Waco, Texas, was 16 when she became pregnant. She went to Planned Parenthood for help:

> My boyfriend put a lot of pressure on me—he really wanted me to do it [get an abortion]. I had been promised confidentiality at Planned Parenthood and I just could not face my parents with my problem. It was too painful; it would hurt them so much.
>
> It seemed so much easier to just get rid of the "mass of tissue" causing the trouble. An "embryo" didn't seem very important. . . . I never knew the truth. . . .
>
> I think I was much farther along than the people at the abortion clinic were prepared for. I was never checked at the clinic to see how far along I was. . . .
>
> I was not prepared for how painful the abortion itself was. We had been shown what they would do and told that some women had pain, but most didn't.

It [the pain] was so bad that I was throwing up. The doctor even asked if I wanted to stop. I just wanted it to be over. . . .

The recovery room had about ten women. All they did to treat us was to ask if we needed an aspirin.[23]

Kathy thought her problems were over. They were just beginning:

When I returned home I had very heavy bleeding and severe cramps for two days. I was so afraid something was wrong. I called Planned Parenthood. They said I was okay, that if I took my pills, I'd be all right. They didn't suggest an exam.

I was trying to go to school and my after-school job to hide that anything was wrong. I was at my after-school job at a dime store three days later when I had to go to the restroom because I was too weak to stand behind the cash register.

That was when I found my baby on my sanitary pad. I was horrified. Until that moment, I didn't know I still had the baby inside me—I didn't know it even was a baby . . .

He had arms and legs with tiny hands and feet; he was only about three inches long. I could make out his little nose and there was a dark spot on his oversized head that I know was his eye.

The feelings of remorse and sorrow overwhelmed me. I was hysterical—there I sat with a tiny dead baby in my hands—what could I do?

I had no "choices"—I wrapped up the whole package and threw it in the trash can. Rather, I laid it gently among the garbage. I stood looking at it for a long time.

What followed were years of turmoil, confusion and emotional death. The boy that I thought loved me couldn't handle what had happened to me. He was the only one in the world who knew about it and he wouldn't listen to me. The relationship dissolved. So did my belief in love. I felt worthless.

I got my own apartment as soon as I was of age, I drank too much, did drugs and entertained any man that would look at me. I was starved for acceptance and any man who found me worthy of affection was welcome.

This self-destructive behavior continued for four long years. I put myself in the most dangerous situations possible. I had a death wish.

I tried twice to do it the fast way—pills once and razor blades, another. But, I couldn't go through with it. So I tried the slow way—drunk driving, going to bars and the lake alone.[24]

OTHER DISSATISFIED CLIENTS

Tina, who says she is "pro-choice," went to a Planned Parenthood facility in Washington state. After receiving a pregnancy test, all the counselor did was provide her with a list of abortionists:

They never asked me if I wanted to keep the baby. They just gave me the names [of abortionists]. They must have just assumed that I wanted an abortion because I was a teenager and not married. They don't counsel. They didn't want to counsel. They wanted to send me to a butcher.[25]

Tina states that she was never asked what she wanted to do. Planned Parenthood asked for a donation, but she left the facility.[26]

Janet went to a Planned Parenthood facility in Norfolk, Virginia, prior to *Roe v. Wade*. As previously noted, abortion was legalized in New York in 1970 and Planned Parenthood began doing abortions the same month it became legal:

I was a nervous wreck and immediately started crying as I told the lady in the office about my situation. She asked me what I wanted to do and I told her I wanted an abortion. She immediately picked up the phone and call [sic] New York City and set up my appointment. I was three months pregnant. I told her I wanted to wait another month in order to get myself together and the money I would need and an excuse to tell my parents. She said, "no problem."

She never once suggested my alternatives to abortion, she just set up the appointment. She did not show me pictures of what a four month fetus would look like, or deal with any emotions that I would have after the abortion. I will never forget her coldness.

. . . I knew right away in my heart that I had done a terrible thing and asked God to forgive me. It took me 14 years to be able to talk about it without crying. I now have problems getting pregnant and the doctor said the abortion could have effected my ability to get pregnant.

The purpose of this letter is to let you know that my experience with Planned Parenthood was horrible and that they offered me no alternatives or help expect a phone call to New York.[27]

A former Planned Parenthood customer from Taylor, Arizona, has become a vocal critic of its brand of counseling:

Planned Parenthood suggested only an abortion. No other options were ever discussed. They said abortion was painless and virtually risk-free. . . .

Planned Parenthood is not telling the truth to girls in crisis pregnancy situations. I have suffered severe emotional problems.[28]

This Planned Parenthood customer was present at a public meeting held to decide whether a family planning clinic would be established in Payson, Arizona. Asked about the woman's story, Gloria Feldt from Planned Parenthood said stories like this are "out and out lies."[29]

A woman from Omaha, Nebraska, reports her experience:

In 1978 I called Planned Parenthood when my period was one week late. They scheduled me for an "endometrial aspiration" which they said would start my period. They offered no counseling. They never said abortion. I didn't even know I was pregnant. . . .

I was shocked to realize I had an abortion. Planned Parenthood deceived me. I was never given a choice. Now . . . I realize I've lost my child forever.[30]

A Minneapolis, Minnesota, woman is less than pleased with Planned Parenthood:

I was pregnant. Marriage was ruled out. Confused and frightened, I called Planned Parenthood. It was awful. None of the alternatives were ever discussed. No encouragement was given to keep or have the baby. Initially, I went to Planned Parenthood for a free pregnancy test. They quickly herded me into the abortion decision. I allowed my baby to be killed, not having been told the truth. I would have grasped any offer for help.[31]

An 18-year-old, who claims she made the right decision in having an abortion, confesses that things are not always good:

Sure, there are days when I have doubts. I'm in college now, and I've noticed something strange. Unconsciously I've been buying all these posters of babies for my dorm-room walls. Looking at them, I can't help imagining how my life would be different if I had one. Sometimes I find myself crying, wondering what my baby would have been like.[32]

While Planned Parenthood claims to have many satisfied customers, it refuses to respond to women who say they have been abused. Planned Parenthood officials either ignore such complaints or claim the women are lying. It is similar to a bad rape trial—ignore the issue and attack the victim's character. It has been reported that some women are paid to keep quiet about complications arising from abortions performed at Planned Parenthood facilities.[33]

One Planned Parenthood publication acknowledges one unsatisfied customer:

For many women, abortion is a great relief, for others it is a crisis. This 28 year old married woman came in shortly after having had a first trimester suction curettage abortion. There had been no medical problems and she had suffered no great discomfort physically. When she came in she felt upset, experienced the pregnancy and abortion as not being real—she felt as if she was living in a nightmare and could not distinguish nightmare from reality. She felt much regret stating that "he probably would have had red hair." My intervention consisted in [sic] helping her express her feelings, helping her see reality and starting her off on resolving her reactions to her feelings of loss.[34]

UNDERCOVER RESEARCH

In July 1989, a Florida woman, posing as a 16-year-old client, went to a Planned Parenthood facility in an effort to gather information for an article she was writing. She went to other facilities that perform abortions as well. The woman describes one of her visits:

First I had to fill out three different forms. One was a medical disclaimer, another was about my last period and birth control and the third was a complete medical history form. It asked so many questions about my medical history and personal ones too! I felt very uncomfortable. I did not sign the bottom of the form stating that the information was accurate because some of it wasn't [name of the woman, etc.]. . . .

The counselor's name was Sue. . . . Sue told me that my [pregnancy] test was negative but that it was not 100 percent accurate and that I should come in for a retest in a week. Then she asked me if I use any form of birth control. I said no. She then told me that I would have to go on the pill. . . . I told her that I couldn't go on the pill because if my mom found out she would kill me. She asked me why I couldn't talk to my mom about such things. I told her that my mother believed sex was wrong before marriage. She said that some people thought that but I should make my own decision. She was very clear in expressing that sex was not wrong and that I shouldn't feel like it was. She said that it was natural and felt good. She remembered being sixteen and how all those emotions get going and you can't stop. . . .

The line that killed me was, "How could something that feels so good be wrong?" She claimed that if two consenting adults wanted to make each other feel good, there was absolutely nothing wrong with it. I, of course, was an adult at 16 because biologically I was mature. I just had to act in a responsible way if I wanted to do adult things. I told her that deep inside I didn't know if premarital sex was right or wrong. I said that sometimes I felt it was good, but people like my mother has [sic] always taught me that it was wrong. I was quite shocked at her rebuttal: "Is your mother always right?"[35]

The woman reports that the Planned Parenthood counselor always referred to her boyfriend as "partner." The counselor did not consider chastity an option. "She even discouraged it," the woman says, "by saying that once you have already had intercourse, there is no way that anyone can expect you to go back to abstinence."[36]

The woman, who had a negative pregnancy test, asked what her options would be had the pregnancy test been positive:

She said that I would have 3 options and asked me what I would have chosen if my test were positive. I told her that I didn't know and I would have wanted her to help me decide. . . . She said that a few months ago I would have had to tell my mom, but the Florida Supreme Court just passed a law. She also mentioned that abortion could be outlawed in the state of Florida soon and how terrible it would be if that right was taken away.[37]

To be sure the experience at the Planned Parenthood facility was not an isolated incident, the woman went to another location in a different Florida city. Her experience was amazingly similar. This time, however, the woman arranged to have a positive pregnancy test:

> After I gave the appropriate responses [to questions regarding the "client's" medical condition], Judy [the Planned Parenthood counselor] told me that my test was positive. She explained that the test was 99 percent accurate. She asked me if my periods were usually regular and then figured out how far along I was. She said that she was glad I came in early enough because I still had time. She asked me what I thought I would do. I just looked completely overwhelmed and fearful and stammered, "I just can't believe this is happening! I don't know what to do!" She told me that this is what happens when you don't use birth control. . . .
>
> She said that I had three options: I could carry the baby and keep it, I could carry the baby and put it up for adoption, or I could have an abortion. She asked me what my feelings on abortion were. I told her that I had always sort of felt it was wrong but it seemed a lot different when it hit home. She agreed with me. She asked me if I could tell my parents. I said no because they were so strict that they would even kill me if they knew I had sex. She said, "so they didn't even give you the liberty to decide when you were old enough to have sex?" I told her that they thought you should only have sex inside of marriage. She said that that would be ideal but that wasn't reality.[38]

The conversation changed to abortion. The counselor told the "16-year-old client" that she had nothing to fear because abortion is "as simple and easy as getting a tooth pulled" and "very safe." The counselor further explained the abortion procedure using exclusively ambiguous terms such as "contents of the uterus." Such rhetoric is used to prevent any value from being placed on the preborn human being.[39]

The counselor told the woman that there are "not really any risks at all until you have had three abortions and then you might be prone to miscarriages." The counselor also told the woman that it is safer to have an abortion than to give birth.[40] The woman asked the counselor about nightmares:

> She said that I might have one or two nightmares because I was in the middle of making a big decision. She said that women have nightmares when they are going to have their baby or even before they get married.
>
> I asked her if it would come back to haunt me later and she said that the only time women ever have problems with it is if they feel that they did the wrong thing. I told her that deep down inside, something told me that abortion was wrong but I didn't know what to do or who to listen to. I told her that I remember people saying it is murder and stuff and I didn't feel very good about it. She said, "Do you REALLY believe that?!" I said that I didn't know. She told me that most of the people who say those things don't understand because they have never been faced with a crisis pregnancy.
>
> She told me that I had to "THINK LONG TERM . . . THINK LONG TERM!" She said, "Can you picture yourself going through high school and college with a baby? How are you going to support it? How would you have felt if your parents brought you into the world with no one to care for you or give you the things you need? I know you know what you need to do . . . "[41]

The strategy of making women feel abandoned, as though their only real choice is abortion, seems common. Little support is offered, emotional or otherwise, to make rejecting abortion seem realistic. Women are led into the abortion decision.

The counselor's rhetoric changed in such a way as to suggest that the woman had made a decision to have an abortion:

> "After you have your abortion, you can come back here for a check up and birth control." She kept emphasizing that having a baby would affect my whole life for the next 18 years . . . She told me that the "mass of cells" in my uterus right now was only as big as my pinky. She said not to think of it as some huge baby.
>
> I asked her what she thought of adoption. She said that it was fine if I could picture myself carrying the baby, going through delivery, and then signing away *my rights* to that baby FOREVER. She emphasized that very few people could do that and it was a very hard thing. . . . She said that considering my age and situation, abortion was the best thing to do for me and "my pregnancy." She said that I would not feel 100 percent sure now but a year from now I will say that I think I did the right thing and two years from now I will say I know that I did the right thing. She gave me the paperwork that I needed to get an abortion . . . and gave me a form that would give me a discount ($225). She emphasized that I needed to make an appointment no later than August 24th [The date of the interview was August 4.] but that I might want to do it this week and just get it over with.[42]

The counselor told the woman to tell her parents about the abortion only if she felt it was best. The woman was also told to make the decision as soon as possible and not to pretend the pregnancy did not exist. The counselor asked the young woman to call her with the decision. "I honestly feel that this woman will get a commission off of my abortion," the woman wrote. "She pushed it so hard!"[43]

In 1991, CBN News sent two 16-year-old girls into a Planned Parenthood clinic. The Planned Parenthood counselor spoke about birth control, including how condoms are used. It was suggested that the teenagers become familiar with the condom so they will know how to use them, even in the dark or in a car. She also said the decision to have sex is a personal one and contraceptives are needed so the teenagers "won't get pregnant . . . won't get any diseases and no one ever has to know." The counselor mentioned mutual masturbation and referred to oral sex as a form of petting. She also told the teenagers they need not speak to their parents about the decision to have sex if they feel their parents will not understand.[44]

Regarding abstinence, the Planned Parenthood counselor told the teenagers it is their choice, but she warned them about the possible consequences of teens with "active hormones." The counselor said the teenagers should not be surprised that their parents would probably object to premarital sexual intercourse. "There's always going to be people who disapprove no matter what you do," she said. "No one's going to disapprove if you abstain—except maybe your boyfriend."[45]

ABORTION BY COERCION

Lavonne Wilenken, a former nurse practitioner at a Planned Parenthood clinic, has many stories about women who have been coerced into having abortions, something denied by Planned Parenthood officials. Nevertheless, Wilenken relies on her personal experiences to support her assertions:

> Once when I was working in the family planning clinic where also the abortuary inhabited the same building, I was in a room with a counselor and a young woman. One of the family planning assistants came—burst in the room and said, "Please, you've got to come quick! She's trying to back out of the procedure and everything's all ready!"
>
> The counselor left hurriedly down the hall and I followed to see exactly what was going on and what I saw in the hall was the counselor, a 17-year-old girl and her aunt, dragging

her into the room as she was hollering, "No, I don't want to go! Please don't make me! Please don't make me do this! I really don't want to do this!"

They very hurriedly shoved her in the room where the procedure was to take place and slammed the door and the counselor came out afterwards with a sort of a, a peaceful, smiling look on his face, and I knew what had happened. I knew that they had aborted her against her will.[46]

Wilenken claims verbal coercion is commonly used by Planned Parenthood counselors:

The counselor would say to the teenager, "Well, where's the $250,000 that it takes to raise a child in society today?," and "What are your parents going to say when they find out that you're pregnant?," and "What is your boyfriend doing? Is he going to help you? Where is he?," and "How are you going to finish your education if you have a baby? Don't you know you can't go to school if you have a baby?" Things like that, very subtle little things that will push the girl over and make her decide.

Then they sort of do a "Mut and Jeff" routine. First will come those questions. Next will come the very motherly, the very soothing, "But we can help you. We can help you out of your problem. Your parents don't have to know. We can help you with money. You don't have to have any money and we can help you out of your situation because we know that you don't want to be pregnant. You just want to be not pregnant and we know that you know that you can't take care of a baby right now. You know that you're not ready and we want you to do these things when you're ready." So they play on the emotions of the young girl who's scared, frightened, doesn't know where to go, but she's been told this is the place to go to get help.[47]

"SAFE AND LEGAL" ABORTION

In a question-and-answer format, Planned Parenthood publishes a document explaining abortion to women:

WHAT IS AN ABORTION? It is the termination of a pregnancy by surgically removing the embryo or fetus from the uterus. . . .

WHEN IS THE OPERATION DONE? The operation should be done as early as possible to reduce the risks to the woman. . . . Planned Parenthood recommends that the woman call for an appointment as soon as possible after her pregnancy is confirmed.

IS IT DIFFICULT TO FIND A DOCTOR? No. Planned Parenthood has a list of doctors who have been approved by its Medical Committee. . . .

ARE THERE COMPLICATIONS WITH ABORTIONS? Rarely, but as with any medical procedure, they are possible. . . .

WILL THE WOMAN BE ABLE TO GET PREGNANT IN THE FUTURE? It is unusual for an abortion to cause infertility. . . .

HOW CAN ANOTHER UNINTENDED PREGNANCY BE AVOIDED? To avoid pregnancy in the future, you need to choose a method of contraception. . . . Planned Parenthood encourages you to return to us for on-going contraceptive care. Any unprotected intercourse following an abortion may result in another pregnancy.

HOW WILL THE WOMAN FEEL EMOTIONALLY AFTER THE ABORTION? The woman's comfort about her choice often affects her feelings afterwards. Women experience a broad range or combination of emotions after an abortion. These may include a feeling of relief sometimes mixed with a sense of sadness, loss or depression.[48]

One question asks how another unintended pregnancy can be avoided. Only birth control is mentioned.[49]

The files at one Planned Parenthood affiliate show that women are clearly victimized. Notations are included by Planned Parenthood personnel concerning 92 abortions performed. Of these, 36 women reported severe or very severe pain. Three women screamed. Ten cried and five complained. Nine women are described by Planned Parenthood personnel as having "overreacted" to the abortion. Six women retched or had nausea and six fainted.[50]

One Planned Parenthood doctor performed an "abortion" on a girl whose second pregnancy test came out negative to "relieve anxiety." Two other "non-abortions" were done, but it was not known until after the procedure was underway that the women were not pregnant. More than 80 percent of the abortions were done on women who said they wanted more children, but now was not the right time.[51]

One study shows that 94 percent of women say they suffered negative psychological effects after getting an abortion, 73 percent of whom say the effects were severe. An astounding 94 percent of the women surveyed said they would not have an abortion if they were able to make the decision over again. Only 2 percent said they would have the abortion again.[52]

A controversy has broken out regarding post-abortion problems faced by women. Several conservative and anti-abortion publications have quoted from a document titled, "Department of Education 3-Year Plan and Long Range Program Goals, 1990–1993." The last page of the document essentially includes an admission on the part of Planned Parenthood that post-abortion problems not only exist, they are at a high level:

> A number of anti-choice studies and surveys (including the Reardon/WIC Study and the Grant Survey) have shown that the incidence of post-procedural trauma for abortion clients may be as high as 91 percent of all cases. While recent unpublished reports from the Alan Guttmacher Institute indicate that the scope of the problem may have been accurately tabulated in these studies, the effect of those same anti-life forces in creating the trauma in the first place has not yet been effectively measured. This volatile political dilemma must be addressed forthrightly by local affiliates. The program is designed to help educators and counselors deal with this sensitive issue.[53]

Looks like a great document, except that Planned Parenthood is claiming that it is a fake:

> PPFA is continuing to look for the source of the phony document titled "PPFA Department of Education Three-Year Plan and Long-Range Program Goals, 1990–93."
>
> The national office now has a copy of the complete document, which has prompted numerous inquiries from affiliates in whose areas it has surfaced.
>
> If this document appears in your area, please try to determine where it originated and how it is being used . . .[54]

There are three likely possibilities: 1) an anti-abortion activist created the document, which is not a smart move; 2) it is an internal Planned Parenthood document and since it includes information abortion foes are not supposed to have, its authenticity is being denied; or 3) the document is a fake but it was done by a Planned Parenthood employee as a hoax to make abortion foes look bad.

While there are a few scientific studies on post-abortion trauma, including what is being called "post-abortion syndrome," the federal government cannot be expected to be of any assistance. President Ronald Reagan had asked then-Surgeon General C. Everett Koop, M.D., to study the matter. Koop said it would take many years and a lot of money to do so. He could not say with any medical or scientific certainly that post-abortion syndrome does or does not exist. It simply has not been studied as much as is necessary.

In a commentary on the non-study, Cristine Russell, the *Washington Post*'s special health correspondent, concludes, "Some would say he dodged the issue, but he came out with an announcement that there would be no report—that he didn't have enough evidence one way or the other to really justify a report that would come out with some strong conclusions."[55] Claims made by supporters of legal abortion that Koop did not find any evidence that post-abortion syndrome exists is accurate, but a half-truth. He did not find that it does not exist either.

Since leaving public life, Koop has chastised abortion foes on several occasions. For example, he is critical of abortion opponents for their view of contraception:

> I've never said this before in public. I believe that the pro-life forces, and I use that in a very broad term and to include everybody that [sic] is pro-life, I think that they have shot their wad in the sense that I don't think there's anything more they can do that will change any more opinion and, therefore, the bottom line is, if you want to get rid of abortion in America there is only one way to do it—you get rid of unwanted pregnancies—and, unfortunately, many of the people who are most vociferous about their anti-abortion stand are the very same people that [sic] have prevented research into contraception and contraceptive advice to the people who most desperately need it. Until we face that issue as a society and get rid of that, we are not going to make progress about the abortion issue.[56]

Jo Ann Gasper reports that some Planned Parenthood clinics are misusing oral contraceptives that are given to women. She cites an example of a "former Planned Parenthood Director, Dr. Jan Petty, [who] has even taught federally funded family planning nurse practitioners to intentionally *misuse* oral contraceptives to 'restart' late periods. These 'restarts' are actually chemically induced abortions."[57]

Lavonne Wilenken tells of her experiences with women who suffered complications at Planned Parenthood clinics. In one incident, Wilenken examined a woman and found a complication. The abortionist was called. He told the woman that she only had a benign tumor and she needed a hysterectomy. A hysterectomy would have removed the evidence of the botched abortion.[58]

Wilenken has other stories. One involves a 17-year-old girl who paid for her abortion and was sent home following the procedure:

> She called in several times complaining of bleeding and cramping. Finally [she] was . . . given an appointment and while waiting for the doctor she went into the bathroom and promptly delivered a 12-week, totally intact, unborn baby in the toilet. This is after her abortion.
>
> Of course, the attempt then was to discredit the patient. That is the way they will always operate. To discredit her or to wear her down. To try to do anything to make her feel like that she's the one who was at fault, and certainly not them or their physicians.
>
> That case was settled out of court for $100,000. What happened is there was a suit and she was paid off $100,000 and asked never to bring this particular incident to the media or the legal people's attention. So that is just another indication of slipshod, sloppy medicine that goes on. I mean, we're talking a factory medicine assembly line that goes on at Planned Parenthood clinics. The name of the game is, "How many patients can you see? How quick can you see them?"[59]

One woman who received an abortion at a Planned Parenthood clinic would concur with Wilenken's assessment:

My experience was a complete horror story at Planned Parenthood. My experience was a back-alley butcher. I felt like I was in a meat market. And this was a controlled, protecting environment for the women? It seems like to me that the back-alley butchers have moved to an uptown environment and they're still butchers but they work maybe at a little nicer looking clinic and they work for Planned Parenthood.[60]

Wilenken explains that she and her co-workers were also told how to speak about the abortion procedure. In such a way that the one not yet born is dehumanized.

Planned Parenthood's Mimi Grinker openly addresses Planned Parenthood's view of preborn human beings:

A six-week-old fetus is not a baby. It's a fetus really: a baby when it's born and this is just a side. I mean, we really don't care what she [the customer] thinks, how she feels about abortion or when she thinks life begins. Our concern is that she make an intelligent choice.[61]

Beverly McMillen, M.D., a former abortionist from Jackson, Mississippi, notes that Planned Parenthood's claims of few complications are unreliable:

Planned Parenthood clinics, and free-standing abortion clinics like them, they claim they have an untarnished record of no complications from their abortion procedures, but what they don't know is that I'm the practitioner who sees their complications. These women don't go back to the clinic where they've had a bad experience. They show up in my office or in my emergency room with their bleeding or with their infections or with their retained placenta, needing another D&C [dilation and curettage].[62]

McMillen reports that many abortionists go from town-to-town and are at different clinics on different days of the week. This helps contribute to poor follow-up. Maybe what women don't know *will* hurt them.

EXCEPTIONS

One of Planned Parenthood's newer strategies is to claim that abortion foes are against abortion for others, not themselves. Its leaders assert that many staunch abortion foes have gone to them for abortions. An article in an internal Planned Parenthood newsletter addresses the alleged practice. "Sally," the article begins, "is one of a growing number of women who came to the affiliate, headquartered in Albany, N.Y., to terminate a pregnancy but who also vehemently declare their opposition to abortion."[63]

It is stated that "these women, some of whom admit to being members of anti-choice organizations, are openly antagonistic and resistant to counseling." The women tolerate the counseling session "while attempting to find some way to rationalize . . . actions with . . . beliefs." According to the article's author, "what separates these women from the majority of abortion patients is their rigid insistence that abortion should never be an option for anyone, that it is always a sin, but that special circumstances in their lives justify the choice." The author makes a point of writing that, "One of the most remarkable aspects of this situation, according to counselors, is that, despite having chosen to terminate a pregnancy, none of these women has altered her basic stance that abortion is wrong and should not be legal."[64]

A drawing of picket signs accompanies the article. One sign reads, "OUTLAW ABORTION (BUT WAIT UNTIL I HAVE MINE)." Another reads, "I AM ANTI-CHOICE (BUT I HAD NO CHOICE, SO I HAD AN ABORTION)." A third sign reads, "(I WAS THE EXCEPTION TO THE RULE) CHOICE IS NOT FOR YOU."[65] Naturally, such assertions are not proven because Planned Parenthood officials can fall back on its confidentiality pledge—an understandable point. This allows Planned Parenthood officials to make statements which cannot be challenged, and they know it.

9

MILLIONS OF DOLLARS

Planned Parenthood's annual report states that, "While some might think that controversy necessarily results in decreased support, Planned Parenthood has found the opposite to be true."[1] Indeed, Planned Parenthood's financial status and growth is without precedent for a nonprofit family planning organization.

A Planned Parenthood five year plan calls for an increase in revenue to Planned Parenthood through a 20 percent increase in clinic income and government funding.[2] In 1990, Planned Parenthood affiliates received at least $32.4 million from abortions[3] and $126.5 million through combined government grants and contracts.[4]

The Planned Parenthood Federation of America is the 12th largest charitable organization in the United States,[5] raising a total 1991 budget of approximately $406.3 million, which includes a $21.6 million surplus for the year for an overall end of the year "fund balance" (surplus) of $207.7 million.[6] The 1991 budget is up more than $22 million from the previous year, $77 million from 1989, and approximately $103 million from 1988.[7] Planned Parenthood is expected to generate nearly $440 million in 1992.

FOUNDATION SUPPORT

In response to the Reagan Administration's decision to withhold funding from the International Planned Parenthood Federation, many private foundations decided to provide support. The following foundations, for example, provided financial support to the International Planned Parenthood Federation because of the policy: the Rockefeller Foundation, the Mellon Foundation, the Ford Foundation, the Carnegie Foundation, Pew Charitable Trusts, the William and Flora Hewlett Foundation, the MacArthur Foundation, and the David and Lucile Packard Foundation.[8]

Have these foundations had any significant impact? The budget for the International Planned Parenthood Federation increased from $61 million in 1987 to $72 million in 1988, despite the Reagan Administration policy.[9] Grants are responsible for the greatest increase in International Planned Parenthood Federation resources.

Planned Parenthood has received funding from many other private foundations, as has other groups supportive of legal abortion. Such donations are possible because the foundations and their leaders are not susceptible to public pressure. Its leaders are responsible to no one.

FUND-RAISING

In a fund-raising letter addressed to "Caring American," Faye Wattleton asks us to take action "*right now* to change one of the most inhumane situations on Earth—the fact that so many children born into this world are *unwanted*." Wattleton urges the reader to consider the tragedy of too many children in drought-stricken Africa and other Third World areas. She suggests that family planning services would "help *far more* of this planet's families" than merely "sending a package of food to an African village, or 'adopting' a little Bangladeshi girl . . . "[10]

After referring to a story of a starving girl from the Sudan, the reader is assured that this child, "Like most of her older brothers and sisters . . . was never really wanted by her parents. They just didn't know how they could control their own fertility. So . . . [the] birth [of the girl] was *unplanned* and *unwanted*." What can be done to help? An "essential" key to improving the "health and quality of life of families throughout Africa and the rest of the developing world" is to give them the right to make a "responsible, rational choice about parenthood . . ." Sending a check to Planned Parenthood would result in "an improved quality of life and a stronger family life" for the people of the Third World.[11]

Over the past three decades, Planned Parenthood fund-raising letters have generated millions of dollars. Many of these dollars are spent on efforts to keep abortion legal.

Planned Parenthood sends many fund-raising letters each year. One which went out with Katharine Hepburn's signature said, "This is when we *must* dig a little deeper and give a little bit more than we ever have before."[12] Hepburn helped to reach a goal of $3.6 million for its Public Impact Campaign.

A common theme in Planned Parenthood fund-raising letters is that the world, or at least the world of Planned Parenthood's philosophy, will crumble unless a great deal of money is raised in a short period of time. A Wattleton fund-raising letter, for example, tells its readers that meeting "the challenge of those who wish to plunge us all back into the 'sex-is-taboo' mentality of Margaret Sanger's day and, at the same time, to maintain our vital ongoing programs, places an enormous demand upon our finances."[13] While not unique to Planned Parenthood, its reliance on such tactics, in conjunction with defending "freedom of choice," is both clever and successful.

Planned Parenthood has placed renewed emphasis on generating income from bequests and other deferred gifts. Its annual reports often highlight how individuals can use this system to donate to Planned Parenthood.

WEBSTER *EQUALS BIG MONEY*

The hearing of *Webster v. Reproductive Health Services* by the United States Supreme Court did much for Planned Parenthood's fund-raising efforts. Ms. reports that many pro-legal abortion groups, including Planned Parenthood, have seen significant financial benefit:

> The renewed threat to legalized abortion is galvanizing grass-roots donors into action—and not a moment too soon, we might add.
>
> According to direct-mail experts, the number of people who gave regularly to reproductive-rights advocacy groups before President Bush opened the assault on choice has jumped from around 1.2 million to between 2 and 2.5 million. The National Organization for Women is getting cash contributions of $80,000 to $100,000 a day from its abortion/ERA direct-mail campaign.
>
> NOW Vice President Patricia Ireland reports that the big surge began last November when Attorney General Richard Thornburgh, in a surprise postelection move, urged the Supreme Court to use the *Missouri Webster* case to overturn *Roe v. Wade*. . . .
>
> The National Abortion Rights Action League's direct-mail intake is running about $20,000 a day, up about 200 percent from last year at this time. Planned Parenthood, which has sent out information on RU 486, AIDS, and teenage pregnancy, has also been getting a bumper crop of responses from its mailings, as has the American Civil Liberties Union, which litigates and consults on about 90 percent of all reproductive rights cases.[14]

While the statistics regarding the National Organization for Women come from the organization itself, they are not going unchallenged. *USA Today* founder Al Neuharth writes:

> NOW admits it has had no growth in 20 years. It now is no more than a frenetic fringe organization kept alive by media hype . . . Many mainstream women . . . consider any association with NOW bad baggage.[15]

While the decision in *Webster* led to modest increases in the fund-raising of groups opposed to legal abortion, this was a short-term increase. Moreover, forces opposed to abortion claim they began from a much smaller base.

Increased funding for groups supporting legal abortion can be attributed to the fear of losing a right that has been seen as secure for more than a decade. That fear has motivated many individuals, who previously were only verbal supporters of legal abortion, to give on a consistent basis. On the other hand, *Webster* has caused abortion foes to become over-confident about the future. Contributions to groups opposed to abortion slightly increased when *Webster* was being heard by the Supreme Court because abortion opponents believed they were on the brink of a major breakthrough. Now that the *Webster* decision has been released, many abortion foes believe there is no reason to contribute. This will likely become a bigger problem after the Supreme Court rules in *Planned Parenthood v. Casey*.

The reversal of *Roe v. Wade*, when it comes, will be a major victory, but it will really be only the beginning. The issue will be returned to the states for decision-making, and more dollars are needed than ever before. Funds are needed to influence state legislation, and to impact public opinion on the state and local levels. Supporters of legal abortion understand this and they are raising funds to be used in each state.

FEDERAL FUNDS

By far, the single largest revenue source for Planned Parenthood has been the American taxpayer. Efforts to cut funding for this advocacy group have been largely unsuccessful due to court decisions and a large, powerful lobby. Naturally, Planned Parenthood seeks federal funding of all abortions as it would guarantee the organization more income. It could then get money to do abortions on women who could not otherwise afford them.

Planned Parenthood officials claim that if abortion is a constitutional right, government should pay for it. This logic is fundamentally flawed. The right to vote, for those over 18 years of age, is guaranteed by the Constitution, but voters cannot bill the government for transportation expenses to the polling place. After all, is it not discriminatory that the poor may not be able to afford such transportation while the wealthy can afford it? Similarly, if there is a constitutional right to own a gun, is the federal government responsible for supplying weapons to poor people? Should the poor be provided with printing presses so they can exercise their right to free speech?

The Public Health Service Act, passed by Congress in 1970, includes the Family Planning Services and Population Research Act, Title X (pronounced "title 10"), the federal family planning program. It is administered by the Office of Population Affairs under the auspices of the Office of the Assistant Secretary for Health within the Department of Health and Human Services. The Department makes grant awards to state health departments or original umbrella agencies that subcontract with local agencies. Planned Parenthood had been the primary recipient of Title X funds, receiving approximately $37 million annually.

While Section 1008 of the Public Health Service Act states that, "No funds appropriated under this title shall be used in programs where abortion is a method of family planning," Title X has provided Planned Parenthood millions of taxpayer dollars. Title X remains an extremely popular program with members of Congress.

Title X requires confidentiality, regardless of age or marital status. Planned Parenthood officials commonly say they are required by law to provide confidential services to minors. Therefore, it is not their fault because Planned Parenthood employees are only obeying the law. This is technically true, but it should be noted that Planned Parenthood leaders have always insisted on the confidentiality provision of Title X. This provision eliminates any rights of parents be part of the process.

Following passage of the Public Health Service Act, federal bureaucrats interpreted Section 1008 to mean that Title X funds could not be used to pay for abortion services, but it did not preclude funds from going to organizations that perform or counsel for abortions. Under the Carter Administration, bureaucrats changed the policy to *require* recipients of Title X funds to refer and counsel for abortions.

Attacks on the Title X program by abortion foes led Planned Parenthood to place full-page newspaper advertisements in defense of this lucrative program. A cut in Title X funding to Planned Parenthood could severely cripple its agenda:

> Our country has a program that reduces teen pregnancies, reduces the need for abortion, and saves taxpayers money. The "Moral Majority" wants it abolished.
>
> It's America's Family Planning Program. For ten years, it's brought comprehensive family planning services to millions of Americans.
>
> It's helped prevent five million unwanted pregnancies. It's helped those who wanted to have children. And it's saved taxpayers money by reducing the need for other services associated with unwanted and unplanned childbearing.

But now some people want to abolish this program. Money isn't really their issue. They are using the need to control federal spending to force their own narrow views of right and wrong on America—their standards of morality on all of us.

We think that is wrong. If you think it's wrong, write your Senators and Representatives to tell them so. And join us in the effort to save America's Family Planning Program. It's vital!

Use the coupon. And please give generously of your time and money.

Helping build a strong America by helping build strong American families.[16]

The need for Planned Parenthood to defend the Title X program steadily increased. It issued a "fact sheet" on the program:

The Need for Publicly Funded Family Planning Programs

- According to a cost/benefit analysis conducted in 1989 by The Alan Guttmacher Institute, without government support for family planning services, an average of 1.2 million additional unintended pregnancies would occur each year to women of reproductive age in the United States.
- Those pregnancies, according to estimates in the studies, would result in approximately 516,000 abortions and approximately 509,000 unwanted births. . . .
- This study also found that taxpayers save $4.40 for every public dollar spent to provide birth control for women who might otherwise not have access to contraceptives.
- The total savings of $1.8 billion a year represents money that would be spent on medical, welfare, and nutritional services (as required by law) for women who would have unplanned pregnancies if publicly funded contraceptive care were not available.
- A 1989 Center for Population Options report set at $19.83 billion the 1988 cost to taxpayers of public services required to maintain families begun by teen mothers.
- Nearly one in four American women using contraceptives each year (exclusive of sterilization) obtain services from publicly funded health care providers.[17]

It is interesting to note that for all of the statistics cited and footnoted in the Planned Parenthood "Fact Sheet," the following organizations and publications are used: The Alan Guttmacher Institute (*Family Planning Perspectives*), the Center for Population Options (which actively supports legal abortion), and, more directly, Planned Parenthood itself.

Under the Reagan Administration, Jo Ann Gasper was named deputy assistant secretary for population affairs at the Department of Health and Human Services. Responsible for administering the Title X program in accordance with the law, Gasper wrote to regional health directors saying that groups advocating abortion are ineligible for Title X funds. Gasper cited Section 1008, but her action was almost immediately rescinded by her superior, Dr. Robert Windom. Gasper was later fired by Dr. Otis Bowen, secretary of the Department of Health and Human Services.

Abortion foes were furious over the Gasper firing. In response, President Ronald Reagan named a successor who held similar views. Moreover, he promised to issue new regulations specifically stating that groups providing abortion counseling and referral as a method of family planning are ineligible to receive Title X funds.

The regulations issued by the Reagan Administration include four key provisions. Title X funds are to be limited to groups and programs that do not: 1) include abortion as a method of family planning; 2) engage in any activities that encourage, promote, or advocate abortion as a method of family planning; and 3) provide counseling and referral for abortion. The fourth provision requires that organizations doing any of the aforementioned prohibited activities maintain physical and financial separation from the legitimately funded Title X activities. The regulations impact Planned Parenthood more than any other group, even though approximately 4,000 clinics would be covered.

It did not take long for Planned Parenthood to begin spreading its version of what the Title X program is and how the regulations amounted to a "gag rule" (a phrase purposefully invented by Planned Parenthood and generally used by the media). Planned Parenthood's Faye Wattleton released a press statement on the issue:

> Nationwide, more than four million women were served, helping to prevent approximately 1.2 million unintended pregnancies and 480,000 abortions. Further, recent studies have shown that for every public dollar spent on family planning, $4.40 in other program costs is saved by taxpayers. . . .
>
> Since . . . [1980], Title X has suffered substantial funding cuts, but managed to withstand several attempts to destroy the program through cruel and counterproductive regulations. . . .
>
> The gag rule prohibits any federally funded family planning clinics from providing their patients with *any* information about abortion, even if a woman requests this information, and even if continuing the pregnancy would endanger her health.
>
> The gag rule unconstitutionally restricts free speech, it violates medical ethics, and it contradicts the established principle of informed consent.
>
> Ironically, Title X does more to prevent abortion than any other federal program, yet it has been a consistent target of anti-choice members of Congress. . . .
>
> The rider requires that abortion providers that receive any federal funds must notify the parents of minors seeking abortions. This applies to all clinics, hospitals and private physicians that receive these funds. (Fortunately, this dangerous and counterproductive measure was dropped yesterday in conference committee.)
>
> If Senator [William] Armstrong really wants to reduce the incidence of abortion, he would support *increased* funding for Title X, rather than his punitive and cruel measure.
>
> It is time for politicians on both sides of the issue to move beyond politics and rhetoric and word towards a realistic goal of reducing the need for abortion. We must work together to increase access to contraceptive services; greatly expand sexuality education; help Americans evolve more positive and realistic attitudes toward human sexuality; and commit increased funding to research to develop new and more effective contraceptive methods.
>
> With responsible leadership, we can achieve all of these goals. Planned Parenthood and the American people call on our elected representatives to provide that leadership.[18]

The Title X regulations were challenged in court. A New York court ruled that the regulations are constitutional and they were upheld in full. A Massachusetts judge, however, invalidated the regulations. The United States Supreme Court agreed to decide the matter.

The Supreme Court reviewed the regulations in *Rust v. Sullivan* and determined them to be both constitutional and a reasonable interpretation of the law creating Title X. Faye Wattleton was quick to attack the decision, calling it "an unimaginable blow to free speech and to the medical profession, as well as to our nation's poorest, most vulnerable women." Referring to the regulations as a "gag rule," Wattleton argued that the Supreme Court gave the government "the green light to impose censorship on doctors and women, and has reestablished separate but unequal justice in America: quality health care for those who can afford it, second class care for those who cannot."[19]

Wattleton argued that the Title X regulations are the result of a "conspiracy to abuse the rights of doctors and the privacy of women by forcing doctors to withhold information from women and interfering with the free speech and ethical responsibilities of medical professionals." Wattleton claimed the regulations would prohibit medical personnel in Title X clinics "from providing a pregnant woman with information on all of her options, including legal abortion—even if her health were at risk, and even if she asked for such information."[20]

The regulations, Wattleton charged, were "invented by the Reagan administration to harass, misinform, and manipulate women" and that the rules constitute "medical malpractice." Wattleton claimed that Title X funds have never been used for abortions so the regulations must be an attempt to "intimidate women." She also argued that the result of the regulations would be an additional 1.2 million unintended pregnancies per year which would result in 516,000 abortions and 509,000 "unwanted births." In addition, "for many women, Title X clinics are the only source of health care, providing preventive services that include pelvic and breast examinations, cancer screening, testing for sexually transmitted disease, and education about all methods of contraception." Wattleton said Planned Parenthood is resolved to continue offering a full "range of family planning services—including counseling and referrals for abortion."[21]

Irving Rust, M.D., medical director of Planned Parenthood of New York City, and the man who brought suit against the government, said, "I just cannot be dishonest. I have to give full information."[22]

One problem faced by Planned Parenthood foes was inaccurate reporting on the part of the media, which may have been fueled in part by Planned Parenthood. Several reports "blamed" the Supreme Court for the regulations. In fact, the Supreme Court had only upheld the constitutionality and legitimacy of the rules. It was the White House which had created them based on the law creating Title X. One example of inaccurate reporting:

> On May 23, the United States Supreme Court outlawed all federally funded abortion counseling. After lengthy debate, the Court's nine justices did not make abortion illegal. What they did, in a five-to-four vote, was forbid certain clinics and doctors—those that receive any federal funding—from giving out advice or information about abortion.[23]

Soon after the Supreme Court's decision in *Rust v. Sullivan*, Planned Parenthood began a campaign to get Congress to reverse the regulations. Planned Parenthood pledged to spend between three and five million dollars in an effort to reverse the rules. Faye Wattleton took a belligerent position. "The government will have to take those funds from us. We're not giving them up," she said.[24]

In its effort to convince the public and, in turn, Congress that the Title X regulations should be reversed, Planned Parenthood placed several full-page newspaper advertisements. The organization emphasized freedom of speech, medical ethics, fairness to women, and similar issues. Abortion foes emphasized the original intent of the Title X program as a preconceptive program, the difference between abortion and contraception, and the financial interest of Planned Parenthood in fighting the regulations. The latter group claimed Planned Parenthood's multimillion-dollar campaign could be viewed as an investment with a $37 million payoff—*per year*.

The campaign to abolish the Title X regulations became one of the most heated in history. Abortion foes made it clear that the vote would be considered an abortion vote. Planned Parenthood claimed the primary issue is free speech, not abortion (its usual strategy).

While it was expected that Planned Parenthood would make effective use of advertising, particularly given its budget, many were surprised to see abortion foes place newspaper advertisements. There were three major advertisements prepared by abortion foes which generally focused on the same issues but with a different headline:

> ***They want to take your tax dollars and refer your daughter for an abortion.***
>
> Planned Parenthood runs the largest chain of abortion clinics in the United States. In 1989, they performed or referred for more than 200,000 abortions—many of them on teenagers, *without their parents' knowledge or consent.*
>
> President Bush's Title 10 regulations make a distinction between abortion and family planning. Family planning providers will continue to receive federal funds, but not to promote abortion. These regulations recognize the difference between abortion, which stops a beating heart, and contraception, which prevents conception.
>
> Planned Parenthood and other abortionists don't like that. They're spending $3 million to $5 million to convince Congress to repeal President Bush's common sense regulations. They want you—the taxpayer—to continue paying them $37 million a year so that they can refer your daughter for an abortion—*without even notifying you!* Planned Parenthood calls this "free" speech. But it isn't free. You and your family pay the price.
>
> You can send a message to the abortionists and the politicians they are trying to influence. Tell them that you don't believe abortion is an acceptable method of family planning, and you don't want tax dollars going to refer our daughters for abortion.
>
> You can make the politicians pay attention. You can tell them that parents are better able to guide their children than special interest groups. After all, *you're* paying their salaries.
>
> Write or call your Member of Congress and say that you SUPPORT President Bush's Title 10 family planning regulations.
>
> **Abortion is not Family Planning.**
> **Tell Your Member of Congress Now![25]**

A second pro-regulations advertisement pictures Carol Everett, a former abortion clinic administrator, with a caption reading, "When I ran several abortion clinics in Texas, I received referrals from a Title 10-funded clinic . . . I know what 'counseling' means: more money for the abortion industry." Bernard Nathanson, M.D., is pictured with a caption reading, "I helped found NARAL [National Association for the Repeal of Abortion Laws/National Abortion Rights Action League], now the nation's leading pro-abortion group, and I presided over 75,000 abortions . . . Now I'm pro-life and I support President Bush's Title 10 regulations." A third photograph pictures Camilla C. Hersh, M.D. Her caption reads, "As a woman and as a doctor, I support President Bush's Title 10 regulations." The headline and text of the advertisement reads:

> ***Do You Think Abortion is Just Another Method of Birth Control?***
>
> *Most Americans don't* . . . A June 1991 National Survey found that 83 percent of Americans oppose using abortion as a method of birth control. President Bush's Title 10 family planning regulations ensure that your tax dollars go to preventive family planning, and not to abortion advocacy.
>
> But Planned Parenthood and other abortion advocates *do* think abortion is just another method of birth control. They're spending $3 million to $5 million to convince Congress that your tax dollars should go to clinics that treat abortion as a method of birth control. Right now, Congress is debating legislation which would overturn President Bush's family planning regulations and fund abortion advocacy.
>
> Planned Parenthood runs the largest chain of abortion clinics, performing or referring for 200,000 abortions each year. Annually, Planned Parenthood receives more than $37 million of your tax dollars from the Title 10 family planning program. No wonder they want to keep "counseling" and "referring" for abortion with Title 10 funds.

Abortion advocates say their fight against President Bush's Title 10 regulations is about "free" speech, but it's really about money. They're demanding millions of your tax dollars to promote abortion. That's not "free" speech. And they want to keep referring teenagers for abortions *without even notifying* their parents. That's not good public policy.

Abortion advocates say this fight is about "medical ethics." We agree. The Title 10 family planning regulations are consistent with medical ethics. Medicine recognizes a distinction between abortion, which stops a beating heart, and contraception, which prevents conception. Additionally, according to Dr. James Mason, head of the U.S. Public Health Service, which oversees the program, "If a woman is found to have any medical problem, the regulation *requires* that she be assisted in receiving the complete and appropriate medical care."

They say poor women will be denied family planning services, but the Title 10 regulations will not reduce family planning funding by *one penny*. The regulations just make sure that your tax dollars go to provide contraception, not abortion counseling and referral.

You can do something to help make sure that abortion is not treated as just another method of family planning with your tax dollars. Call or write and let your Member of Congress know that you SUPPORT President Bush's Title 10 regulations.

Abortion is not Family Planning
Tell Your Member of Congress Now![26]

A third advertisement concentrates on the financial investment being made by Planned Parenthood:

When Planned Parenthood Says "FREE" Speech You Pay . . . $37,000,000

Under the guise of "*free speech*," Planned Parenthood and other abortion advocates want to take millions in taxpayer money—money intended to help low income women *prevent* unintended pregnancies—to also counsel and refer for abortion as a routine method of birth control.

This despite the fact that a national survey found that 83 percent of Americans oppose abortion as a method of birth control. Appropriately, President Bush's Title 10 family planning regulations ensure that your tax dollars go to preventive family planning and *not* to abortion advocacy.

But, right now, Congress is under intense pressure from the abortion lobby to change the Title 10 family planning program into one which would also provide abortion counseling and referrals. Planned Parenthood *alone* is spending $3 million to $5 million on a campaign to see that Congress does that.

That's because Planned Parenthood not only runs the nation's largest chain of abortion clinics, but also receives the largest share of Title 10 funds: $37 million out of the program's total $144 million budget, according to the *New York Times*. Spending $5 million to get $37 million a year in taxpayer subsidies may be a good deal for Planned Parenthood, but it is a bad deal for the rest of us.

Abortion advocates pretend to want the government *out* of the abortion debate. But when it comes to *subsidizing* abortion, they insist that the government get involved—on their side. They are working in Congress now on a bill to force taxpayers to fund their agenda that includes abortion as the equivalent of any other family planning method.

A $144 million taxpayer subsidy for programs promoting abortion as birth control—even though Americans overwhelmingly reject abortion as birth control. This is "free" speech?

Planned Parenthood's speech isn't free. You're paying for it!

Help stop the proposed federal subsidy for abortion. Let your members of Congress know that you don't want your tax dollars going to support the work of special interest groups that treat abortion as family planning.

Abortion is not Family Planning
Tell Your Member of Congress Now! [27]

A fourth advertisement pictures Camilla C. Hersh, M.D.:

"As a woman and as a doctor, I support President Bush's Title 10 regulations."

I'm a practicing obstetrician-gynecologist, and I'm a member of the American College of Obstetrics and Gynecology, the American Medical Association, and the American Fertility Society. I support family planning, and I don't consider abortion a method of family planning.

I strongly support President Bush's Title 10 regulations, which separate abortion from the nation's family planning program. They do not violate free speech rights or medical ethics.

Distinguishing between abortion, which stops a beating heart, and family planning, which prevents pregnancy, makes sense to most Americans, but abortion promoters want to continue using Title 10 funds to counsel and refer for abortions. With *our* tax dollars.

Abortion promoters say their fight against the regulations is about "free" speech, but it's really about money. They're demanding millions of our tax dollars to keep promoting abortion. That's not free speech, and it doesn't respect our rights as taxpayers.

Abortion advocates say this fight is about "medical ethics," and that the regulations won't let them help a pregnant woman whose life is threatened. In fact, the regulations *require* that women with health problems receive complete and appropriate medical care. These regulations are consistent with medical ethics.

Most Americans—like me—don't consider abortion a method of family planning.

Why should we have to fund that philosophy with our tax dollars?

You can do something to help make sure that abortion is not promoted as just another method of family planning with your tax dollars. Call or write and let your Member of Congress know that you SUPPORT President Bush's Title 10 regulations.

Abortion is not Family Planning
Tell Your Member of Congress Now! [28]

Despite the unprecedented effort, expense and cooperation of anti-abortion groups, and after months of wrangling, Congress passed a bill which would have effectively nullified the Title X regulations. President George Bush vetoed the legislation.

In one advertisement published by Planned Parenthood following the veto, the phrases "freedom of speech," "fairness to women," and "medical ethics" have the word "VETO" stamped across them. The advertisement pictures a female doctor with a gag which reads "CENSORED." The caption reads, "A pregnant woman needs her doctor's advice. Not the government's opinion."[29] The advertisement continues:

Stop George Bush's veto.
Call Congress immediately.

President Bush promises to veto legislation designed to overturn the Gag Rule and preserve a woman's right to quality medical care.

If he prevails, a woman who goes to a federally funded family planning clinic and asks an urgent question about abortion won't get a straight answer—even if pregnancy is dangerous to her health.

That's the Gag Rule in action. A shocking Bush Administration rule that censors what health professionals can say in answer to a woman's questions about safe, legal abortion.

They can't tell her abortion is one of her options. They can't tell her abortion is a private decision for a woman and her doctor.

They can't even tell her abortion is legal.

All they can say is what the President himself dictates—"abortion is not an appropriate method of family planning." This is no substitute for timely, impartial medical information.

The Gag Rule violates basic medical ethics.

It also unfairly denies poor women medical information that is available to affluent women, creating a system of separate and unequal birth control services.

Millions of women depend on publicly funded clinics for their health care. You can make sure they continue to get the answers they need.

The same answers you expect from your doctor.

Congress has one last chance to protect women's access to medical care.

It must vote to override the President's veto.

The veto can be overridden by a two-thirds vote in both the House and Senate.

Call your elected representatives in Washington immediately at 1-202-224-3121 and tell them the Gag Rule must be overturned before it's too late.

> Time is running out. Please, make sure that women have the last word on abortion. Not the man in the White House.
>
> ***Override the Gag Rule veto. Call 1-202-224-3121.***[30]

Donations are requested for the Planned Parenthood Action Fund.[31]

Narrowly failing to override the President's veto, the Department of Health and Human Services prepared to enforce the regulations. Planned Parenthood officials were left with a choice: adhere to the rules, lose federal dollars, or find a way around the regulations (a loophole) while simultaneously working in Congress in another attempt to nullify the rules.

Rebecca Bumsted, board president of Planned Parenthood of Lancaster County (Pennsylvania), said, "In June [1991], we made a decision to remain true to our mission of providing complete medical and ethical care for our patients." However, Bumsted also said that Planned Parenthood would "deny no one service because of their inability to pay."[32] This was said despite Planned Parenthood's claim throughout the Title X fight that millions of poor, vulnerable women would go unserved. How could this be?

According to Nancy Osgood, director of Planned Parenthood of Lancaster County, the group is asking donors to increase the size of their gifts either by doubling them or by giving on a monthly basis. It has also been seeking new donors through monthly phone-a-thons. Moreover, as a direct result of the Title X regulations, Planned Parenthood of Lancaster County received a $15,000 challenge grant which is contingent on the agency raising an equal amount in new donations or increases.[33]

Planned Parenthood clinics across the country have instituted similar programs to restore funding. As one article on the issue stated:

> Planned Parenthood clinic directors from New York to New Mexico say they will reject money rather than accept it and comply with a ban on abortion counseling at federally funded family planning clinics.
>
> The result: 4 million poor women could be denied medical services ranging from AIDS-virus testing to cancer detection because clinics—heavily dependent on federal money—will have to cut back all services.[34]

Despite such doomsday statements, mass closings and turning away of customers has simply not materialized.

USA Today reports that hundreds of family planning clinics "have figured out ways to skirt the law that prevents them from counseling" women on abortion:

> A family planning clinic counselor just "hands the (pregnant) client off to another worker in the office who is not funded by Title X.
>
> How can that happen? [Brad] Hughes [of Kentucky's health department] says it's a matter of how the Title X regulations are interpreted. And according to Kentucky's interpretation, handing off patients is perfectly fine.[35]

The newspaper reports that "some clinics in some parts of South Dakota, Texas, Kentucky and Nevada—all places where Title X regulations were not blocked by lower court rulings—have found them relatively easy to circumvent." For example, in Kentucky, Hughes says the state does not inspect clinics to see if they are adhering to the ban. Clinic directors need only sign a statement stating they will comply with the Title X regulations. The same is true in other states.[36]

Jim Guest, president of Planned Parenthood of Maryland, said, "We'll just keep doing what we've been doing until the feds knock on our door and tell us to stop. . . ." He also called the regulations "hypocritical" because when Planned Parenthood affiliates give up the Title X money, it will "prevent women from getting the birth control they need, which will lead to more unwanted pregnancies and more abortions.[37] Abortion foes point to such statements to prove that Planned Parenthood is more interested in protecting its abortion business than in delivering real health care to women.

In March 1992, in an apparent attempt to clarify the rules, President Bush announced that doctors may discuss abortion with women, but counselors and nurses may not. Since more than 95 percent of such counseling is not done by doctors, the change will have a negligible effect, but it is unclear how the clarification is justified under the intent of the legislation which created Title X. However, they do reflect political and effectual reality.

Hearing of the clarification Faye Wattleton criticized the President for trying to make it appear as though he had softened his position. "Mr. Bush has tried to distort and obfuscate the entire debate about the gag rule," Wattleton said. "America entered a dangerous era with the release of President Bush's guidelines for the enforcement of his draconian 'gag rule,'" she alleges. "The guidelines affirm the president's intent to gag all medical professionals at federally funded family clinics, preventing them from fully informing poor women about all of their reproductive options." Wattleton was referring to the White House and congressional supporters of the regulations when she said, "Those who have sentenced women to the back alley, by playing politics with our lives, will be held accountable."[38] Planned Parenthood advertisements virtually always emphasize and picture "gagged" medical professionals, primarily doctors, but the fact is that almost all abortion counseling is done by non-medical personnel who are trained almost exclusively by Planned Parenthood.

The intensity of the battle over the Title X regulations proved to be a vast learning experience for many anti-abortion leaders. In an effort to shape public opinion, some abortion foes are saying it is time to reach a new level in communication. Learning from Planned Parenthood, while maintaining honesty and integrity, groups opposed to abortion decided to take on Planned Parenthood on its own, heretofore largely exclusive, turf.

When the battle over the Title X regulations began to increase in its intensity, the reality of the situation became clear. Led by abortion foes such as Greg Erkin of the Knights of Columbus, Marjorie Dannenfelser, executive director of the House Pro-Life Caucus, and John Walker of the Family Research Council, anti-abortion groups are now playing hard-ball. These leaders have realized they, too, must play the media game.

"Any battle based on the facts, we will win," explains Walker, "but right now the battle isn't geared toward facts, it's geared toward political rhetoric. Whoever wins the rhetorical battle will win the abortion war." Walker is not happy about the way things are, but he understands reality. "The vast majority of the public doesn't want to take the time to find out the facts and their position on the issue is based on a 15-second sound-bite and a catchy slogan." Walker cites "gag rule" as a prime example of such a slogan.[39]

It seems Walker, Dannenfelser, and Erkin are on the right path. Not only have anti-abortion groups carefully chosen their rhetoric in more recent legislative battles, they have also developed their own sound-bites and catchy slogans. The phrase repeated in the Title X battle was "abortion is not family planning." In the battle to prevent unborn human beings who are intentionally aborted from being used for experimentation, the phrase "fetal experimentation" has been abandoned and replaced with "baby harvesting."

The Title X regulations confrontation surprised Planned Parenthood when a coalition of anti-abortion organization joined to form "The Abortion Is Not Family Planning Coalition." While Planned Parenthood had threatened to spend nearly $5 million in defense of its position—a sum supporters of the regulations could not hope to come even close to, much less match—the Coalition placed several advertisements in influential newspapers. Christian radio stations were also urged to spread the Coalition's message. As previously noted, in the end, legislation to overturn the Title X regulations was passed, but abortion foes were successful in sustaining President Bush's veto. Walker notes that he and his colleagues continue to learn more about the way to approach these issues.[40]

Robert J. Conrad, Jr., a Charlotte, North Carolina, attorney and member of the 1987 Mecklenburg County (North Carolina) Adolescent Health Task Force, argues in a guest editorial that programs like those funded by Title X are part of the problem, not part of the solution. Conrad writes that "statistical research showed that teenage family planning program participation was associated with higher rates of both pregnancy and abortion." He argues that Planned Parenthood is simply a duplication of already available services that are "better and without the ideological baggage."[41]

UNITED WAY

In some areas, Planned Parenthood receives funding from the United Way. All United Way giving to Planned Parenthood is determined at the local level. Contrary to common belief, there is not a national United Way organization which supports charitable groups.

Most United Way organizations use a system called "negative designation" or "donor choice." Under negative designation, persons donating to United Way may list organizations the donor does not want to receive any part of his or her money. The problem with this system is that agencies receiving United Way funds are usually budgeted a specific amount of money. If many people say they do not want Planned Parenthood to receive funds, bookkeeping records could show that twice as many dollars are taken from a donor who did not use the negative designation. Planned Parenthood ends up with the budgeted amount regardless of how many people say they do not want *their* money going to the organization.

The *Chronicle of Philanthropy* confirms that, in most cases, donors are allowed to specify certain charities which should not receive their funds. However, the practice is somewhat controversial within the United Way organization.[42]

Under donor choice, Planned Parenthood receives only the amount of funds designated by the givers. This is not great, but it is much better than traditional systems. The *Chronicle* reports that the organization most often designated by givers for not receiving funds is Planned Parenthood. A full 64 percent of dollars donated with a negative designation list Planned Parenthood. The second most frequent negative designation is listed by a mere 6.1 percent of donors.[43]

Another system being implemented to appease abortion foes is forcing Planned Parenthood to operate its abortion facility with a separate checking account, books, and advisory board (not board of directors). This is merely a matter of bookkeeping and other paperwork. Under the plan, Planned Parenthood receives funds from United Way as it has always done.

Those in the media who support Planned Parenthood are hailing the system as an acceptable "compromise," but it does nothing but create more paperwork. Note the editorial printed by one newspaper which strongly supports Planned Parenthood. The *Democrat and Chronicle* argues that, until the "compromise" was reached, United Way of Greater Rochester (New York) had "been caught between a rock and two hard places." The two hard places are the supporters of Planned Parenthood who said they would stop supporting United Way if Planned Parenthood did not get its way and opponents who said they would stop supporting United Way if Planned Parenthood continued to be part of the agency.[44] What was the rock?

> The rock was last year's decision by Planned Parenthood to set up an abortion clinic for poor women.
>
> Such a clinic is vital: Each month, 60 or 70 women are told they can't get a Medicaid abortion in Rochester.
>
> Since no local hospital has been willing to take over the problem, Planned Parenthood has had no choice but to solve it, or betray its obligation to serve those most in need of help.[45]

According to the newspaper, everybody is a winner. "Planned Parenthood has met its obligation to serve poor women. United Way has met its obligation to serve the community," the editorial states. "Both understood that compromise is not a dirty word. It need not mean compromising one's principles."[46] This is true for Planned Parenthood. It gets to do what it wants and still collect its United Way funds. There seems to be no one to stand in its way (see chapter 16).

PLEDGE-A-PICKET

One of Planned Parenthood's most innovative methods to earn revenue is through the Pledge-A-Picket program. The program has two purposes: raise money for Planned Parenthood and discourage picketing of its facilities.

Pledge-A-Picket involves asking supporters to pledge money for each protester at the Planned Parenthood facility. Planned Parenthood officials believe they win either way. They will have more money and for fewer picketers. While Planned Parenthood may win either way, it is important to remember that such a win is on a limited and generally unimportant scale. The debate over abortion will surely not be decided by such a program.

A September 6, 1988, letter from the executive director of Planned Parenthood of Central and Northern Arizona explains the Pledge-A-Picket program in detail:

Dear Friend,

For many years now we have endured anti-choice pickets at our Planned Parenthood sites. Picketers have harassed clients, insulted staff and attempted to interrupt our ability to provide family planning services to Arizona families. Here's an example of the kind of incident that frequently occurs:

- Not wanting to be rude, the young couple walking toward the Planned Parenthood clinic took what the picketer so insistently shoved at them. To their horror, they were being handed grisly photos of dismembered stillborn fetuses.
- "Don't kill your baby!" the picketer shrieked as the couple tried to cross the parking lot. The picketer followed, shouting, "It's murder! God will punish you!" Unable to bear the abuse any longer, the young mother of two stopped and turned, "Leave me alone!," she cried desperately. "I can't take care of another baby!" she sobbed.
- A Planned Parenthood staff person rushed to help her and her companion into the waiting room. Relieved to find herself in caring hands at last, the young woman trembled and wept quietly as she waited to see the doctor. An already troubling time was made immeasurably worse by the harassment she'd experienced outside.

For years we have restrained ourselves in responding to picketers. We have not wanted to lower ourselves to their level. When their tactics broke the law, we filed suit. But otherwise, we have ignored them.

Well, it's time for us to stop being passive. We don't intend to break the law or to limit their right of self-expression under the Constitution. *But we do intend to fight back.* PLEASE JOIN US. It's easy and convenient.

We invite you to become part of the Planned Parenthood Picket Pay Back Plan. This plan allows you to pledge a certain amount of money to Planned Parenthood for each picketer who appears at our centers, or to make a one-time contribution.

Your donation gives us a way to respond to the picketers, while continuing to provide vital services to women and their families.

OUR PLAN: We will give a "thank you" card to every picketer everytime they show up at a Valley Planned Parenthood clinic. (I have included an example of the card.)

We believe this strategy will seriously deflate the picketers' self-righteous egos—and may even lessen the number of picketers who consistently harass our clients.

But this plan won't work without you!

What can you do?

Indicate on the enclosed pledge card the amount you will contribute to Planned Parenthood for each picketer each day, beginning October 1, 1988 and ending September 30, 1989, or make a one-time donation. Sign the card and mail it to us today.

Your active participation in the Picket Pay Back Plan will help raise needed funds for the continuation of family planning services and will discourage picketers from continuing to harass our staff and clients.

Yes, you can set an upward limit on the amount you would like to contribute. Remember, every dollar you pledge helps us serve more women who depend on us for family planning services.

What will we do?

Every time picketers show up at a Planned Parenthood facility, we will personally hand them a "Planned Parenthood Pay Back Thank You" card.

We also will post our "Picket Pay Back Thank You" poster close to the picketers so everyone can see how their presence is promoting family planning in Arizona.

Please return your pledge card as soon as possible. I'll be pleased to report to you—and to the picketers—how much money we raised because of picketing activity.

It will be wonderful to turn the unpleasantness of the picketers' harassment into something as positive as increased funds for our vital work—which, by the way, is the only thing that will reduce the need for abortion. Thank you for your continued support.

Sincerely,

Gloria Feldt
Executive Director

P.S. The picture on our envelope, showing the "Clowns for Life" picketing we endured in July is an example of the kinds of harassment we experience. Please be generous in contributing to this exciting chance to turn incidents like this into reasons to celebrate.

The Planned Parenthood
Picket Pay Back Plan
Thank You Card

Thank you for being here today. Your presence assists Planned Parenthood in raising funds to carry out our programs. With your help, we can raise the funds necessary to promote family planning and expand all of our programs and services.

Not only do we agree with your right to demonstrate, we applaud it. Because, with your help and hard work, we will raise more than $30,000 this year on our Planned Parenthood Picket Pay Back Plan. This money can be used to:

- Pay for abortions for needy women.
- Pay for birth control for men and women who cannot afford it.
- Pay for Planned Parenthood's community education programs.

Once again, thank you for your continued presence and support.[47]

Pledge-A-Picket has been successful in raising limited dollars for Planned Parenthood, but it seems to have little effect on picketing. The general attitude of Planned Parenthood critics seems to be that the organization will not be successful at limiting picketing, regardless of any programs that are implemented.

MARKETING CONDOMS

The Planned Parenthood Federation of America entered the contraceptive market with its own brand of condoms, which were to be distributed through its affiliates. While there were no immediate plans to sell Planned Parenthood brand condoms in drug stores to compete with other brands, the idea was not ruled out.

The revenue raised from the sale of Planned Parenthood brand condoms was expected to "help meet the family planning needs of those who cannot afford private care" and would "be put toward education programs . . ." It has been estimated that the sale of Planned Parenthood brand condoms would raise more than $50,000 in the first year alone. Moreover, if the condom sales proved profitable, one could have expected to see Planned Parenthood begin to market other contraceptive devices.[48]

Planned Parenthood did market its own condoms, but decided to discontinue sales because of problems in getting its affiliates to push them. It is possible Planned Parenthood will resume the sale of its condoms, but it will be done under another brand name.

FINANCIAL ACCOUNTABILITY

Planned Parenthood claims to be a public charity. However, a study of records at one Planned Parenthood affiliate show that 90-95 percent of all non-Medicaid clients who receive government assistance to visit a Planned Parenthood clinic are not needy and are able to pay for their visit. In other words, all families are being taxed to pay for Planned Parenthood services—even for its wealthy clients.[49]

While government family planning programs are largely intended to provide services to the poor, it is not required that the clients be poor. In 1973, Planned Parenthood records show that 17 percent of the clients were welfare recipients. In 1983, only 13 percent were on welfare and 32 percent of this 13 percent figure was for clients under 20 years of age.[50]

The most shocking information to come to light is that Planned Parenthood has been accused of milking the taxpayers whenever the government pays for a service. For example, when a client pays cash for a pregnancy test, the average cost is $16.36. When the government is billed, the average cost for the same pregnancy test is $57.93. This is even more amazing when one considers that the average pregnancy test costs less than $3.00.[51]

Congressman Jon Kyl, R-Arizona, informed the inspector general of the Department of Health and Human Services of the abuses alleged against Planned Parenthood. An assistant to Kyl reports that a subsequent investigation concentrated on Planned Parenthood clinics in New York and New Jersey.

The investigation apparently caused some people to get nervous. Planned Parenthood officials in New York and New Jersey reportedly asked their counterpart in Arizona to complain to Kyl about the "harassment." Kyl refused to ask that the investigation be halted because it is his duty to report allegations of fraud regardless of the source.[52]

The ensuing investigation was done in an interesting manner. "We performed work in the State of New Jersey to determine if the problem did indeed exist and if additional work, such as a nationwide audit was warranted," writes Inspector General Richard P. Kusserow. "We found no evidence to substantiate the allegation that Planned Parenthood overcharges patients on Government aid. . . . Patients paying cash and those receiving Government aid were treated equally and charged according to a fee schedule based on income levels. . . . Clinics billed Medicaid directly and at the prevailing rate, in accordance with Government regulations."

Kusserow reports that it was determined that no rules or regulations were being violated "in the State." Therefore, in the opinion of the Inspector General's office, "grantees were in compliance in carrying out their responsibilities under grants for family planning services. Regulations and requirements established by grantees for subgrants were also being followed by delegate agencies. Therefore, we determined a nationwide audit was not necessary."[53]

The report which accompanied the Kusserow letter gives additional detail regarding the investigation:

> The author alleges that Planned Parenthood organizations routinely overcharge the Government for family planning services provided to Medical Title X and Title XX beneficiaries. . . .
>
> Our review found no instances of overcharges by Planned Parenthood to Government agencies. The Federal Government is not directly charged for client services. Under Federal grant programs, awards are made to grantees who in turn make subawards to such organizations as Planned Parenthood to subsidize the costs of providing services to all clients. Customers are charged according to fee scales based on income levels. Federal and State regulations require that third-party payers like Medicaid pay at the top of the sliding-fee scales or at the prevailing reimbursement rate. The Planned Parenthood organizations were properly charging all clients in accordance with these fee scales.
>
> We also concluded that Department rules or regulations with respect to Federal funding of family planning services were generally being followed. Grantees were carrying out re-

> sponsibilities under grants for family planning services, and, as far as we were able to determine, regulations and requirements established by grantees for subgrants were also being followed by delegate agencies. . . .
>
> We selected this site for our field work because the Office of Inspector General already had ongoing related audit work in the area. . . .
>
> Our review disclosed no instance of improper charges to individuals on Government assistance by Planned Parenthood organizations.[54]

Some basic questions come to mind: Why was the "investigation" conducted in a state not alleged to be the site of the problem? Would the time laps between the writing of the book in which the allegations were made allow Planned Parenthood to alter or even hide its activities? Why were the documents obtained for the original allegation never checked? Planned Parenthood surely knew an investigation was taking place for other reasons in New Jersey. Would Planned Parenthood make an effort to make sure everything was in order in that state?

10

PUBLIC POLICY ADVOCACY

Planned Parenthood's stated mission includes bringing about "the virtual elimination of unwanted pregnancy in the United States" and acting as "the nation's foremost agent of social change in the area of reproductive health and well-being."[1] These goals seem to have become the most important of all to Planned Parenthood leaders.

USA Today reports that Planned Parenthood would choose to give up a $20 million federal grant rather than stop advocating abortion. The Agency for International Development, which allocates the funds, does not give grants to groups that encourage abortion. However, Planned Parenthood did not give up without a fight. The newspaper reports that, "Planned Parenthood launched a media blitz—part of a $1.5 million campaign being waged in courtrooms and Congress—against the policy."[2]

Planned Parenthood has been active in public policy through school boards, the courts, state/provincial legislatures, city and county councils, Congress/Parliament, and other areas for many years. In a 1975 article, Planned Parenthood officials summarize one school of thought with regard to the group's political advocacy. "If we are idealists in a cause," the position holds, "how can we enter the political arena of compromise."[3]

STATE/PROVINCIAL AND LOCAL POLICY

Planned Parenthood's dollars have been a key factor in shaping public policy. It has even targeted local school boards for public policy advocacy. Consider the words of Planned Parenthood's Andrea Wemette:

> There are many school board members and we need to examine where they are coming from. Many are Planned Parenthood supporters. If that's the case, then we can slip a lot past the boards without real approval.[4]

An example of Planned Parenthood's attempt to influence state lawmakers is not hard to find. In a January 1981 Planned Parenthood letter sent to members of Congress and state legislators nationwide, it was announced that the Planned Parenthood Federation of America would launch a $3.7 million "massive legislative and public education program to preserve individual freedom and civil rights in America." Two main priorities were announced for the year: "Continuation and expansion of Title X [taxpayer] funding . . . and defeat of attempts to pass a constitutional amendment that would severely limit every woman's right to choose to have an abortion."[5]

Several local full-page advertisements were printed in national publications around the time of the 1984 elections. Many urge readers to contact candidates and elected officials to express support for legal abortion. The issue of teen pregnancy is raised in one advertisement. It is suggested that putting sex education in schools and giving information on birth control and abortion would solve the problem. The advertisement slogan is "Planned Parenthood: For the Love of Children."[6]

Another affiliate advertisement tells readers that, "A happy baby is the best argument for birth control," because unintended pregnancies "too often" end up in "neglect and abuse for children." It continues, "That's why Planned Parenthood believes every child should be a wanted child." Again, readers are urged to contact candidates and elected officials.[7]

The Planned Parenthood Federation of Canada has intensified its efforts to become active on the national, provincial, and local levels. However, such activism is far behind that experienced in the United States. A local and provincial approach is being emphasized.

FUND-RAISING AND FEDERAL POLICY

The chief goal of Planned Parenthood is made clear in a fund-raising letter signed by Katharine Hepburn. She writes that "reproductive freedom is a basic, personal issue . . ." Hepburn continues:

> My mother . . . knew even then [over 50 years ago] that no woman . . . can ever truly be free without the right to personal control over her own reproductive life. . . .
>
> [L]egislation now pending before Congress would completely destroy all of her tireless work. . . .
>
> Thanks to your generous support and involvement, Planned Parenthood's Public Impact program has begun to mobilize public outrage against the HLA [Human Life Amendment]. Americans are frightened by this attempt to legislate "when life begins." The chances of the HLA passing Congress are now fading.[8]

Hepburn writes that Planned Parenthood is the "most respected family planning service and advocacy organization in the country . . . "[9]

In another letter signed by Hepburn, readers are warned about the Human Life Statute and the Human Life Amendment. She writes that if either of these pieces of legislation were to pass, "you and I will lose one of our most fundamental individual rights. There is only *one* way to stop this from happening. The American people must be shown *quickly* that the threat is real, that tragedy will follow for millions of innocent women, men, and children, and that our Constitution was not intended to be used by the Moral Majority or any other group to foist its particular religious beliefs on the rest of us."[10]

Faye Wattleton, former president of the Planned Parenthood Federation of America, states in a fund-raising letter that Planned Parenthood is resolved to "STOP the insane headlong rush toward a Constitutional Convention by *awakening all Americans to the real threat it poses to us all.* We must create a groundswell of grassroots opposition that will silence the rantings of the anti-choice minority and the right-wing fanatics." It also refers to a "firm resolve" to "*STOP* the return of the 'dark ages' of back-room and self-induced abortions, by establishing an emergency loan program which will help finance safe, professional abortions for women in financial need who have been ruthlessly denied federal and state funds."[11]

A publication of the Alan Guttmacher Institute deals with the issue of public funding of abortions. "A holding by the Court that restrictions on medically necessary abortions are constitutional would be a crushing blow to poor women seeking access to publicly funded abortions," the article reads. "A ruling that these restrictions are unconstitutional would be a major victory for poor women and the pro-choice movement."[12]

Planned Parenthood even urges its customers to lobby for its legislative goals. Some have raised objections to this practice, saying it interferes with the right to privacy.[13]

A Wattleton fund-raising letter attacking the Title X (pronounced "title 10") regulations urges readers to take action to stop the regulations. It was sent shortly after the Reagan Administration issued the rules. There are two actions requested:

> *ACTION STEP #1 Please sign the enclosed Petitions to your Senators and Representatives.* Let them know that you wholeheartedly support family planning and want them to take appropriate action to block President Reagan's regulations affecting Title X.
>
> *ACTION STEP #2 Please help Planned Parenthood meet the extraordinary costs of our PUBLIC IMPACT CAMPAIGN by making as generous a contribution as you possibly can.*[14]

An almost identical fund-raising letter was sent to Planned Parenthood supporters following the election of President George Bush:

> *ACTION STEP #1* Please sign the enclosed petition to President Bush. Let him know that you wholeheartedly support family planning and want him to take appropriate and enlightened action to remove the restrictive regulations.
>
> *ACTION STEP #2* Please help Planned Parenthood meet the extraordinary costs of our PUBLIC IMPACT CAMPAIGN aimed at bringing pressure on both the new administration and Congress by making as generous a contribution as you possibly can today.[15]

A full-page advertisement that appeared in the *New York Times* is likely to have a strong impact on public policy. Headlined, "Some Women Are Silent on the Horrors of Illegal Abortion. The Rest of Us Can't Be," the advertisement pictures a graveyard:

> Some women are silent on the horrors of abortion.
>
> The rest of us can't be.
>
> Not now. Not when every woman's right to choose a legal and safe abortion is threatened.
>
> Yesterday, the Justices of the Supreme Court heard government attorneys argue that states should have the power to interfere in a woman's most personal and private decisions.
>
> Tomorrow, no matter what the Court decides, we all could be faced with a decision on the so-called Human Life Amendment to the U.S. Constitution. It would give an embryo legal status from the instant of fertilization. And would make any abortion, by definition, murder.
>
> Today, we are forced to remember what happens when abortion is criminalized.
>
> Women die.
>
> By the thousands, they are maimed and killed.
>
> It was true in America before 1973.
>
> In nations where abortion is still illegal, unsafe and clandestine procedures are among the leading causes of death for women of childbearing age (the global death toll is over 200,000 a year).

Those who ignore this horror, or choose to forget it, pretend that outlawing abortion will stop it.

The [Bush] administration argued in the Supreme Court to take away your right to decide for yourself. The President himself calls for the Human Life Amendment. But Bush's administration has taken no leadership on reducing the need for abortion by supporting increased funds for family planning, sex education and research into new birth control.

His administration must be held responsible for the growing threat to women's lives.

Some women are silent on the horrors of illegal abortion. But those of us who survive them can't be silent. We must speak out. We must act.

Mail the coupons below. Thank you.[16]

Planned Parenthood urges readers of the advertisement to send a coupon (part of the advertisement) to President George Bush. Like the rest of the advertisement, the coupon demonstrates a public policy agenda:

Dear Mr. President:

Your support for the so-called "pro-life" campaign is a dangerous betrayal of basic American values: freedom of conscience, respect for privacy, tolerance of differences. You have no mandate to upset the national consensus on abortion rights. If you want to stop abortion, help people prevent an unwanted pregnancy.[17]

Richard Thornburgh, who at the time of the advertisement was attorney general of the United States, was to receive a coupon (also part of the advertisement) as well:

Dear Mr. Thornburgh:

Your experience as Governor of Pennsylvania showed you that the so-called "pro-lifers" are insatiable in their demands. I strongly urge you to combat their campaign of violence and intimidation . . . and uphold the Constitutionally-protected right of women to decide for themselves.[18]

As is often the case, a third coupon is included. It reads, in part, "I believe the abortion decision is a personal and private question for a woman and her doctor. Blockades, bombings and other threats to safety and health of women are outrageous." The coupon concludes by requesting a tax-deductible contribution. The name of the advertisement series is, "Don't wait until women are dying again."[19]

Planned Parenthood uniformly makes use of cliché, inflammatory, and unsubstantiated rhetoric. Nevertheless, the use of such language has done much to make Planned Parenthood one of the most successful organizations in the world with regard to raising funds and impacting public policy. Abortion foes have yet to learn that, with regard to influencing public policy, they need to work more on sound bites, rhetoric, and image than on facts and figures. So far, anti-abortion groups have concentrated more on details while Planned Parenthood has emphasized image. Which group has won the most battles?

In March 1991, Planned Parenthood placed a full-page advertisement in the *New York Times*. Headlined, "For Millions of Women, the 20th Century Began on a Quiet Brooklyn Street in 1916," the advertisement features a photograph from early in the century of women with baby carriages:

THE FREEDOM TO CHOOSE whether and when to have children makes our other life choices possible.

Yet until 1916, when the first family planning clinic in the U.S. opened its doors on a quiet street in Brooklyn, that freedom was out of reach to all but a few.

In the three generations since, Planned Parenthood has worked long and hard to bring the benefits of freedom to people world-wide, regardless of their circumstances.

> Today, thanks to the understanding and support of contributors across the country, our 26,000 staff members and volunteers serve 4 million Americans in 49 states and the District of Columbia. Women and men in 22 other nations receive voluntary family planning aid through our international division.
>
> We are proud to have pioneered new ways to make safe, responsible choices available to the young, the low-income, the disenfranchised—those who are so often denied the options the rest of us enjoy.
>
> For many, Planned Parenthood is their primary source of medical care.
>
> From birth control to cancer screening, treatment of sexually transmitted diseases, abortion services, infertility counseling, and prenatal care, our 171 affiliates offer a comprehensive range of reproductive health options.
>
> Yet none of us is free to take freedom for granted.
>
> Through education, public advocacy, and legal action, Planned Parenthood continues to enhance and safeguard the private choices basic to women's health and equality.
>
> We have made three-quarters of a century of progress in the face of constant, increasingly violent challenges. But the quiet revolution is still not over.
>
> We invite you to celebrate Planned Parenthood's 75-year tradition of choice.
>
> We also ask you to defend it.[20]

The advertisement includes the Planned Parenthood slogan, "A Tradition of Choice for 75 Years," and a coupon soliciting contributions.[21]

JUDGING THE JUDGES

Since the inauguration of President Ronald Reagan in January 1981, Planned Parenthood has expressed concern about nominations made to fill vacancies on federal courts. While the Reagan Administration claimed it did not have a litmus test for court nominees, virtually all were advocates of "judicial restraint." According to the Reagan Administration, and many legal scholars, the judicial branch has abused its authority by inventing laws, not interpreting them. It is this practice that led to the *Roe v. Wade* decision.

Planned Parenthood said little about Reagan's nomination of Antonin Scalia and Sandra Day O'Connor to the United States Supreme Court. However, his third nominee became the victim of one of the biggest injustices ever foisted upon the system of checks and balances. Robert Bork is a constitutional scholar of unequaled caliber. He has written extensively on many issues. As a strong advocate of judicial restraint, Planned Parenthood became convinced that Bork would provide the deciding vote in overturning *Roe v. Wade*.

Planned Parenthood could no longer get by with verbal attacks on nominees to the nation's highest court. The organization teamed up with many of the most liberal interest groups to mount an unprecedented campaign against Bork. Planned Parenthood led the fight.

In one newspaper advertisement, Planned Parenthood paints the nominee as a right-wing extremist and judicial ideologue:

> If your senators vote to confirm the Administration's latest Supreme Court nominee, you'll need more than a prescription to get birth control. It might take a constitutional amendment. Robert Bork is an extremist who believes you have no constitutional right to personal privacy. He thinks the government is free to dictate what you can and can't do in highly personal and intimate matters such as marriage, childbearing, parenting. If he wins a lifetime seat on the Supreme Court, Bork could radically change the way Americans live.[22]

The scathing advertisement points to the fact that four members of the Court support the "moderate and balanced consensus protecting Constitutional rights and liberties" and the other four members "generally vote against expansion of our basic freedoms." Robert Bork, according to Planned Parenthood and its cohorts, would "throw the Court out of balance" and would lead to "state-controlled pregnancy." Such state control could include a ban on birth control, the imposition of "family quotas for population purposes," outlaw abortion, and even force men and women to be sterilized.[23] One man, Robert Bork, could make this happen?

The United States Senate narrowly rejected the nomination of Judge Bork, whose scholarly writings, in which he took a stand (even if they were well-reasoned), proved to be a key factor in making a case against him. Anthony Kennedy was later confirmed to fill the vacancy. While Planned Parenthood opposed the Kennedy nomination, it had already fired its big gun and confirmation came easy.

Cases brought before the Supreme Court of concern to Planned Parenthood show that the organization will fare about as badly with Kennedy as it would have with Bork, except that Bork would likely have voted to overturn *Roe v. Wade.* The decision in *Planned Parenthood v. Casey* shows this is not the case with Kenedy who, along with O,Conner and David Souter, voted to reafirm *Roe*.. Nevertheless, in attacking Bork, Planned Parenthood and its allies in the Senate managed to harm a man's reputation, make a mockery of justice and the process, flex its political muscle (which made cowards of many United States Senators), and make headlines.

Subsequent nominees to the Supreme Court, made by President George Bush, have also been opposed by Planned Parenthood. The nomination of David Souter was confirmed with little opposition, due largely to the nominees relative obscurity. Souter was nominated, in fact, because of his obscurity. The Bork Affair taught those involved in the nomination process a great lesson: appoint someone who has done little writing. Therefore, those who write scholarly works, regardless of how brilliant they may be, can expect to stay off the United States Supreme Court. Those who write little or nothing, be it because of an inability or unwillingness to do so, may serve on the High Court.

Planned Parenthood revived its attack campaign with the nomination of Clarence Thomas. However, as an African-American, the target was not easy to hit. Even after Thomas was accused of sexually harassing a former employee, Planned Parenthood's attacks failed to produce the essential alliance of anti-Thomas groups. The nominee was narrowly confirmed, but his reputation had been damaged. Senator Dennis DeConcini, D-Arizona, played a pivotal role in Thomas' confirmation.

Anita Hill, who made the accusations, is a strong supporter of Planned Parenthood. Jesse Jackson, speaking of Hill at the April 5, 1992, Washington, D.C., rally in support of legal abortion, compared her to Jesus Christ. Both were crucified on a hill Jackson said, and Hill, too, will be resurrected.[24]

CANADA

So far, Planned Parenthood facilities in Canada do not perform abortions. When James Dobson, Ph.D., did a radio program highlighting Planned Parenthood, the

Canadian division of the International Planned Parenthood Federation called to complain, saying it resented being linked to the abortion industry.

Dobson's organization, Focus on the Family, one of the most influential and reputable Christian-based groups in the country, investigated. It discovered that while the Planned Parenthood Federation of Canada does not own and operate abortion facilities, it has been active in abortion. Dobson reports the results of the investigation in an October 1989 broadcast. "Planned Parenthood in Canada has been on record as advocating that abortion be removed from the Criminal Code. In other words, allowing unlimited access to abortion," Dobson states. "They agitated for that very early."[25]

Dobson discusses a 1977 survey which shows that the Planned Parenthood Federation of Canada is the largest abortion referral agency in the country. Furthermore, in 1986, Planned Parenthood in Ontario asked the provincial government to allow free-standing clinics to perform abortions, rather than requiring that hospitals do the procedure. In 1988, the same Planned Parenthood affiliate co-sponsored an abortion facility application. Dobson summarizes the Planned Parenthood Federation of Canada's activism by saying, "I think it's pretty clear. Planned Parenthood actively refers and lobbies for abortion in Canada and . . . they're not far away from being in the business themselves."[26]

Canada has essentially had abortion-on-demand since 1969. The Parliament has been unwilling to impose any meaningful restrictions on abortion since the Supreme Court of Canada struck down the weak abortion laws which did exist in 1988.

The Planned Parenthood Federation of America presents a Margaret Sanger Award, as do most of its affiliates, once per year. The 1989 recipient was Henry Morgentaler, M.D., "whose leadership and courage in challenging Canada's repressive laws on abortion have inspired millions of reproductive rights advocates worldwide."[27] Morgentaler largely ignored and flaunted Canada's abortion law when it did exist.

With the election of the New Democrats in some Canadian provinces, Canada's anti-abortion movement has a lot to do. The governments pay for abortions and are willing to go to great lengths to allow them without restrictions. In Ontario, the government pays all expenses including transportation and lodging. The party seems to be attempting to put American supporters of legal abortion to shame in that their neighbors to the south are not rabid enough.

The increasingly open and aggressive approach of the Planned Parenthood Federation of Canada is found in an advertisement it joined in placing in a Canadian newspaper:

> ***His Choice or Hers?***
> ***We think the choice is hers. And we know that most of you agree with us.***
>
> In recent months, Canadians—both men and women—have been shocked to see young women dragged through the courts by disgruntled ex-boyfriends seeking to prevent abortion.
>
> The privacy of women has been grossly violated. Women's most intimate acts, thoughts and decisions have been exposed to everyone.
>
> This demeaning carnival of publicity is a somber warning of what a minority in Canada intends to inflict on all of us.
>
> The next woman singled out for humiliation—and for a medically dangerous delay—could be your sister, your daughter, your friend . . . or you.

> ***Our freedom of choice is in danger.***
>
> The Canadian government is now considering whether to put abortion back in the Criminal Code. We don't need a new criminal law. Pregnant women are not criminals. Their intimate decisions are not a matter for the public courts.
>
> The Supreme Court of Canada has spoken. Last year, Canada's highest court ruled that each woman controls her own child-bearing. Any rule requiring her to seek the consent of any party (aside from her doctor) is a violation of her constitutional right to personal security, liberty and freedom of conscience.
>
> And, in fact, the Court did *not* invite the government to make a new law. We don't need one because 99.6 percent of all abortions in Canada are performed before the end of the 20th week of pregnancy.
>
> ***What do we need?***
>
> We need a truly adult and responsible approach to reproductive health care. The government should act decisively to provide:
>
> - access to women's health care (including abortion) across the country
> - more family planning counselling
> - more education
> - more birth control centres—prevention is better than abortion
>
> ***Help us mount an effective, grassroots lobby across Canada.***
>
> We need your generous contributions to work toward safeguarding choice. And we urgently ask you to write or call your Member of Parliament. We must act swiftly, before Parliament tries to strip away our rights to reproductive dignity, health and freedom.[28]

The Planned Parenthood Federation of Canada joined with 17 other Canadian organizations, including the Canadian Abortion Rights Action League, the Humanist Association of Canada, and the Canadian Labour Congress, in placing the advertisement.[29]

The Planned Parenthood Association of British Columbia published a June 1989 newsletter which attacks anti-abortion civil disobedience. It asserts that, "The goal may be admirable, the method is not. It carries ugly connotations of mob rule, and takes a short-term, limited approach to what is clearly a long-term problem."[30]

Specifically referring to Operation Rescue activities, the writer of the article suggests that, "If the time and energy being used in the 'rescues' were spent trying to improve programs such as day care, low cost housing, and education in contraception, thereby removing some of the factors that lead women to seek abortions, the number of abortions would decrease dramatically." Simply put, "breaking the law cannot be justified on the basis of garnering headlines. . . . This practice comes down to taking the law into one's own hands, a practice that has no place in a democratic society."[31]

Two comments are necessary here. First, why do people always have to tell their active opponents how they could better spend their time? In other words, the writer is saying, "You could spend your time more productively if you would leave me alone so I can be about my business unchallenged." Second, the writer assumes that rescues are done only to generate headlines. Saving those not yet born must just be the excuse. Margaret Sanger would be ashamed of such an attack on civil disobedience.

The writer quotes from a report by the Anglican Church which states the "need for better educational programs on sexuality that include contraception and birth planning services by public health units and voluntary organizations such as Planned Parenthood. . . . 'The church must not forget her primary calling to be a reconciled people, ministering to those caught in the pain and brokenness of abortion,' the report to the churches concludes."[32]

The Planned Parenthood Association of British Columbia newsletter also discusses the organization's aims:

> The success of last year's Long Range Planning encouraged us to approach its up-date with renewed energy. . . . With your help the following mission statement was developed:
>
> Within three years, P.P.A.B.C. will be a cohesive organization with men and women actively involved at every level, including Board, staff and clients. We will also represent the diversity of the community at all levels.
>
> We will be highly visible to the media and the general public, as well as professional organizations. There will be an active media watch in every branch and a standardized response mechanism for media inquiries.
>
> Board members and other volunteers will have a complete orientation and training to ensure maximization of our human resources. We will have an overall financial strategy to meet current and future needs.[33]

The newsletter states that, "The Society's main objective is to promote the provision of family planning services in British Columbia as a fundamental right of all people, as an aid to responsible parenthood and as a means of improving the quality of life." It is noted that the organization "is a member of Planned Parenthood Federation of Canada. It is affiliated with the International Planned Parenthood Federation which supports family planning activities in 114 countries."[34]

In an effort to reach the minority population in the province, the Planned Parenthood Association of British Columbia applied for and received a grant to hire two "ethnic educators" who will "work with the immigrant community."[35] Some things never change.

GENERAL POLICY ADVOCACY

In "'Til Victory is Won . . . An Action Agenda for 1982-84," six goals are listed. Under each goal, with the exception of the last, "objectives," "direct medical services," "advocacy and public information," and "research and demonstration" headings are followed by specific strategies.[36]

The first goal mentioned in the document is the desire to "address the unmet need for fertility regulation services in the United States regardless of age or ability to pay." The strategies listed under "advocacy and public information" are of interest:

- Increase and strengthen statewide public affairs programs.
- Seek expanded funding for unmet needs from the public and private sectors.
- Solidify public and professional opinion behind the premise that unmet family planning needs are a national health problem deserving of increased public funding.
- Encourage physicians, health agencies, hospitals, and others to provide or expand family planning services.[37]

To meet the goal of reducing "the incidence of unwanted pregnancies and births among adolescents," Planned Parenthood lists two strategies:

- Define and promote community objectives and public policies for dealing with adolescent sexuality and pregnancy.
- Assure the continued availability of services to adolescents with complete confidentiality and privacy.[38]

For the goal of preserving and assuring "access to safe, legal abortion services and counseling for all women, regardless of age or ability to pay," Planned Parenthood's advocacy plan sets five strategies:

1. Increase the number of statewide public affairs programs.
2. Sustain the 1973 Supreme Court decisions on abortion.
3. Eliminate, where necessary and possible, restrictive legislation at the local, state, or national levels which impedes access to abortion or in any way violates the letter or spirit of the 1973 decisions.
4. Work to modify governmental policies which prohibit or restrict financial support for legal abortions.
5. Solidify the national majority constituency that supports free reproductive choice.[39]

Goal number four is to "further biomedical and behavioral research in fertility regulation methods":

- Build a strong constituency to advocate scientific and financial support to pursue biomedical research in human reproduction. The constituency could encompass a wide range of consumers and professionals.
- Devote increasing attention to safety issues involving present contraceptive methods.[40]

Goal number five is to "address the unmet need for fertility regulation services around the world." Planned Parenthood has one strategy listed under "advocacy and public information":

- Raise the level of awareness, both at home and abroad, about the magnitude of the population problem, the role that the United States must play in meeting it, the relationship between population growth and the role of women, and the need for increased support for these programs.[41]

Planned Parenthood's last goal is to "affirm human sexual learning as a life-long educational process which influences personal development, social responsibility, and community well-being."[42]

While Planned Parenthood has publicly emphasized voluntary family planning, several of its publications have suggested a possible need for government intervention in family size. *Planned Parenthood News*, the newsletter of Planned Parenthood-World Population, refers to a report issued by a panel of the White House Conference on International Cooperation. "A plea for a 'new sense of urgency' to stem the rapid growth of world population ran throughout the report," the newsletter article reads, "which warned that the dangers were so great that this 'may be the last generation which has the opportunity to cope with the problem on the basis of free choice.'"[43]

Similarly, *Family Planning Perspectives* refers to a United States Census Bureau report which revises downward the projected population growth in the country through the year 2000. Despite the projected change, mention of coercion is made in the report and referenced in the Planned Parenthood-World Population publication. It is noted that the authors of the report state that "coercion in the regulation of family size is likely to be unacceptable to the American people."[44] Yet earlier in the publication it is suggested that alternatives to a voluntary system should be considered:

- The elimination of unwanted fertility is an important goal in human terms as well as in terms of its potential impact on future U.S. Population growth. Social policies to accomplish this would include:

- Significant expansion of research to develop more effective means of fertility control.
- Development of more efficient systems of distribution of contraceptive methods among all Americans, including those low-income couples who have not had access thus far to effective family planning.
- Legalization of abortion on request as a back-up measure in cases of failed contraception, and appropriate policies to make abortion available to all who need it, regardless of socio-economic status.

If the fertility patterns of the last decade continue, these three measures by themselves might reduce U.S. population growth considerably. They would not require any change in the number of children couples appear to want now, and thus, would not require governmental policies designed to change family-size norms. No alternative population control measures which have been proposed appear to hold out as much promise of a reduction in U.S. population growth. It seems apparent therefore, that a major program along these lines would be a significant element in any national program to reduce population growth.[45]

PARENTAL INVOLVEMENT

Planned Parenthood has increased its anti-parental consent and parental notification activity. Many Planned Parenthood affiliates distribute literature urging clients to become involved in stopping "anti-choice laws." One such pamphlet says, "Planned Parenthood encourages family involvement whenever possible but believes that *no* law or rule should *require* parental consent or notification."[46]

Polls show that a strong majority of people, including many who consider themselves "pro-choice," support such laws. Consequently, Planned Parenthood has already begun verbal engineering, dubbing such legislation "teen endangerment bills."[47]

Planned Parenthood has prepared a brochure regarding parental consent and notification. The brochure states that such laws "thrust the government into the heart of extremely private family decisions." It asserts that, "These laws may sound good at first . . . However . . . for the teens who feel they *can't* tell their parents the laws are terribly damaging."[48] The brochure gives eight reasons for opposing parental consent and notification legislation and laws:

1. For most teenagers, such laws are unnecessary. . . .
2. Forced communication can destroy families. . . .
3. The laws present troubled teens with unacceptable alternatives. . . .
4. "Judicial bypass" invades family privacy by giving parental authority to judges. . . .
5. "Judicial bypass" threatens teens' health and increases their emotional and financial burden. . . .
6. "Judicial bypass" discriminates against disadvantaged teens. . . .
7. "Judicial bypass" is illogical. . . .
8. Experts agree that the laws are useless and damaging. . . .[49]

In the brochure it is argued that "family communication can't be legislated." People are urged to write to their lawmakers and to get involved in other activities.[50] While several states have passed parental consent or notification laws, Congress has consistently failed to do so.

Faye Wattleton saw parental notification and consent laws as counterproductive. She argued that there are no laws requiring consent for her daughter to get pregnant and have a baby, so why should there be laws requiring consent for an abortion?[51]:

> . . . I believe more today than I did when my daughter was five, that parental notification and consent laws are nothing more than an attempt to punish her for not conforming to the double standard of sexuality in our society. They require parental involvement for young women but parents will not be informed about the sexual activity of their young men.
>
> I wonder how many of you have asked or will ask your parents . . . for permission to become sexually active. These are very private matters.
>
> Parental notification laws are also out of step with the national trends. Of course, you will argue that a young woman has to have her parents permission to have her ears pierced and I will argue back that ear piercing is a little bit different than having a baby. But even so, the law doesn't require it and it doesn't require parental involvement on a whole host of other decisions that minors can make on their own without their parents' knowledge.
>
> But if the Supreme Court upholds the parental notification provision in the Pennsylvania law, and if my daughter lived in Pennsylvania, she would not need my permission to get prenatal care and to have a baby, but she would need my permission not to have a baby. It simply doesn't make sense.
>
> If I have not built a family structure sufficiently strong to weather the difficulties of my child growing up through adolescence then no government law is going to erect one for us. My daughter will not share her personal life with me. The only thing the government can force her to do is to circumvent the law and to fall into the hands of those who could threaten her safety and her life.
>
> Just as attempts to enforce restriction on abortions led to censorship of speech, the same slashing zeal could lead to limits on the fundamental right of travel. . . . And so we must reject these laws. We must say no to laws that interfere with our most personal and private decisions of women [sic]. Regardless of our age, regardless of our economic station in life, women are not property of politicians. We are not property of the courts and young women are not chattel of their parents.[52]

In her book, *How to Talk with Your Child About Sexuality*, Wattleton acknowledges that there are cases where children should not be allowed to make their own decisions:

> Making their own decisions is another way youngsters develop a sense of competence. It pays to encourage them whenever it's appropriate. Obviously an eight-year-old can't be allowed to decide whether she will go to school or not on a given morning, but she can decide which outfit she will wear. Becoming comfortable with making decisions helps children take the next step—to accept responsibility.[53]

The obvious question is: Why can't the child decide whether she will go to school on a given morning?

In an interview about smoking conducted with Michelle Bloch, M.D., of the Advocacy Institute, Timothy Johnson, M.D., medical editor for ABC, asks about free choice:

> Now, one of the themes that comes out of the women's movement in relation to this issue [smoking] is the freedom-of-choice issue. You will hear both the tobacco companies and defenders of the tobacco companies in the women's movement say, "This is a freedom-of-choice issue. We can make up our own minds. We should not be told what we can read or what we can see or hear." How do you respond to that?[54]

Bloch responds by saying, "You know, adults can choose, but children need to be protected."[55] Contrast Planned Parenthood's attitude with that of one school district which now requires a signed permission slip in order for a student to hear an anti-abortion guest speaker in school.

Amy Polka, a teenager from Belleville, Illinois, had an abortion in 1989. "My parents, who raised me and cared for me, certainly love me more than abortion clinic workers and the abortionist 'cared' about me," Polka states. "That seems so logical now, but in my time of crisis I hadn't thought of that simple fact."[56]

STRATEGIC PLAN

The Planned Parenthood Federation of America has distributed a "confidential" document titled "A Ten-Year Strategic Plan for Securing Abortion Rights." The plan was prepared by Hamilton and Staff, a consulting firm.[57]

The authors argue that the public is "still developing" an opinion on abortion. It is admitted that "much of the public remains skeptical about [the] current use of abortion, feeling that there is a need for the option as a safety valve as long as it is accompanied by a philosophy encouraging prevention of unwanted pregnancies. Development of a true and consistent majoritarian view on the abortion rights issue must be nurtured."[58]

The authors write that those groups supporting legal abortion have "been playing catch-up with the anti-choice forces in terms of state/local grassroots infrastructure" since the United States Supreme Court decision in *Webster v. Reproductive Health Services*. It is noted that "parity" has been achieved in many places.[59]

The report makes four assumptions: 1) abortion is now in the political arena primarily at the state level; 2) the pro-legal abortion message needs to be polished and communicated in a manner that will achieve a consistent positive response from a majority of the people; 3) it will be a long-term battle that will require a specific plan of action; and 4) the battle will cost a lot of money to be used primarily for public affairs.[60]

The report states the following goal for Planned Parenthood with regard to abortion: "build and support expanded and effective grassroots organizations in as many states as possible; these organizations need to have the flexibility to influence legislative activity, initiative campaigns, and candidate campaigns (with the legal restrictions on PPFA/PPAF [Planned Parenthood Federation of America/Planned Parenthood Action Fund]."[61]

The board of directors of the Planned Parenthood Federation of America has identified four programs to be used in protecting and defending legal abortion:

1. A "national consultancy to advise, monitor, encourage and upgrade the national political action program and the grassroots lobbying efforts of PPFA and its affiliates."[62] The consultancy consists of Planned Parenthood staff and other experts who give "political, strategic, and technical advice" to local affiliates. The group works as an emergency team when an immediate response is needed in a state where legal abortion is being challenged. The consultancy also assists in targeted states with the development of state political action plans and will provide all affiliates with training in politics, campaigning, and grassroots lobbying. The document includes more specific duties for the consultancy. Cost of the program is expected to exceed $1.5 million per annum.[63]
2. A "national education/persuasion campaign to increase public support for the overall position of the pro-choice movement."[64] The campaign supports

"increased lobbying and electoral activity in key targeted states where abortion rights are threatened." It also educates citizens to believe that abortion should remain legal. Emphasis is placed on "pro-choice leaners and part of the muddled middle" who either do not consider abortion to be an important issue or who oppose the position because of one or two specific policy issues. The report instructs that "intrusive communication" must be used if success is to be achieved. More specific recommendations are also included in the report. Cost of the program is estimated to be $8.85 million.[65]

3. A "national grassroots network, identified and utilized to further the efforts of the pro-choice movement by both PPFA nationally and each affiliate."[66] A voter identification survey will be conducted, by telephone, identifying at least one million voters who support legal abortion. At least 10 percent of these voters will become part of a National Alert System and they will write or call lawmakers upon request. The national headquarters and affiliates will have access to the survey. More specific recommendations are also included in the report. Cost of the program is estimated at $1.5 million.[67]
4. A "model state political action program, which could be implemented in target states to more effectively influence legislation, initiatives, and candidate campaigns at the state level."[68] Those involved in the program will launch initiative campaigns, conduct grassroots lobbying efforts, and build strong rapport with lawmakers. More specific recommendations are also included in the report. Cost of the program is estimated at $480,000 per state, with an additional $702,000 needed for the "Model State Initiative Campaign" which would be conducted in a maximum of four states per year.[69]

The report estimates that the entire plan, for all ten years, will cost in excess of $201 million.[70] A warning is also given:

> The decade of the nineties will be a tough one. The campaign to secure abortion rights will be expensive, it will be hard work, and constant vigilance will be the watchword. The opportunity for securing abortion rights exists; so does the danger of losing these precious rights.[71]

POLITICAL PARTY POLICY

Planned Parenthood advocates support the position of the Democratic party with regard to abortion. However, while platforms of the Democratic party have, in recent years, strongly supported unrestricted legal abortion, there are some Democrats who have objected. In mid-1989, 50 Democrats in the House of Representatives signed a letter sent to Ronald Brown, chairman of the Democratic National Committee, objecting to the ardently pro-legal abortion stance of their party:

> We . . . want to take this opportunity to express our deep concern over an issue which in recent years has divided both the Nation and the party—the issue of abortion.
>
> As you know, the current party platform states:
>
> "We believe . . . that the fundamental right to reproductive choice should be guaranteed regardless of ability to pay."
>
> This plank not only defends abortion as a "fundamental right" but also calls for the public funding of abortions. As you know, abortion is one of the most important public

policy issues of our time. We, along with millions of our fellow Democrats, believe that the principle and practice of abortion on demand is wrong. Consequently, we believe the platform plank is bad public policy. We, as good Democrats, simply cannot accept that plank as part of our Democratic heritage and philosophy.

Moreover, it is also poor politics. A good case can be made that the last three presidential elections have turned, at least in large part, on the loss of traditional Democrats who have broken with the party over so-called social issues, particularly abortion.

On the night of this last election, ABC summed up its exit poll results as follows:

"Despite all the TV ads and speeches on prison furloughs and the Pledge of Allegiance, few voters cited those as key issues. The number one issue? Abortion! Cited by nearly a third of voters interviewed by ABC news. And those who cited abortion went for Bush."

The Democratic party is seen more and more as the party of abortion—a sure recipe for losing irretrievably a significant segment of our traditional base of support. . . .

This issue is not going to go away. Nor is it likely that public attitudes on this issue will change significantly given the mere passage of time. We, therefore, think it politically wrongheaded for our party to be on record as favoring the use of taxpayer dollars to fund an alleged "fundamental right" which is so strongly opposed in conscience by millions of Americans and by ourselves.

We sincerely urge you to take appropriate steps to alter the party's course.[72]

Brown refuses to take any such steps. He strongly supports the position held by the Democratic party.

Governor Robert P. Casey, D-Pennsylvania, sees the strong tie to abortion as damaging to his party:

Interest groups that take the most extreme pro-choice view have too much control over the party. I believe it's a major reason why the Democrats have lost every national election since 1964—except Jimmy Carter . . . It's cost the party support.[73]

The Republican party platform has included anti-abortion language since the election of President Reagan in 1980. However, Planned Parenthood officials are not giving up on the Republican party. William W. Hamilton, Jr., director of the Washington, D.C., office of the Planned Parenthood Federation of America, writes that, "Those who support reproductive rights can't afford to write off the Republicans. Rather, we have to identify the pro-choice activists among them—and there are many—and encourage them to restore reason to the Grand Old Party."[74] Hamilton notes that some leading Republicans attended a meeting of a group called Republicans for Choice at the 1988 Republican National Convention:

Among then [sic] were some pretty well known Republican leaders: former national Chair Mary Louise Smith of Iowa, former United Nations Representative Shirley Temple Black of California, U.S. Senator Nancy Kassebaum of Kansas, Congressmen Jim Leach of Iowa, Bill Green and Sherwood Boehlert of New York, Congresswoman Nancy Johnson of Connecticut, and ex-Governor Dick Snelling [now deceased] of Vermont. Plenty of people there were close friends and supporters of now-President Bush and will, we hope, keep reminding their friend in the White House that he, too, used to make sense of issues such as abortion and family planning . . .[75]

Efforts concentrating on reversing the Republican platform plank against abortion have intensified. Several prominent Republicans met in Virginia in mid-1991 to discuss plans to neutralize the Republican platform on abortion. Ann Stone, leader of Republicans for Choice, says, "We've been civil and silent and while we may remain civil, we ain't going to be silent anymore." Republicans for Choice has one goal: recruit and elect Republican candidates and convention delegates who support legal abortion.[76]

Abortion foes in the Republican party are not ignoring the fight. Phyllis Schafly has founded the Republican National Coalition for Life. Its aim is to retain the strong anti-abortion language in the platform.

AFRICAN-AMERICANS

Planned Parenthood has launched a campaign called African-American Men for Choice. It is promulgated as "a new Planned Parenthood effort to involve an important constituency in the struggle for reproductive rights."[77] The program is the idea of the former chairman of the Planned Parenthood Federation of America, Kenneth C. Edelin, M.D., who described his reason for suggesting formation of the group: "Its purpose is to get more African-American men involved in the pro-choice movement, as defenders of the rights of all women, but in particular, African-American women, who will suffer the most if reproductive freedom is lost."[78]

Joe Louis Barrow, Jr., chairman of Planned Parenthood's minority caucus, explains that the organization hopes to make abortion an issue for African-American men who are currently uninterested. "When we contacted African-American fraternities and organizations for black businessmen we discovered that choice was not in the forefront for them, that it was not even on their agenda," Barrow states. "We want to involve these men, generate a level of enthusiasm from them, and keep the choice issue before them."[79]

Planned Parenthood developed an advertisement for placement in the December 1991 editions of several African-American-oriented magazines such as *Black Enterprise*, *Emerge*, and the eastern edition of *Ebony*. The advertisement pictures Edelin, Barrow, Earl G. Graves of Earl Graves Ltd., actor Ossie Davis, musician Wynton Marsalis, Gordon Parks who is a photographer, writer, and director, Alvin Poussaint, M.D., attorney Victor Dates, and Earl Monroe, president of Pretty Pearl Records. The advertisement text reads as follows:

> Today, we are taking a stand side by side with women to guard their most fundamental right.
>
> The right to choose.
>
> We have not forgotten that, before the Supreme Court's 1973 ruling in *Roe v. Wade*, it was African-American women who suffered the most from cruelly restrictive abortion laws.
>
> It's also painfully clear that any law designed to undermine *Roe v. Wade* and limit a woman's right to choose will inevitably hit hardest at the women we care about the most . . . the sisters, mothers, and daughters of the African-American community.
>
> Already, millions of African-American women are suffering from limits placed on their reproductive choices.
>
> As African-American men, we share a compelling responsibility to secure the health and safety of our people.
>
> To stand up and be counted in local and national battles for reproductive freedom.
>
> And to support organizations such as Planned Parenthood which defend women's lives and health every day.
>
> We invite you to join us now. All you have to do is call, toll-free.
>
> Call 1-800———. Because freedom and courage have always gone together.[80]

The advertisement urges African-Americans to call the toll-free telephone number to "voice their support" for legal abortion. The caller listens to a recorded message and is asked to leave his name, address, and telephone number on tape.

The information is sent to the Planned Parenthood affiliate nearest the caller's home. The affiliate contacts the caller and urges him to become involved in Planned Parenthood efforts, including having the men "help in role-model programs for young men or male responsibility education programs."[81] It is expected that names will be gathered, donations solicited, and chapters formed.

Several influential African-American men have reportedly joined African-American Men for Choice. While the advertisement targets men, Planned Parenthood officials realize women will also be impacted.[82]

While Planned Parenthood seeks to increase its support among African-Americans, some have been speaking out against abortion, calling it a form of "genocide." Mildred Jefferson, M.D., Erma Clardy Craven, Dick Gregory, James H. Meredith, and Kay James have spoken and written about the subject for many years.

As a strong advocate of legal abortion, Jesse Jackson participated in pro-legal abortion marches in Washington, D.C., in 1989 and 1992. In 1977, however, he had a different position:

> There are those who argue that the right to privacy is of higher order than the right to life . . . that was the premise of slavery. You could not protest the existence or treatment of slaves on the plantation because that was private and therefore outside your right to be concerned . . . the Constitution called us three-fifths human and the whites further dehumanized us by calling us "niggers." It was part of the dehumanizing process . . . these advocates of taking life prior to birth do not call it killing or murder they call it abortion. They further never talk about aborting a baby because that would imply something human . . . fetus sounds less human and therefore can be justified.[83]

Some Americans who are not of African descent are speaking out as well, including liberal columnist Nat Hentoff, who has said the genocide attack used to strike him as "foolish hyperbole." Hentoff now says he is "not so sure."[84] Conservative columnist Joseph Sobran theorizes that Hentoff's new attitude may be well-grounded:

> He [Hentoff] is probably less sure, as I am, after hearing the House debate on federal abortion financing the other day. Congressman Steny Hoyer, a Maryland Democrat, conjured up a vision of a woman being impregnated by Willie Horton. We've moved well beyond "Would you want your daughter to marry one?" An anti-abortion Republican told me he was heatedly asked in private, by a pro-abortion colleague: "What if your daughter were raped by some black?"
>
> Our elected representatives don't seem equally worried about black women who get pregnant by white rapists, which I guess tells us something or other. Maybe that some unwanted children are more unwanted than others.
>
> I hope non-white Americans in general are paying close attention to this debate. They will learn, if they don't already sense it, that a great many of their white fellow citizens regard them as social pests whose offspring should be nipped in the larval stage.
>
> Some whites are "right-wing" . . . but they are just as likely to be known publicly as liberals.[85]

Sobran suggests the debate includes using abortion "as a method of controlling the minority population. This is hardly a question the pro-abortionists will enjoy discussing in public, however freely they may talk about it in private." He also writes that, because one study has shown that up to 43 percent of those aborted have African-American parents, they "are the most strongly anti-abortion group in the country."[86] This is true despite what most African-American "leaders" believe.

In 1990, only 58 percent of Planned Parenthood's abortion clients were Caucasian.[87] However, the relative opposition to abortion among African-Americans has generally not translated into support for anti-abortion candidates for political office. As with many Catholics, African-Americans tend to support Democratic candidates, either ignoring or diminishing the importance of the politicians stand on abortion. If this were to be reversed, anti-abortion candidates would easily out poll supporters of legal abortion in most elections where there is a significant African-American population.

Planned Parenthood does not seek only to activate African-Americans. It has also created an organization called Physicians for Choice. A "Dear Colleague" letter states, "We are organizing pro-choice physicians to reflect the strong medical support of individuals' reproductive freedom . . . "[88]

THE ABORTION PILL

Planned Parenthood has become the most vocal advocate for the worldwide manufacture and distribution of RU 486 (Mifepristone). In fact, David A. Grimes, M.D., who serves on the board of directors of the Planned Parenthood Federation of America, made a presentation during a seminar called, "New Birth Control in the Next Century." RU 486 was the subject of his speech.[89] Louise B. Tyrer, M.D., then-vice president of Planned Parenthood's medical division, and Allan Rosenfield, M.D., a former member of Planned Parenthood's national board and dean of Columbia University's School of Public Health, also made presentations.[90]

Developed in France, use of RU 486 has been restricted to Europe. It is manufactured by Roussel-Uclaf, which holds the patent on the drug. Roussel-Uclaf's parent company is Hoechst. The United States Food and Drug Administration issued an import ban on the drug for abortion-related research and personal use. The drug may be imported for testing unrelated to abortion.

RU 486 induces abortion when taken during the first months of pregnancy by blocking the pregnancy hormone (progesterone), starving the preborn human being. The drug makes the body believe it is not pregnant. When used alone, RU 486 reportedly has an 80 percent efficacy rate. When used in conjunction with a prostaglandin, the efficacy rate increases to 90 percent. It is recommended that RU 486 be used as early in pregnancy as possible. One reason for this recommendation is that efficacy decreases as the pregnancy progresses. In addition, the less the woman weighs, the higher the efficacy rate of the drug. RU 486 may not be used beyond eight weeks gestation.

Planned Parenthood and advocates of legal abortion see RU 486 as giving easier access to abortion. Easy access has been a closely guarded cornerstone of the right to abortion.

Before leaving Planned Parenthood, Faye Wattleton said the organization will "do whatever it can to support the development and availability of RU 486, which offers women another choice."[91] In the summer of 1992, a California woman, Leona Benten, calimed to be pregnant (not independently confirmed) and went to Europe where she obtained the abortion pill. In order to create a test case, Benten had contacted the Food and Drug Administration, telling them she would bring the drug to the United States. Upon her arrival in New York, the drug was confiscated.

A judge ordered RU 486 returned to Benten, but said she did not prove the import ban violated the Constitution. An appeals court overturned the judge's order. The decision was appealed to the United States Supreme Court on an emergency basis. It was claimed Benten had to take RU 486 by July 18, 1992, for it to be most effective. On July 17, the United States Supreme Court voted 7-2 against returning RU 486 to Benten and against lifting the import ban on the drug. Justices John Paul Stevens and Harry Blackmun were the dissenters.

Interestingly, Louise B. Tyrer, M.D., who was generally identified as Benten's gynecologist, often appeared with Benten. Of course, Tyrer has served as vice president of the Planned Parenthood Federation of America's medical division. One can expect an increase in RU 486-related activity by Planned Parenthood and like-minded organizations.

The chairman of Roussel-Uclaf, Dr. Edouard Sakiz, does not see the role of abortion foes in the distribution of RU 486 as standing in the way of progress. "If they consider that there is a real ethical problem and the possibility to increase the abortion rates in the world and they are against abortion, it's a logical attitude," Sakiz says.[92] However, Dan Weintraub of the International Planned Parenthood Federation has a different point of view:

> We're talking about abortions performed with sticks and stones and ah, a piece of wire. I've even seen people inject bleach. That's the kind of life that many women live in these [Third World] countries. RU 486 has the potential to alleviate an incredible amount of human suffering in these countries.[93]

Lynn Sherr, an ABC News correspondent for "20/20" who reported on RU 486, states that Weintraub told her that he "thinks the drug has been blocked by political acquiescence to a small but vocal group." Sakiz has said such pressure, if true, would have "global consequences."[94] He seems surprised by such a statement:

> If because, as you say, this [is a] small vocal group, why [is] you[r] president is making [sic] declarations on the same side? It's [political pressure] coming from [the] United States. It's not coming from France. The pressure, worldwide, today, is coming from your country.[95]

Sakiz claims he is no longer receiving letters opposing RU 486 from French citizens. All of the opposition, according to Sakiz, is coming from the United States.[96]

"It is a medical scandal and a national shame," argues Planned Parenthood's David Andrews, "that a small self-interested group of extremists has been permitted to intimidate a major health care company." Andrews says "there is a need for the American people to understand the issues. In this country it [RU 486] would be a terrific advancement for American women."[97]

Sherr notes at the end of her report that Roussel-Uclaf has an agreement with the World Health Organization that any country which requests RU 486 may get it, but none have requested the drug. Planned Parenthood officials claim the countries fear the United States will cut funding to the World Health Organization if it becomes more involved in abortion.[98]

Planned Parenthood claims, "RU 486 has many potential uses beyond pregnancy termination." The organization claims the drug "is being tested for possible treatment of breast and prostate cancer, Cushing's syndrome, glaucoma, and infertility."[99]

Planned Parenthood associates and other supporters of legal abortion seem to be claiming that RU 486 will cure everything short of homelessness and driving drunk. There is no evidence to give anyone cause to believe that RU 486 will be useful for anything other than killing human beings who are *in utero*.

Advocates for legal abortion see an advantage to claiming that RU 486 may have medicinal uses. Their goal is to get RU 486 into the United States. If people become convinced, families who have relatives suffering from or who have died from the various diseases mentioned will become active in promoting the drug. Unfortunately, this is nothing more than a cruel hoax in that it gives these people false hope. Evidence which shows RU 486 may aid in treating disease is equal to that which shows a 357-Magnum may aid in the treatment of a headache.

It should be noted that organizations which oppose RU 486 have not objected to doing research on the drug. Such research is taking place with private funds inside the United States. Foreign governments, as well as private sources, are funding research being done in other countries. In decrying the amount of federal funds spent on contraceptive research, Planned Parenthood claims the Department of Defense spends in 15 minutes that which is spent on researching birth control methods in one year.[100]

Planned Parenthood claims that RU 486 is "safe and effective." It must be conceded that the drug is effective in killing preborn human beings. However, in April 1991, the French government announced a ban on RU 486 for women who are "regular smokers" and those who are over 35 years of age. At the same time, the government ordered that the amount of prostaglandin used in conjunction with the drug be reduced. The announcement was made after it was discovered that the hormone can cause the development of heart problems.[101]

One month earlier, it was reported that a 31-year-old woman had died after taking RU 486 in conjunction with an injection of prostaglandin. It was the first death reported following use of the drug.[102] Other safety and side effect issues relating to RU 486 include incomplete abortion, hemorrhaging brought on because of an incomplete abortion, adrenal impact, nausea, vomiting, and pain.

Despite the problems associated with RU 486, several politicians have moved to bring the drug to the United States. Congressman Ron Wyden, D-Oregon, chaired a subcommittee hearing in which only two opponents of the drug were allowed to testify. No other members of Congress attended the hearing. Wyden, known as a strong supporter of abortion, used the hearing as a vehicle to ensure the importation of RU 486. Its impact was designed more for public relations than for actual legislation. Wyden had held a similar hearing some months earlier in which he blasted pregnancy counseling centers. Once again, Wyden was the only member of Congress to attend the subcommittee hearing, at which *no one* from a pregnancy counseling center was allowed to testify (see chapter 14).

The New Hampshire state legislature passed a resolution urging corporations which may want to test RU 486 to do so in the state. The same legislature has also passed other legislation which supports the pro-legal abortion movement.[103] Faye Wattleton referred to the passage of the RU 486 resolution as "a very courageous and important action, and a refreshing one."[104]

In 1989, the Planned Parenthood Federation of America presented its annual Arthur and Edith Wippman Scientific Research Award to Dr. Etienne Emile Baulieu, who developed RU 486.[105] (The 1990 winner was Sheldon J. Segal, Ph.D., a developer of Norplant.[106])

Abortion foe Bernard N. Nathanson, M.D., argues that RU 486 is now an outdated drug. "We now have abortion pills. And if you think RU 486 is state of the art, you're five years behind the times," Nathanson says. "RU 486 is history"[107]:

> There is a new pill which is being developed just now called Lilopristone. It doesn't cause an abortion; it causes the pregnancy to disappear, to simply vanish with no trace. There is no bleeding, no passage of a baby. There is no suctioning. The pill simply makes it vanish.[108]

Peg Yorkin, ex-wife of television producer Bud Yorkin, is described in press reports as being "fed up with what's happening to women's rights."[109] To rectify the situation, she gave the Feminist Majority Foundation $10 million to be used for the establishment of the Feminist Empowerment Center. The first priority of the Center is to bring RU 486 into the United States.[110] The Feminist Majority Foundation is headed by the former president of the National Organization for Women, Eleanor Smeal.

Writing in *USA Today*, Diane Culbertson, operations director for the newspaper's editorial board, refers to the $10 million gift by saying she is "pleased because it could do a lot of good."[111] This is before Culbertson discusses the restricted use of the grant:

> Could they have picked a more divisive, unneeded cause? They may as well throw the money in the trash. . . .
>
> The already too-easy availability of abortion has wreaked havoc on this nation. The family as an institution has been weakened. Too many men have regarded abortion as the solution to a "mistake" and have walked away from their responsibilities as fathers. Too many women have casually looked at abortion as just another form of birth control . . .
>
> The women's movement has opened many doors for both women and men in the last few decades. But now, it seems to have a single-minded devotion to protecting and spreading the "right" to abortion while ignoring the rights of the unborn and the many still-unrealized rights of women.
>
> Nationwide abortion protests . . . show that much of the public refuses to fall in line with the so-called feminist majority.
>
> To many, the group is becoming a fringe minority.[112]

Many supporters of legal abortion, journalists, and politicians believe RU 486 will bring an end to the "abortion war." Prolific writer George Grant has written *The Quick and the Dead: RU-486 and the New Chemical Warfare Against Your Family*, in which he awakens those who believe RU 486 or any of its sister drugs will end the abortion debate:

> [T]hey [the abortion pills] have been lauded by sundry war-weary politicians and journalists in both Europe and America as a possible peaceful compromise on the issue of abortion. No such luck. Though quickly embraced by the World Health Organization, the Population Council, Planned Parenthood International, and the United Nations Council on Population Affairs, multiplied revelations of disturbing risks, side effects, and complications plus serious questions about practical complexity and tangible effectiveness, along with unrelenting opposition by pro-life organizations and medical ethics associations, have thrown the drugs into a boiling cauldron of ideology, technology, sociology, and theology.[113]

Indeed, the conflict has merely been expanded.

NO COMPROMISE

Planned Parenthood officials like to paint their opponents as uncompromising lunatics who just cannot listen to reason. What these leaders do not say so publicly is that they want abortion to be legal and unrestricted throughout pregnancy. Planned Parenthood considers *Roe v. Wade* to be "the compromise." This argument works with people who do not understand the Supreme Court decision as it relates to *Doe v. Bolton*.

A commentary in the *Wall Street Journal* points to Planned Parenthood rabid support for absolutely no abortion restrictions:

> Only about 5 percent of all abortions involve the so-called "hard cases" of rape, incest, or a serious threat to the woman's health.
>
> The "right to choose" provides a powerful slogan. But the public also knows that some women will make irresponsible choices. Americans overwhelmingly disapprove of abortion as a form of birth control. Yet today some 40 percent of all abortions are repeat procedures, and thousands of women have undergone four or five abortions. At least a few parents use abortion as a means of ensuring a child of the "appropriate" sex. And 16,000 abortions each year—or roughly 45 every day—are performed after the 20th week of pregnancy.[114]

Despite these facts, the writer notes that "the 'pro-choice' movement has obdurately resisted any restriction, however symbolic, on legalized abortion."[115] The fear among abortion apologists seems to be that acknowledging that any prenatal life deserve to be protected will cast doubt on their position regarding all prenatal life.

POLICY BY DECREE

Planned Parenthood's influence in the courts has been extensive. It has been involved in virtually every major abortion case. Until the late 1980s, every meaningful restriction on abortion had been struck down as unconstitutional by the courts.

Some of the most celebrated cases in which Planned Parenthood took an active role include: *Planned Parenthood v. Ashcroft, City of Akron v. Akron Center for Reproductive Health, Planned Parenthood v. Danforth, Planned Parenthood v. Belotti, Planned Parenthood v. Alexander, Planned Parenthood v. Kempiners, Webster v. Reproductive Health Services, Rust v. Sullivan,* and *Planned Parenthood of Southeastern Pennsylvania v. Casey*.

Planned Parenthood turned to the judicial branch to attain what it was unable to get from the legislative branch. Gloria Feldt, executive director for Planned Parenthood of Central and Northern Arizona, writes, "Public policies have been changed for the better . . . because of Planned Parenthood's willingness to challenge unjust laws which prevent people from exercising their reproductive choices."[116]

In light of *Webster v. Reproductive Health Services* and subsequent decisions, along with the hoped for dismantling of *Roe v. Wade*, Planned Parenthood will have to change its approach. If the elected representatives of the people are re-empowered to determine abortion law, one can expect Planned Parenthood budgets for advertising and the influencing of public opinion to skyrocket. This will be especially true in initiative and referendum states where the people will be able to vote directly on proposed legislation. It will be difficult for those opposed to abortion to endure the coming campaigns which will require millions of dollars and thousands of volunteers. When Planned Parenthood and its allies lose, they will return until they win. The challenge to abortion foes is great. The most committed will win in the long, long run.

11

BEYOND NORTH AMERICA

Planned Parenthood is an international, national ,and local organization. The International Planned Parenthood Federation, founded in 1952, is involved in at least 114 countries and is headquartered in London, England.

Though the International Planned Parenthood Federation works on the pretense of family planning, what is its long-range agenda? Frederick S. Jaffee, director of the Center for Family Planning Program Development of Planned Parenthood-World Population, notes more than two dozen ways in which population can be controlled, including:

- encouraging increased homosexuality;
- adding fertility control agents to the water supply;
- introduction of a child tax and a substantial marriage tax;
- reducing or eliminating paid maternity leave or benefits;
- compulsory abortion of out-of-wedlock pregnancies;
- limitation or elimination of public-financed medical care scholarships, housing, loans and subsidies to families with more than the "allowed" number of children (usually two or fewer);
- compulsory sterilization of all who have two children, except for a few who would be allowed to have a third child;
- confinement of childbearing to only a limited number of selected adults;
- payments to encourage contraception, sterilization and abortion; and
- abortion and sterilization on demand.[1]

AFFILIATION

The Planned Parenthood Federation of America is the United States affiliate of the International Planned Parenthood Federation. The Canadian affiliate is the Planned Parenthood Federation of Canada.

All levels of the Planned Parenthood organization—local, national, and international—are connected through affiliation standards and a common agenda. Such affiliation allows the respective groups to use the Planned Parenthood name and logo, if they wish to do so. Local affiliates pay dues to their respective national organization which, in turn, pay dues to the International Planned Parenthood Federation.

Many in Planned Parenthood attempt to disassociate themselves from others within the organization. This is done when someone says or does something the others find an embarrassment. They will claim, "But that's not us!" This is somewhat similar to the local Chrysler dealership disassociating itself from Chrysler, except that the association between the International Planned Parenthood Federation and the various national and local affiliates is much more strict than in the business world.

The affiliation standards of the Planned Parenthood Federation of America state, under "program requirements," that, "The program emphasis shall be prevention of unwanted conceptions and births."[2] It also states that, "Each affiliate shall . . . Conform to all policies adopted by the Membership and insure that all Affiliate Board members are fully advised of the Bylaws, objectives and policies of the Federation, including these Standards of Affiliation."[3]

In November 1978, the International Planned Parenthood Federation adopted a policy statement which requires that "membership in IPPF [International Planned Parenthood Federation] imposes a responsibility upon FPAs [family planning associations] to perform in the best interest of the Federation, both in their activities at home and their contribution to the international movement . . . "[4] In addition, the Standards of Affiliation of the Planned Parenthood Federation of America reads, "Each Affiliate shall publicly support the purposes and policies of PPFA [Planned Parenthood Federation of America] and shall develop a program to further those purposes and policies."[5]

Another International Planned Parenthood Federation document reads, "Membership of the IPPF reflects the consonance of a membership association's aims and objectives with those of the IPPF. All IPPF members must conform to the fundamental principles laid down in the IPPF Act."[6] Consequently, all Planned Parenthood organizations, regardless of their level of work, adhere to the same philosophy, despite denials by some Planned Parenthood leaders.

BLACKMAIL OF THE THIRD WORLD

In August 1974, the World Population Council, a group sponsored by the United Nations, met in Bucharest, Romania. Unlike earlier worldwide conferences on population, delegates at Bucharest had the authority to commit their respective governments to a plan adopted by the Council.

First World countries went to Bucharest prepared to write into the plan such proposals as setting a 1985 deadline for universal access to birth control and having the small family become the accepted norm universally. Japan, the United States, and Great Britain strongly supported such proposals. From the beginning of the conference, however, Third World delegates from all parts of the ideological spectrum resisted Western efforts to impose their population control values on their developing nations.[7]

Western nations at Bucharest were essentially lobbying for Planned Parenthood's objectives. As a result of the objections raised by Third World delegates, the plan deals more with supporting the redistribution of the world's resources than with controlling population growth. Those who support the Planned Parenthood approach left the meeting disappointed.[8] It appears the delegates from Third World nations seek positive solutions to their problems, not the elimination of their peoples.

The International Planned Parenthood Federation pressures Third World governments and their peoples to comply with its wishes. These methods are explained in the publication, *Human Right to Family Planning*:

> The state has a right to expect responsible fertility behavior within national population policies. IPPF [International Planned Parenthood Federation] should press upon governments the realization that only after they have demonstrated a genuine concern for the living conditions for the individual, and after they have provided universal access to fertility regulation information, will they be entitled to ask their citizens to adhere to specific population policies. International Planned Parenthood Federation and other non-governmental organizations should give high priority to building up community support for social change, including responsible fertility behavior. If abortion is denied by national law, then you would have to adopt a gradual approach to promoting full choice of fertility regulation methods. IPPF and family planning agencies should exert pressure on governments to expand the choice of methods [of fertility regulation] available . . . [9]

The International Planned Parenthood Federation supports the use of incentives and disincentives to get compliance:

> Incentives given to communities as a whole, particularly those which are related to development schemes, are increasingly used, especially in parts of Asia . . . Disincentives to individuals and families should not be applied retroactively for reproductive behavior which is now to be discouraged . . . Incentives and disincentives which create community support for desired reproductive behavior should be considered.[10]

The International Planned Parenthood Federation has spent many years seeking to popularize its population control activities overseas, especially in the Third World. The Planned Parenthood three year plan includes a section called, "Direct Demand Creation." Under this heading fall several tactics by which Planned Parenthood's own cultural outlook might be imposed upon indigenous peoples.[11]

Massive propaganda campaigns would be ineffective without concurrent legislative change. The three year plan examines various tactics for effecting Planned Parenthood inspired laws:

> Pressing national and local authorities to meet the family planning needs of the people, through advocacy at the political level and by conducting public information and education campaigns.
>
> Studying the legal and other obstacles which limit full and free access to family planning services, and fighting for their removal . . . International Planned Parenthood Federation will support FPA's [family panning associations] which find it necessary to fight for abortion law reform.[12]

The International Planned Parenthood Federation urges its supporters to ignore laws opposing its programs as if it has a right to proclaim itself the international judge of national law:

> While ultimately necessary . . . legal change is not a prerequisite for the promotion of family planning. A vigorous service programme for which there is a demonstratable need can precede, and indeed, stimulate legal change. Especially in countries where anachronistic legislation is not enforced, an outright confrontation with the law and a premature move for legal change could be counter-productive, at least in the short run.

> Family Planning Associations [International Planned Parenthood Federation affiliates] and other non-governmental organizations should not use the absence of law or the existence of an unfavorable law as an excuse for inaction; action outside the law, and even in violation of it, is part of the process of stimulating change. They should take full advantage of existing legal or quasi-legal instruments such as decrees, regulations and policy statements, which can be constructively interpreted to support the provision of fertility regulation services or specific methods.[13]

The International Planned Parenthood Federation also suggests that family planning associations "examine their national constitutions and international documents ratified by their governments to identify those principles and provisions which constitute a legal base for promoting the right to family planning and for seeking to redress its violation."[14] Furthermore, those associations and organizations promoting such a legal right "should include in their strategies the extension of the scope of this right to the greatest possible number of fertility regulation methods."[15]

The International Planned Parenthood Federation is using American dollars to lobby foreign governments. Third World governments have a difficult time opposing Planned Parenthood given its willingness to pour vast finances and services into their countries. While Planned Parenthood's tactics have been largely successful in dealing with the Third World, the countries have only reluctantly accepted the programs. Such programs were originally regarded as impositions, not welcomed charities. Planned Parenthood programs were presented along with coercion, not care.

Planned Parenthood has presented Margaret Sanger Awards to several Third World family planning activists including 1985 awards to Guadalupe de la Vega, founder and first president of Mexico's association of private family planning agencies, and Mechai Viravaidya, deputy minister for industry and a family planning leader in Thailand.[16] In 1990, a Margaret Sanger Award was given to Mufaweza Khan, executive director of Concerned Women for Family Planning in Bangladesh, who operates a door-to-door family planning service in rural and urban communities.[17]

CONDOM AIRLIFT

In 1989, the International Planned Parenthood Federation orchestrated an airlift of 40,000 condoms to Romania after the fall of dictator Nicolae Ceausescu. The airlift was reportedly to "end the family planning emergency" created by Ceausescu's strict laws against contraception and abortion.[18]

Ceausescu's policies were not based on a moral defense of human life, but on a desire to increase the population of Romania. Children were essentially property of the state and those not adopted were forced to serve in the military. Planned Parenthood officials, however, make use of the fact that one of the first actions of the Romanian government following Ceausescu's downfall was to legalize birth control and abortion. The Planned Parenthood hierarchy seems to forget that in a 1959 Planned Parenthood Federation of America newsletter, it is written that while most communist countries "encourage contraception and abortion," Romania is an exception because of its "predominately Greek Orthodox population,"[19] not exclusively because of Ceausescu's desire to increase the population for nationalistic reasons.

The Planned Parenthood Federation of America has had its hand in Romania. Under its Family Planning International Assistance program, Planned Parenthood "began an outreach effort that led to its providing a $22,000 grant in 1990 for the purchase of abortion equipment for use in that country." Discussions have also taken place with family planning providers in other eastern European countries.[20]

MEXICO CITY POLICY

A Reagan Administration policy, announced at the 1984 International Conference on Population in Mexico City, states that the United States will not allow its monies to go to foreign groups that promote abortion as a method of family planning. The Mexico City Policy, as it is called, is strongly opposed by Planned Parenthood, the world's leading advocate of birth control, sterilization, and unrestricted abortion. The Reagan Administration issued a letter claiming that "too many governments pursued population control measures . . . rather than sound economic policies that created the rise in living standards historically associated with declines in fertility."[21]

"To have succeeded," wrote former United States Senator James L. Buckley who led the American delegation at the conference, "would have required that a significant number of delegations acknowledge the responsibility of their own governments for much of the misery experienced by their people." Buckley noted that this was the reason for the swift and resoundingly negative reaction to the Mexico City Policy.[22]

Planned Parenthood was quick to attack the policy and to find loopholes in it. It filed a lawsuit to stop enforcement, claiming the policy is a violation of a "First Amendment right to advocate abortion" and that it interferes with the "rights of privacy of people seeking family planning information." Faye Wattleton, former president of the Planned Parenthood Federation of America, also attacked the policy as "a clear infringement on the constitutional rights of not only the plaintiffs involved, but of all Americans. . . . Planned Parenthood has refused to abide by the Reagan Administration's 'gag rule' and will continue to do so."[23]

A Planned Parenthood newspaper advertisement referring to the policy is headlined, "The Reagan Administration is Promising the World to the Anti-Abortionists." The advertising campaign is titled, "The Government Should Protect Your Rights. Not Take Them Away":

> The Reagan Administration couldn't get enough Americans to agree with their personal views on abortion in the United States.
>
> So they're trying to impose their views on the rest of the world. Where they don't need a majority.
>
> The White House has proposed a policy that would take away all U.S. support from private organizations that—with their own funds—advocate the right to abortion or provide abortion services in other countries.
>
> It's unconstitutional. The government cannot deny U.S. organizations the right to make decisions about how they use their own non-governmental money.
>
> It's inhumane. It amounts to depriving millions of people all over the world of desperately needed family planning services. Not to mention depriving them of their fundamental human rights.

And it's dangerous. In a world where hundreds of thousands of women die every year from illegal abortions, family planning offers the best hope of preventing the need for abortion in the first place.

Since 1962, every U.S. Congress and every U.S. President has supported voluntary family planning programs worldwide. The government has wisely relied on private organizations to provide those services abroad. Working with local groups, in accord with local customs and meeting local needs.

But now, the White House intends to reverse that policy in order to do abroad what it couldn't do at home—impose its own views on abortion. To satisfy a small but vocal minority.

Write your congressional representative in Washington, D.C. And urge them to support more—not less—U.S. funding for family planning overseas.

It is critical that we, the majority, make our voices heard.[24]

The advertisement ends with a coupon which requests a donation and asks for verification that the reader has written to his or her member of Congress.[25] The verification can be used to augment Planned Parenthood's mailing lists and fund-raising campaigns.

An advertising series in the *National Journal,* a relatively small but politically influential weekly in Washington, D.C., is called, "A Kinder, Gentler Nation Begins With Family Planning," a reference to statements made by George Bush during his presidential campaign. One advertisement in the series pictures a young girl from a Third World country. The headline reads, "How Can You Explain That Her Mother Died of Politics?":

MORE THAN HALF OF THE WOMEN in the developing world still have no access to family planning services.

For them, pregnancy itself is a matter of life and death. . . . Desperate women resorting to illegal, often self-induced abortion run terrifying risks as well. Hospital records alone show that 200,000 women die from such non-clinical abortions worldwide—each year the real total is estimated to be much higher.

Many of the dead are worn out from eight, nine or ten pregnancies in as many years. The young children who survive their mothers may not survive for long.

This reality impels many local family planning organizations to make safe abortion or referral part of their program. Where abortion remains illegal, many groups place a high priority on lobbying for reform.

In 1970, U.S. law forbade the use of taxpayer funds for abortion services abroad, a limitation our own top-rated international program has scrupulously observed. Life-saving referrals to non-U.S.-funded clinics were still possible.

But then White House extremists made a demand outside the law. To curry favor with anti-family planning forces in the U.S., they rewrote international aid contracts to ban any foreign family planning group from doing anything except discourage safe, legal abortion. Referrals were forbidden even if no U.S. funds were used to make them.

Failure to inform a woman about all of her reproductive health options clearly violates medical ethics. Imposing such gag rules on local providers would be not only irresponsible but illegal here at home.

The "Mexico City Policy," as it is known, is not set in law or codified as regulation. It is a remnant of the ill-considered extremism that did no credit to the previous Administration and has no place in the new one.

Precious time has been wasted playing politics with America's international family planning program. We look for a new era of professionalism under President Bush and Mr. [James] Baker at the State Department.

And a return to the policy and practice of allowing the countries we aid to choose their own family planning directions.[26]

Faye Wattleton announced that Planned Parenthood would surrender $20 million available from the United States Agency for International Development because the agency does not give grants to groups that encourage abortion, as required by the Mexico City Policy. Wattleton said Planned Parenthood would give up the federal grant "rather than stop encouraging abortion." She also announced that Planned Parenthood would launch a new media blitz in response to the policy.[27]

Wattleton said the decision to halt funds to Planned Parenthood "could result in nearly one million deaths from illegal abortions each year." She said the consequences of the action would be "hundreds of thousands of more unwanted pregnancies, hundreds of thousands of more unwanted children, hundreds of thousands of more families thrust that much deeper into poverty. Why? Why would anyone single out the most vulnerable people in the world and deprive them of one of their sources of hope?" Wattleton asked. "The answer is that the decision from the White House has nothing to do with foreign policy, with national security, with compassion or with rationality. It has to do with rabid right-wing ideology and with the appeasement of single-issue voters."[28]

Planned Parenthood's first advertisement attacking the Mexico City Policy appeared in February 1987. It shows a woman from the Far East with two lean and grim children. The advertisement is headlined, "Why We're Suing Peter McPherson" (administrator of the Agency for International Development), and refers to "extremists" who, because they failed to stop abortion in the United States, want to eliminate international family planning.[29]

Another Planned Parenthood advertisement in the series is headlined, "The Right-Wing Coup in Family Planning." It deals specifically with the withdrawal of federal funds for Planned Parenthood programs. The advertisement tells readers that, thanks to family planning, the primary defender of which is Planned Parenthood, "Millions of children have been spared the ravages of hunger." It continues, "Where there was only desperation, we [Planned Parenthood] have brought hope."[30]

The advertisement goes on to say that "a handful of extremists at the White House and the Agency for International Development (A.I.D.) aim to destroy America's international family planning program—and Planned Parenthood in particular." It says that since the White House and the agency have been unsuccessful at imposing their "fanatical anti-family planning agenda on the American people," they have "decided to victimize people who can't fight back." The advertisement includes a claim that, "The very survival of women and children is at stake in this battle."[31]

Another advertisement in the series is titled, "White House Extremists and the Clause that Kills." It tells readers the White House and the Agency for International Development are "trying to eliminate the reproductive options for women in developing nations." It says the agency is requiring organizations like Planned Parenthood "to act as overseas 'thought police' for the fanatical right-wing forces in the US [United States]." The advertisement also says "similar attempts to suppress pro-choice viewpoints have already been ruled illegal" by courts in the United States.[32]

Planned Parenthood refuses to agree to restrictions for the use of the federal money as a "matter of ethics and principle."[33] The name given to a series of advertisements is, "If the extremists win, the whole world loses. Help us fight back."

It was reported that seven more advertisements would run in newspapers and magazines. The advertisements are designed to influence the public to push for a change in the agency policy before the grant was up for review.[34]

Planned Parenthood's advertising campaigns, attacking many of the Reagan Administration's policies with regard to international family planning, have been successful in gaining some public sympathy for its cause. Its efforts, made possible by its vast financial resources, will continue. Moreover, Planned Parenthood's impressive financial empire makes refusing to cooperate difficult for Third World countries.

Despite intense lobbying and attempts to gain public sympathy, the Bush Administration announced that the Mexico City Policy will be continued. Several attempts have been made in Congress to reverse the policy. On June 3, 1991, the United States Supreme Court refused to hear an appeal by the Planned Parenthood Federation of America of a lower court ruling which upheld the constitutionality of the Mexico City Policy.

COERCION IN CHINA

With regard to People's Republic of China, where many have decried the barbaric practices of infanticide and coerced abortion, Planned Parenthood officials tell us, "Despite false reports which sometimes circulate outside China, there is no element of compulsion to any aspect of the family planning program. It is entirely based on education, national discussion and the free availability of all methods [of fertility control]."[35]

Planned Parenthood has had a profound impact on family planning policies worldwide. Are its officials correct when they say there has been "no element of compulsion" with regard to family planning policies overseas? Is the Chinese government's program really based on "education" and "national discussion?" Have the incentive and disincentive policies encouraged by Planned Parenthood been adopted by Chinese officials?

Dr. Quan B. Li was a citizen of the People's Republic of China who traveled to the United States to pursue a doctorate in mechanical engineering at Arizona State University. The Chinese government, in line with its usual practice, did not allow Li's family (his wife and son) to travel with him to the United States. This policy was designed to ensure that Li would return to China following his studies.

In an unusual move, Li's wife, Ping Hong Li, was later granted special permission to study in the United States along with her husband. A nurse, Ping Hong Li was a member of the Communist Party in China and the factory where she worked endorsed the travel application. Ping Hong Li, and her son, joined Quan Li in Phoenix, Arizona, three years after he had arrived.

The Li family was looking forward to returning to China as their additional education would guarantee high placement. However, Quan Li became frightened when he learned that his wife was pregnant for the second time. Li was concerned about China's one child per couple policy. He contacted Arizona Right to Life seeking help. I was working for the organization at the time and soon took a personal interest in the case. For the first time, the Chinese population control policy meant something to me personally.

Quan Li expressed his fear that if he returned to China, his wife would be forced to kill their preborn child. While Li feared for the life of his preborn baby, he also feared for the lives of his relatives if his story was to become public. (He later agreed to limited publicity in an effort to awaken the world to China's policies.) To authenticate his fear, Li brought forth several documents he had received from China.

Li and his wife received several letters from Ping Hong Li's mother who, along with other relatives, was being harassed and threatened by factory and population control officials to put pressure on her to have an abortion. One letter reads, "You'd better have this baby aborted now . . . "[36]

The Lis initially refused outright to have an abortion and later they simply stalled. At one point, they wrote that the abortion had been done when in reality it had not. Ping Hong Li received a letter from her employer saying she must get an abortion or suffer the consequences. The letter is authored by Li Gao of the Walfantia Bearings Company:

> I reported your situation of being pregnant to the supervisory cadre [party officials who work in the factories] who is currently in charge of the birth control program at our factory and asked for her opinion. The answer from her is as follows: Our country has set this birth control program for controlling the population growth. Our government has emphasized and reinforced the birth control policy again and again that one family is only allowed to have one child. How much effort for keeping this policy has been a very important criterion for evaluating and reviewing a unit.
>
> Second child is absolutely banned. If somebody insists to have a second child, promotion of the factory and salary raise of all employees of the factory shall be banished. All of us, from the lowest staff to the president of the factory, shall be punished for that. All related units and departments shall be disqualified for any public contest. The responsible individual shall be paid for only the minimum living expenses. She shall also be placed under probation. I think that you absolutely cannot afford these political and financial losses.
>
> In order to send this letter to you, we visited your mother and asked her to mail it out. We also informed your mother [of] all the consequences you may have to take as mentioned above. Your mother then told us that the district officials came to her many times for checking this . . . Finally, I hope you [will] not . . . lose any time and fix your problem as soon as possible.[37]

A second letter from the company gives more detail about what the Li family could expect if the abortion were not performed:

> Birth control is one of our nation's basic policies. It is known to every family and every person that one couple is only to have one child . . . Recently, one case of [a couple] having a second child occurred at [another company] regardless of warning. Afterwards, both of the couple were officially disqualified for any employment and put under probation for one year. They are given only 30 yuans for living expenses. They were ordered to pay back the subsidy they received for the health care and nursery reimbursement for their first child. All leaders of different levels at their units lost their bonuses for several months.
>
> Our factory is now working on company's expansion. We have already passed all the evaluations and reviews. If we have a second child case on our birth control program, it would stop [our company] from being expanded from low level to high level. The effort that 20,000 employees worked hard for would become vain. The whole factory would be disqualified for any contest. The bonuses and benefits for all employees would be directly impacted. From the president to the middle level leaders and the cadres in charge of the birth control program, all of us would be punished. The consequences are unimaginable.

> You shall be condemned by all staff and workers of the factory. How could we afford these losses?[38]

A third corporate letter expresses frustration regarding the urgency of the matter:

> Have you received our last express-mailed letter? Have you decided what to do? The factory officials are anxious to know your decision. Since this would affect the benefits of all employees of the factory as well as the company's future, the punishment to this kind of violation is very severe. We advise you absolutely not to take any chances. If you really cannot have an abortion done abroad, the factory president orders you to return immediately. You must not delay. Otherwise you will be punished according to the rules and regulations for all the consequences. There is nothing ambiguous about it! Hope you make up your mind immediately.[39]

Quan Li's sister, a population control official, wrote to encourage him to have his wife get an abortion. However, she made a point of separating her professional and personal opinions:

> Some "illegal" pregnant women were forced to have induced abortion when the pregnancies were 8-9 months, or even just about mature. In some cases people were physically pushing and pulling or even had some other violent means of forcing the pregnant women to have abortion . . .
>
> Some families were fined up to 5,000 yuans after they escaped out of town and later came back with their "illegal" children already born . . . As your sister, though I am in charge of the birth control program here, my heart is same as that of everybody else. I also wish you to have another smart child and add one more to our family's next generation.[40]

One writer quotes from what is called an "official document to define the punishment to those individuals who insisted to have [a] second child." This is in direct contrast to those who admit that such events occur, but who claim the practice is not an official government policy.[41]

While the Li family worked to stall Chinese government and factory officials, Ping Hong Li gave birth to a girl, Mahwae Rose Li, the English translation of which is "America." Quan Li sent a photograph of the baby to some of those working on the asylum request.

While still in Arizona, I placed a call to Steven Mosher, director of the Asian Studies Center at the Claremont Institute, to inform him of the situation. Mosher had written about the Chinese population control program in the past and had visited China. He wrote articles about the Lis' predicament which were published in many newspapers and magazines. The articles served to bring the issue to the attention of millions of people.

Unfortunately, a rift developed between Mosher and Arizona Right to Life regarding the process and the best way to handle the situation. Arizona Right to Life had already established a plan, concentrating on political asylum, yet Mosher wanted to do things differently, even though it was Arizona Right to Life which brought the matter to his attention in the first place. Mosher, on the other hand, apparently felt Arizona Right to Life was unqualified, largely due to inexperience, to deal with the matter. For example, Mosher attempted to veto plans made by Arizona Right to Life, and the organization's involvement and work were ignored in articles written by Mosher. He also attempted to veto related projects organized by a national anti-abortion organization which had, with the consent of Quan Li, scheduled a related event.

Due to the disagreement, the parties generally operated independently, but the conflict actually led to complimentary work. While Mosher worked to bring the issue to the attention of millions of people through his articles, Arizona Right to Life and the Christian Action Council worked the political asylum route. Clearly, one effort without the other would have made success much more difficult.

A letter seeking assistance was sent by me to Congressmen Jon Kyl, R-Arizona, and Christopher Smith, R-New Jersey, and Senators John McCain, R-Arizona, and Dennis DeConcini, D-Arizona. Kyl wrote to the Immigration and Naturalization Service urging political asylum be granted to the Li family.[42] Nevertheless, the application was rejected. Tim Glazewski, an aide to Kyl, was particularly helpful.

Smith wrote to his colleagues in the House of Representatives drawing their attention to the issue:

> Despite consistent public denials by Chinese officials and their apologists here in the United States, the evidence continues to mount that the government of the People's Republic of China is systematically employing coercive measures—including forced abortions at late stages of pregnancy—to implement their restrictive "one-couple, one-child" policy.[43]

Smith points to the Li case as evidence:

> Dr. John Aird, formerly the Senior Research Specialist on China at the U.S. Bureau of the Census, has recently confirmed that China has tightened its enforcement of the "one child" policy. Clearly, the Chinese program continues to violate internationally recognized principles of voluntarism and respect for human rights. I hope you will keep these ongoing human rights violations in mind during future debates on U.S. policy towards China and international population control organizations which participate in China's program.[44]

Following the failure of the Immigration and Naturalization Service to grant political asylum, four members of Congress authored a letter to then-Attorney General Edwin Meese III, requesting that the Justice Department grant political asylum to the Li family.[45] An Immigration and Naturalization Service official wrote to the Justice Department urging the denial of asylum.

Since my contacts with members of Congress had been limited while working in Arizona, my move to Washington, D.C., turned out to be most helpful. While attending a meeting of conservative leaders, a Meese associate, Becky Norton Dunlop, thanked the group for its support of the embattled attorney general. She then said, "If there's anything the Attorney General can do for you, he would like to know about it." While I was new to this group of "movers and shakers," I saw an opportunity I could not let pass. I raised my hand, explained that I had been working on the case for almost a year, and I would like the Attorney General to act favorably. Dunlop asked that I send the appropriate documents to her office, and she would make sure the matter came to the personal attention of the Attorney General.

Follow-up calls were frustrating. Dunlop reported significant opposition to political asylum within the Justice Department. The reasons varied. Some did not want to anger the Chinese government. Others simply support the Chinese policy.

The primary person responsible for blocking approval of the political asylum application was being considered by the Senate Judiciary Committee for permanent appointment as an assistant attorney general. DeConcini, a member of the committee, agreed to question the nominee on the matter at his confirmation hearing. Senator Jesse Helms, R-North Carolina, also a member of the committee, was outraged at the delay. Dunlop quoted the Senator as saying, "If he [the Justice Department official] doesn't do the right thing, his nomination will rot on the calendar."

Becky Norton Dunlop called on August 2, 1988, to say the Attorney General had decided to grant political asylum, and it was simply a matter of days before the announcement was made. I was offered the honor of contacting the Lis with the news, which I immediately did. Political asylum was officially granted by Meese on August 5, 1988.

In November 1989, Congress passed the Armstrong-DeConcini Amendment which would have ordered the Immigration and Naturalization Service to look favorably upon requests for political asylum when threats of persecution can be proven. The bill included several somewhat unrelated issues as well. Due to pressure from the Chinese government, President George Bush vetoed the bill that included the Armstrong-DeConcini Amendment.

Dr. Julia J. Henderson, a member of the board of the Better World Society and former secretary general of the International Planned Parenthood Federation, argues that there is no coercion in the Chinese program. Speaking for the Better World Society on a television program on which the China Family Planning Association was presented with the Population Medal (an annual award presented by the Society), Henderson argues that the term "coercion" is used too loosely in the Western press:

> It makes it sound as though there's a government official beating people over the head or arresting them and sending them to jail if they don't conform to the policy. This is not true. I think they are getting the willing cooperation of the large part of the population and they're doing that by persuading people in the first place that it's better for the health of the mother and the child.[46]

The China Family Planning Association was created to help implement China's one child per couple policy. Wang Wei, vice president of the Association, accepted the award.[47] The deputy director of the China Family Planning Association, Ambassador Zhou Boping, serves on the board of the Better World Society.

The *Washington Post* ran an article on the Chinese policy in January 1985. Writer Michael Weisskopf explains how the Chinese policy has led parents to eliminate children of the "wrong" gender. In Chinese culture, as in many others around the world, males are preferred over females because of economic security and pride. Nevertheless, the cultural requirement that a man produce a son, and a political policy which limits couples to one child, has led to the deaths of countless female newborns:

> The baby girl became another victim of the ugliest side of China's war against overpopulation—female infanticide.
>
> Official population statistics indicate a loss of more than 230,000 baby girls in 1981, a casualty list that is said to have grown dramatically in more recent years as the Communist government tightened its nationwide policy limiting Chinese couples to one child . . .
>
> Failure to have sons can ruin a woman's life. While this dilemma for Chinese women is as old as China, it is intensified by the one-child policy. In the old days, women kept trying until they had a son. Now they have one chance. Unsuccessful wives have been poisoned, strangled, bludgeoned and socially ostracized, according to official reports.[48]

It has been reported that Chinese families having one daughter will be allowed a second chance to conceive a boy if they obtain a permit to do so. Infanticide of baby girls has been causing "a catastrophic demographical imbalance."[49]

Contrast this startling information with the statement by the former president of the National Organization for Women. Molly Yard (Garrett) said, "I consider the Chinese government's policy among the most intelligent in the world."[50]

Human Numbers, Human Needs, a publication of the International Planned Parenthood Federation, scolds the Chinese people. The International Planned Parenthood Federation argues that if Chinese parents had taken action sooner to end population growth, "it would have been acceptable for them to have two children." It is noted that the need for the one-child policy is only due to the resistance of the Chinese people to population control policies.[51]

The Chinese are preparing to mandate abortion and sterilization of the mentally handicapped. The law is already being enforced in the Gansu province and will likely become national policy. It requires sterilization of mentally handicapped couples as well as abortion for the children of individuals who are mentally handicapped.[52]

Public officials in the Gansu province stress that the policy is designed to raise "the quality of the population" while assisting in the elimination of poverty. Li Yong, an official of the State Family Planning Commission, says, "The arrival of this law is an advance for eugenics. We think it reflects progress and civilization. This local law will have a profound influence on the country for the elaboration of a national law on eugenics."[53]

While the Chinese had considered eugenics programs for more than a decade, they had previously been slow to adopt such policies for fear that "China would come under attack from abroad for human rights violations, particularly from the United States." One Western diplomat notes, "Most of the time, the Chinese do not take moral issues into consideration when they tackle these problems. Because of this, they are very sensitive to observations made on the subject by foreigners."[54]

It is estimated that China has 50 million physically and mentally handicapped people among its population of over one billion. Four million physically and mentally handicapped children were expected to be born between 1986 (one year after the estimates of the numbers of physically and mentally handicapped individuals were made by Chinese officials) and 1990. The official Chinese newspaper, *China Daily*, has said euthanasia has been carried out by some doctors and that a majority of the Chinese people favor the practice.[55]

Faye Wattleton wrote, "We have never . . . advocated any sort of compulsory reproductive behavior . . . "[56] She used Norplant as an example as her comment refers to domestic policy. Yet Wattleton would not condemn the programs of the People's Republic of China. Due to the country's high population, it seems to be a special case where the extreme measures are considered "necessary."

Does the International Planned Parenthood Federation really believe there is no element of coercion in the Chinese program? In light of the official policies of the International Planned Parenthood Federation, is it at least partially responsible for such practices? How can the Better World Society deny these practices occur when there is so much evidence to prove otherwise? The People's Republic of

China is a modern-day example of what can happen when any government embraces the ideology of Planned Parenthood and its founder.

Dr. Alan F. Guttmacher's statement that, "Each country will have to decide its own form of coercion, determining when and how it should be employed," is coming to pass. Guttmacher continues, "The means presently available are compulsory sterilization and compulsory abortion."[57]

UNITED NATIONS POPULATION FUND

Planned Parenthood is a strong supporter of the United Nations Population Fund, commonly referred to as the UNFPA. (When the organization's name was changed to United Nations Population Fund, the acronym was retained.) An international "population control" agency, the Fund had enjoyed the support of American taxpayers for many years. The United States ended its support in 1985 because of the Kemp-Kasten Amendment which provides that American funds may not be used by "any organization or program which, as determined by the President of the United States, supports or participates in the management of a program of coercive abortion or involuntary sterilization." The decision to withhold funds is also in line with the Mexico City Policy. The United Nations Population Fund supports the coercive abortion and sterilization policies of the People's Republic of China.

Congress has moved to restore funding to the United Nations Population Fund, but such efforts have been rebuffed by Presidents Ronald Reagan and George Bush. Congressman Peter Kostmayer, D-Pennsylvania, and Senators Barbara Mikulski, D-Maryland, and Paul Simon, D-Illinois, have led efforts to restore financial support to the Fund. Legislation provided that up to 20 million American dollars be given to the Fund with stipulations that, as one amendment put it, "none of the funds made available under this heading . . . be made available for programs in the People's Republic of China," the American contribution be kept in a separate account, and the funds be returned to the United States Treasury if the United Nations Population Fund "provides more than $57 million for family planning programs in the People's Republic of China."[58]

The language of the amendment to the Foreign Aid Appropriations bill was designed to placate members of Congress and anti-abortion organizations. Proponents claim that ample safeguards are included to prevent American funds from aiding China's program, but it is simply a matter of bookkeeping. If the United States were to give $20 million to the United Nations Population Fund, with the stipulation that it not be used to support China's coercive program, the Fund would use the monies of another country to support it. It would simply be necessary to keep records which follow the American funds to another program.

Another problem with the amendment is that the funds are to be returned if more than $57 million is spent on China's program over a five year program. While it had been argued that the figure represents the current funding level provided by the Fund to support China's program, it would actually have represented an increase. Moreover, it would have legitimized the program—something the Chinese government desperately wants to see happen.

In an effort to increase opposition to funding of the United Nations Population Fund, I asked President Bush to meet with the Quan B. Li family at the White House. It was hoped that the meeting would serve two purposes. First, it would educate the President regarding the program. After all, the Li story is a powerful one. Second, it would strengthen the President's opposition to supporting the Fund. If the President were to actually meet with a victim of the program, it would not be easy to decide in favor of supporting the Fund.

Quan Li agreed to meet with the President because, as Li explains, it is important to keep others from experiencing the same pain. It was decided that Ping Hong Li and their baby, whose life had been saved, would also attend. The Lis would fly to Washington, D.C., meet with the President and several members of Congress, discuss their experience and passionately urge the President and Congress to oppose support of the United Nations Population Fund.

President Bush decided against meeting with the Li family. Instead, as with most duties relating to abortion, the chore was assigned to Vice President Dan Quayle. However, as plans began to be firmed up, the Lis became increasingly nervous. Quan Li, who had been in contact with Steven Mosher, notified me that his wife and children would not be joining him. Fears were expressed about the response of the Chinese government including possible penalties which might be imposed upon relatives still living in China.

The Vice President's staff was not happy. In fact, the Vice President's office had been most excited to hear that Ping Hong and Mahwae Rose Li would be in attendance. When the staff learned that only Quan Li would be present, it was made clear that the "deal" had been significantly altered. Nevertheless, the meeting would take place.

Quan Li called once again to say he did not want the media to be present at the meeting. Upon hearing this news, the Vice President's staff became even more upset as plans had called for a public event.

A few days before the meeting was to take place, Steven Mosher called to say Quan Li could not go to Washington, D.C. My response was to be expected. An immediate telephone call to Li confirmed that he would be in Washington, D.C., for the March 12, 1991, meeting with the Vice President.

Due to timing problems in confirming Quan Li's trip, and because there were few days from the time the meeting was scheduled to when it was held, efforts to convince members of Congress to meet with the Vice President and Li were largely unsuccessful. Six men were present at the meeting: Vice President Dan Quayle, Dr. Quan B. Li, Senator Jesse Helms, R-North Carolina, Senator Dan Coats, R-Indiana, Bill Gribbon, an aide to the Vice President, and myself.

Helms was his usual warm and personable self. He showed intense interest and spoke with care and conviction. This was especially true when Quan Li produced several photographs of his daughter. It did not take long for the Senator to ask if he could have one of the photographs. Li gladly agreed to the request. Helms turned out to be both smart and bold as he got first pick of the photographs. While Coats was more subdued, he, too, showed an acute interest.

The response of the Vice President was quite encouraging. He expressed an interest in supporting the cause for which Quan Li had traveled to Washington, D.C. He seemed thrilled to receive a photograph of Mahwae Rose Li. The decision of the three leaders was unanimous, Mahwae Rose Li is a beautiful little girl and her life would have been extinguished had China's program been allowed to run its course.

In an act of kindness, Congressman Christopher Cox, R-California, agreed to a personal meeting upon Li's arrival at his office, even though an appointment had not been made. Li also met with staff members at several congressional offices.

Mention was made of the meeting between the Vice President and Dr. Li by some lobbyists while working against passage of the Foreign Aid Appropriations bill, but it passed anyway—with the United Nations Population Fund amendment attached. Even several members of Congress who have anti-abortion voting records voted for the bill, apparently believing the amendment included sufficient safeguards. The White House, however, continued to assert its opposition to the bill because of the amendment. Perhaps the meeting was worth the trouble after all.

We may have a hint as to the attitude of some members of Congress who support the United Nations Population Fund. One key anti-abortion member of Congress, when he heard of my work with the Quan Li family, told me about a conversation with the chairman of a congressional subcommittee which considered the bill giving American dollars to the Fund. In a conversation with another member of Congress, the chairman explained his support for the bill and concluded by saying, "There are too many Chinese anyway."[59]

12

ATTACKING THE CRITICS

As one would expect, the leaders of Planned Parenthood do not have many nice things to say about those opposed to their programs. This is most evident when they write or speak about their most vocal critics—those opposed to abortion, whom they portray as enemies of everything good.

THE MOVEMENT

In the Planned Parenthood pamphlet *Defend Your Freedom to Choose*, we are told that those who oppose legal abortion "call it murder of the unborn. That is what they called contraception, ten years ago."[1] The pamphlet lashes out against the anti-abortion movement in other ways:

> The [right to life] movement includes several white supremacist organizations, several fundamentalist religious groups, and some sincere people concerned with the theological issues of their own religion.
>
> Right To Life is opposed to your right to choose abortion. Many of its members are also opposed to equal rights for women, intellectual freedom, and contraception. Some of them say that we need lots and lots of babies so that we will have cheap soldiers for war and cheap labor for continued "progress".
>
> Right To Life wants to do your choosing for you.[2]

While it is implied that the movement opposing legal abortion includes only racists, religious bigots, and confused religious people, no person who supposedly holds the views mentioned in the pamphlet is named or quoted.[3]

Planned Parenthood's former president, Faye Wattleton, referred to her opponents as "an increasingly vocal and at times violent minority" who want to "deny all of us our fundamental rights of privacy and individual decision-making." Wattleton asserted that those who oppose what she believes also "want to pass laws that reflect their view of morality. And they don't believe in separation of church and state."[4]

When accepting the Humanist of the Year Award, Wattleton referred to abortion foes as "those who would impose upon us all their bigoted views, their moralistic codes, and their inhumane policies."[5] She continued to attack those who disagree with her philosophy:

> They are the apostles of ignorance. They represent the kind of fanaticism that once caused people to hang witches and to burn books. They are, as Abraham Lincoln described them, "people who believe the realm of truth always lies within their own vision."[6]

Name-calling was a Wattleton trademark. However, whether she uses name-calling or not, the ruthlessness of the attacks is not diminished:

> There is a great inconsistency in the anti-abortion effort in that they also want to restrict the availability of contraception . . . You have to look at the deeper rationale in that movement. There is a lack of compassion for women and for the unwanted children already born.[7]

Wattleton referred to her opponents when she wrote in the *Rockford Register Star*:

> My concern is that self-righteous zealots, who presume to have all the "right" answers, are increasingly intent on imposing their narrow, dogmatic beliefs on the rest of us. American democracy rests on the pillars of liberty from persecution, tolerance for differing viewpoints and freedom to determine one's own destiny. If women are denied our most basic right—the right to become parents by choice and not by chance—then our great nation will indeed take a giant step toward the fascist regime . . . [J]oin Planned Parenthood, and the millions who support us, in preserving the American Way.[8]

Abortion opponents are accused of trying to brainwash the American public. In "The Facts Speak Louder: Planned Parenthood's Critique of *The Silent Scream*," the introduction states, "Those who seek to restrict or eliminate access to safe, legal abortion in this country have launched another attack in their desperate attempt to win the hearts and minds of the American public."[9]

In a fund-raising letter, Planned Parenthood says its rivals are a "self-righteous minority" who are "trying to impose its own view of morality on the rest of society."[10]

A Planned Parenthood fund-raising and lobbying advertisement says "there's an increasingly vocal and violent minority that wants to outlaw abortion for all women, regardless of circumstances. Even if her life or health is endangered. Even if she's a victim of rape or incest. Even if she's fifteen and not ready to be a mother." The advocates for those in the womb are accused of "attacking the Constitution."[11]

A similar advertisement asserts that abortion foes "oppose birth control and sex education—ways of *preventing* abortion." This advertisement makes a clear point about Planned Parenthood's most vocal critics. It says anti-abortion activists have "resorted to threats, physical intimidation and violence." The advertisement ends with a plea for money in order to keep the anti-abortion movement in check.[12]

Another Planned Parenthood advertisement refers to "an increasingly vocal and violent minority that doesn't trust women to decide [for or against abortion] for themselves."[13] The advertisement gives details:

> They want to outlaw all abortions for all women. Even if her life or health is endangered by a pregnancy. Even if she's a victim of rape or incest. Even if she's too young to be a mother. Many are fanatics who even object to birth control and sex education. They believe there's only one place for women. At home, in the kitchen and nursery.[14]

Another advertisement takes a similar approach:

> They have strong support from a variety of right-wing groups (for example, the John Birch Society . . .), some of them political extremists, whose opposition to the [Supreme] Court's abortion decisions is often linked to their views on a variety of other political issues, including opposition to equal rights for women, school desegregation, sex education, civil rights legislation, and unionism.[15]

More recently, a workshop was presented by Marie Bass at the 1990 Planned Parenthood Federation of America annual meeting titled, "New Birth Control in the Next Century." An outline of the workshop lists issues to be covered including a "Discussion of the anti-abortion lobby. Many are also anti-contraception, anti-sexuality and anti-woman."[16]

In a full-page advertisement appearing in the *New York Times*, Planned Parenthood writes that "having failed to convince the public or the lawmakers, certain of these [anti-abortion] people have become violent extremists, engaging in a campaign of intimidation and terror aimed at women seeking abortions and the health professionals who work at family planning clinics." The advertisement consists of reasons for keeping abortion legal.[17]

The attacks do not end there:

> The anti-abortion leaders really have a larger purpose. They oppose most ideas and programs which can help women achieve equality and freedom. They also oppose programs which protect the health and well-being of women *and* their children.
>
> Anti-abortion leaders claim to act "in defense of life." If so, why have they worked to destroy programs which *serve* life, including pre-natal care and nutrition programs for dependent pregnant women? Is this respect for life?
>
> Anti-abortion leaders also say they are trying to save children, but they have fought against health and nutrition programs for children once they are born. The anti-abortion groups seem to believe life begins at conception, but it ends at birth. Is this respect for life?
>
> Then there are the programs which diminish the number of unwanted pregnancies *before* they occur: family planning counseling, sex education and contraception for those who wish it. Anti-abortion leaders oppose those too. And clinics providing such services have been bombed. Is this respect for life?
>
> Such stances reveal the ultimate cynicism of the compulsory pregnancy movement. "Life" is not what they're fighting for. What they want is a return to the days when a woman had few choices in controlling her future. They think that the abortion option gives too much freedom. That even contraception is too liberating. That women cannot be trusted to make their own decisions.[18]

A companion advertisement, published in the *New York Times* the following day continues the attack:

> Public opinion polls show that a strong majority of Americans favor preserving safe, legal abortions, but there is still a vocal minority which does not. They want to make abortion a crime, robbing women of their right to decide for themselves when or whether to have children. Lately, some of these people have been accosting women who enter family planning and abortion clinics. Others have been planting bombs.[19]

The companion advertisement, which pictures a woman with a child, goes on to accuse those who oppose abortion of being uncaring:

> The anti-abortion movement is increasingly hostile to the actual concerns of real people. They fail to acknowledge that lives are being ruined every day. Not by legal abortion, but by lack of education and access to contraception, by the lack of more effective, safer contraceptives, by men who refuse to share responsibility, and by society's inattention to the fundamental needs of young people.[20]

One advertisement that appears in the *National Journal* is headlined, "Poverty Doesn't Come Cheap." The advertisement urges support for Title X (pronounced "title 10"). It also refers to "a small group of extremists" who have attacked Title X. The "extremists" are accused of "proposing rules that would violate medical ethics and cripple an effort already eroded by inflation." The advertisement also says, "Closed-mindedness is a luxury we cannot afford."[21]

An advertisement in the, "A Kinder, Gentler Nation Begins With Family Planning," series is headlined, "To Stop the Spread of Sexually Transmitted Diseases,

Just Say KNOW." It argues that teens need sex education. It also says "it's time the 'Just Say No' campaign was supplemented by a 'Just Say KNOW' curriculum." Planned Parenthood argues that, "The idea of comprehensive sex education, including instruction on the use of contraceptives, is backed by 89 percent of all American adults—as broad a consensus as you are likely to find." The advertisement says the Bush Administration has "an opportunity to clear out the [Reagan Administration's] closed-minded ideologues who have obstructed such common sense, life-saving public policies for far too long."[22]

Planned Parenthood's Gloria Feldt says there are obstacles which "prevent . . . families from having full access to reproductive health care, information, and choices . . ." The first obstacle listed is the anti-abortion movement. "Our successes brought a political backlash which spawned anti-choice organizations . . . These people are guerrilla fighters who sabotage our positive agenda by intimidating legislators," Feldt writes.[23]

According to Feldt, "Physical and emotional harassment of patients and staff—pickets, bomb threats, and the like—are everyday occurrences."[24] Officials with Arizona Right to Life decided to follow-up on the charges. In checking with Phoenix police, it was learned that there have been no reports of bomb threats "and the like."[25]

Faye Wattleton compared the anti-abortion movement to the Ku Klux Klan and other segregationists. She objected to those who compare the anti-abortion cause to the civil rights movement:

> The only association that I can see is with the Ku Klux Klan and other segregationists who were willing to go to any extreme to force their will. Oh, yes, they are the Ku Klux Klan of the reproductive rights controversy, which is essentially a human rights protection movement—people who go into court and will not give their names, just as the Klan hooded their heads; who speak from the Bible and seek their justification from Christian dogma; people who talk about protecting the race, as did the Klan during the civil rights movement. This is the beginning and end of their similarity to the civil rights movement.
>
> They are willing to terrorize, willing to violate the privacy of women, willing to show themselves ugly. They stand in front of abortion clinics, preaching from the Bible and condemning women to hell. That women have to go through these lines of chanting hysterics—being attacked by people who don't even know their names, let alone care about them—that is outrageous. The ugly meanness of their movement is frightening, and people, regardless of their position on the abortion issue, basically don't like their tactics.[26]

It is common knowledge that Wattleton wanted people to believe that those opposed to abortion are a small minority of the American people:

> I see them as a fringe element. There seems to be a small group of hard-core organizers who come into a town and link up with a few people who have been agitators for many years, who have persistently picketed and vandalized abortion and family planning clinics. They can turn out two or three hundred people, and you could say, "Wow, this massive well organized movement is growing all over the country," but you have to keep it in perspective. They have been given far more attention than their numbers deserve. At least now their violent nature has been brought home to the American people. I think that the Supreme Court has created such an enormous backlash of anger and resentment, real rage, that people who have never come out on this issue are now coming out.[27]

Referring to Operation Rescue, Faye Wattleton stated that she refers to the group as "Operation Guerrilla Warfare."[28] She also compares Operation Rescue to another organization:

> Despite their claims to the contrary, their only resemblance to the civil rights movement is their resemblance to the Ku Klux Klan, they are driven by a religious fervor run amok. Like the Klan, they march and terrorize in the name of Christianity.
>
> And like the Klan, which attacks blacks because they are black, they attack women because they are women. . . . We will no longer tolerate the tyranny of the radical fringe![29]

A commentary printed in the *Wall Street Journal* sheds some light on Planned Parenthood's argument that rescues hurt the image of the anti-abortion movement:

> In the aftermath of the 1963 protest marches in Birmingham, a Gallup poll found a solid 60 percent majority of citizens complaining that such demonstrations hurt the cause of the civil rights movement. Yet, within months, the marchers had attained their main objective: the passage of the Civil Rights Act.[30]

It seems rather strange, however, that Planned Parenthood and its allies claim that rescues are a waste of time and harm the image of the anti-abortion movement. If this is true, why does Planned Parenthood oppose them? Oh, yes, to "protect" their customers.

The Planned Parenthood Federation of Canada produces fund-raising letters remarkably similar to those written by its American counterpart:

> Planned Parenthood Federation of Canada is under attack again.
>
> That's why I'm writing to you now. I need your help to counter threats which, left unchallenged, will cut off access to family planning services and put an end to all our vital work.
>
> Small numbers of well-financed, reactionary groups operate across the country. These "anti-choice" organizations are currently engaged in an organized and highly vocal campaign to close down Planned Parenthood. They want their personal beliefs forced on everyone. Not everyone knows that if these misguided goals are realized, women will be robbed of their right to decide if and when they will have a baby, and deprived of access to counselling, education and birth control information.[31]

The "well-financed" comment is hilarious. All anti-abortion organizations would gladly compare combined finances with those of Planned Parenthood, never mind its allies, at any time. The fund-raising letter, which is signed by Katherine McDonald, treasurer of the Planned Parenthood Federation of Canada, does not end there:

> These groups claim that Planned Parenthood encourages and promoted abortion. The truth is "*Our Intention Is Prevention.*"
>
> It is tempting to dismiss these *so-called* "right to lifers" as fanatical and therefore ineffectual. But, we cannot afford to ignore them when adequate family planning services are unavailable or have been withdrawn from one end of the country to the other.[32]

Canada is a prime target for expansion of Planned Parenthood's influence. The Planned Parenthood Federation of Canada is actively working to establish affiliates throughout the country. This is evidenced in a brochure used by Planned Parenthood Alberta. The publication mentions the goals of the organization, as well as its desire to open more offices:

> P.P.A. [Planned Parenthood Alberta] believes that when every pregnancy is an intended pregnancy the chances for improvement in the quality of life are enhanced.
>
> Planned Parenthood Alberta seeks to carry out its mission by working in concert with our national office, our provincial affiliates, governments, like-minded individuals and community organizations and services agencies to ensure there is improvement towards:
>
> - equality of access to reliable information
> - freedom of choice in decisions relating to pregnancy

- informed consent by individuals to decisions bearing on their reproductive health
- equality of access to services for all Albertans . . .

Planned Parenthood Affiliates

- Planned Parenthood Association of Edmonton
- Calgary Birth Control Association
- Community Resource Centre—Banff

Planned Parenthood Alberta encourages the formation of new affiliates and associations throughout the province.[33]

The Washington, D.C., Planned Parenthood affiliate placed an advertisement in the *Washington Post* shortly after the re-election of President Ronald Reagan. In the advertisement, Planned Parenthood referred to "[a]nti-choice terrorists" who "want to deny women their right to family planning and abortion. And they will use any means to accomplish it."[34]

THE PEOPLE

Planned Parenthood has taken on some of its most recognized opponents. Two separate full-page advertisements placed in *Time* picture Pro-Life Action League leader Joseph M. Scheidler and Operation Rescue founder Randall A. Terry.

The advertisement featuring Scheidler pictures him speaking into a bullhorn. It is headlined, "Should a Woman's Private Medical Decisions Be Made By a Man With a Bullhorn?" The advertising series is titled, "It's Time to Go Public for Privacy." The advertisement quotes a *Chicago Tribune* article which alleges that Scheidler hired a private detective "to track down a 12-year-old girl scheduled for an abortion." The newspaper reports that Scheidler "harangued her mother" through his bullhorn, "demanding to see the child alone."[35]

The advertisement featuring Randall Terry is headlined, "I Don't Think Christians Should Use Birth Control." This advertising series is titled, "Don't Wait Until Women Are Dying Again." The advertisement quotes Terry as saying he opposes birth control and implies that the entire leadership of the anti-abortion movement opposes true contraception.[36] (See Appendix C for an analysis of several Planned Parenthood advertisements.)

Randall Terry has even become the subject of a t-shirt. A Planned Parenthood publication reports that Teed-Off Shirts, a Los Osos, California, company, is selling t-shirts which read, "I Wish I Had Been Randall Terry's Mother."[37]

What do abortion foes really support? The vast majority of organizations support a ban on abortion except when necessary to save the physical life of the mother. Given the significant increase in medical technology since 1967, such cases are virtually non-existent, however. Alan F. Guttmacher, M.D., former president of the Planned Parenthood Federation of America, commented on this fact when he wrote, "Today it is possible for almost any patient to be brought through pregnancy alive unless she suffers from a fatal illness such as cancer or leukemia and if so, abortion would be unlikely to prolong, much less save life."[38]

Opponents of abortion seek only to make *abortion* illegal, *not* contraceptives. Supporters of the movement do not believe the Constitution, when properly interpreted, makes abortion a right. They support parental involvement in contraceptive decisions with regard to minors.

Planned Parenthood makes good use of name-calling and misinformation. Its primary technique is to lump together all opponents of legal abortion. Planned Parenthood officials believe that if one abortion foe is, in their view, inconsistent in philosophy, that makes all that they believe invalid.

Advocates for the preborn human being do not oppose sex education unless it includes the teaching of values that do not respect human life and dignity. Such education is often called "value neutral." While not traditional in nature, "values" *are* taught in such courses.

All legitimate groups which oppose abortion, without exception, have strongly condemned the use of threats, intimidation, and violence. They also support legislation that will provide women with the care needed to carry a pregnancy to term. Public opinion polls show that, like those who oppose abortion, most Americans do not support the current abortion law.[39] Polls also show that most people have a gross misunderstanding of the abortion law and that women are more anti-abortion than are men.[40]

Until my second book, *Inside Planned Parenthood,* became well-known, my comments regarding Planned Parenthood went virtually unanswered. My traveling throughout the country speaking about Planned Parenthood, along with the book, were bound to catch up with me—making me a target of Planned Parenthood defenders.

In a speech in Reading, Pennsylvania, in early 1992, I noted that Planned Parenthood generates approximately $400 million per year. However, the local newspaper printed, "He said the non-profit organization makes about $400 million a year in abortion services."[41] Needless to say, this led to many letters to the editor taking me to task. Some excerpts:

> The preposterous assertion made by Doug Scott . . . that Planned Parenthood makes $400 million a year in abortion services cannot go unchallenged. . . .[42]
>
> In America it is acceptable for each of us to determine if he is pro-choice or pro-life on the abortion issue. But those who speak in a public forum have an obligation not to distort the facts when they oppose an idea or practice. . . .[43]
>
> Contrary to the false accusations made by . . . Doug Scott, Planned Parenthood devotes itself to the prevention of the need for abortion.[44]

Planned Parenthood's local leaders could not let the rare opportunity to ridicule me pass. Note that the following statistics are from their own organization, yet the writer makes them appear to be neutral and from an outside, independent group. This is followed by the usual "join us" line:

> According to studies done by the Alan Guttmacher Institute, for every dollar spent by the government to prevent unintended pregnancy, $4.70 is save in future welfare, medical and social service costs, and approximately 1.2 million unintended pregnancies are prevented.
>
> These studies also show that at least four in 10 of these pregnancies would end in abortion.
>
> Surely this is a successful and cost-effective program which those who want to eliminate the need for abortion should be happy to support. I think the Christian Action Council should join with Planned Parenthood in trying to prevent unintended pregnancies so that the need for abortion can be reduced.[45]

Just in case the comments of the board member were not sufficient, the president of the organization takes her turn:

> In the wake of repeated attempts to discredit the work of Planned Parenthood, one important point needs to be reasserted: Planned Parenthood does more than any other organization to prevent the need for abortion. . . .
>
> What is especially troubling is flagrant disregard for the truth which can mislead the public to believe false information.[46]

Strangely enough, the error allowed Planned Parenthood to escape the other comments I had made. For example, my references to Margaret Sanger, reported in the newspaper, were ignored. The Planned Parenthood leaders often theorize that if they can discredit a person, maybe they will not have to address the issues.

Soon after printing the letters to the editor, the *Reading Eagle* published the following statement: "*CORRECTIONS:* Planned Parenthood operates on $400 million yearly budget, said Doug Scott . . . A February 1 article in *a.m.BERKS* incorrectly quoted Scott as saying the non-profit organization makes about $400 million a year in abortion services."[47]

Of course, by this time the damage was done. What would Planned Parenthood supporters have written had the newspaper not made this error? Surely it would have been more of the "we are about more than just abortion" dribble.

An announcement of a trip to Normal, Illinois, gave people a chance to read *Inside Planned Parenthood* before my arrival. Several letters to the editor were published which trashed me and the book before I even stepped foot in the town.

One letter-writer argues that my objection to Planned Parenthood's painting all pregnancy counseling centers as being unethical "is humorous since Scott's book is a practice in the same methodology."[48] It is inferred, then, that all of the examples cited by me are exceptions. The comparison is ludicrous. It is clear from the original sources that they are representative of the entire organization. This is clearly not the case for pregnancy counseling centers.

The letter-writer also states that most of the book consists of quotations from "various individuals from the pro-choice movement and represents them as speaking for the entire pro-choice movement." It is argued that, "The book is full of such double standards. Scott complains they are too forward with their positions, they are in essence too honest about their philosophy."[49]

Not quite. Planned Parenthood officials are quoted far more than leaders of any other group. Margaret Sanger and Faye Wattleton are the most frequently quoted former leaders. Once again, these are not comparable situations. Planned Parenthood leaders, regardless of their level (international, national, or local) are involved in the same organization. Quoting Randall Terry, Joseph Scheidler, Judie Brown, Jack Willke, or Doug Scott is quoting five different people representing five different organizations. Moreover, supporters of legal abortion maintain more strict control over their spokesmen than do abortion foes.

As for being "too honest," a case is simply being drawn for those who do not believe Planned Parenthood is involved in the abortion industry. I am not condemning Planned Parenthood's honesty, it is just surprising given the organization's history.

The writer continues:

> The reader [of the book] is encouraged to woo the media, elected officials and school personnel on the committee. The reader is also instructed not to make their affiliation with anti-choice groups or their anti-choice philosophy known to the committee members.
>
> Is it 1984? Is truth bad and lying good and Christian?[50]

Lying is certainly not suggested. It is not even an issue. Planned Parenthood foes woo the media. Why should Planned Parenthood be the only group to do so? Is the writer suggesting there is something wrong with this? What successful group does not do so?

With regard to affiliation with anti-abortion groups, the point is to not make abortion the issue. Therefore, affiliation in anti-abortion groups, the Boy Scouts, or the Elk's Club, is irrelevant.

A student newspaper column really goes after me. Unfortunately, it shows the youth of the writer in its rhetoric and lack of basic information. I should have realized what I was in for when I read, "Doug Scott, the pro-life/anti-choice advocate who attacks Planned Parenthood as a means of promoting his anti-abortion stance, makes my stomach turn."[51] There's more:

> He blasted the organization with a number of very unfavorable and unsubstantiated claims.
>
> As I understand it, Planned Parenthood does not perform abortions. They do, however, provide abortion referrals and discuss abortion as an option with clients who request the information.
>
> I asked a friend of mine who did volunteer work at the Planned Parenthood in Bloomington, and she told me the same thing.
>
> The organization has two departments. One performs medical exams and dispenses birth control, and the other provides counseling on a variety of topics.
>
> Additionally, the organizations have programs in many schools, like the "No Touch" program they bring to elementary schools to teach children what kind of touching is acceptable behavior from adults, what is not and how to deal with a situation involving sexual touching.[52]

Boy, someone does not have the facts. Maybe the Planned Parenthood in Bloomington (which borders Normal) does not do abortions, yet, but the implication is simply wrong. The writer is not finished with me:

> I also do not give much credence to the "statistics" he cited about how many abortions Planned Parenthoods [sic] perform each year because I, and everyone else in the audience, have not seen these statistics.
>
> Scott attacked Margaret Sanger, founder of Planned Parenthood, and even called her an advocate of civil disobedience, a trait which I personally admire. So do many other Americans, apparently, based on the celebration of Martin Luther King Jr. Day.[53]

Okay, we give no credence to statistics we have not personally seen. They are easy to find. Just call Planned Parenthood for an annual report.

My comments about Sanger were in relation to Planned Parenthood's current disdain for civil disobedience. The organization has a double standard.

The author of a letter to the editor uses arguments similar to those used in Reading, Pennsylvania:

> One of the complaints that Scott had with Planned Parenthood was that their informational materials are upfront regarding the support of a woman's right to choose from among all of her legal options, including abortion. For some reason, the idea of an agency honestly presenting its services and philosophy is disturbing to Scott.
>
> I suppose I shouldn't be surprised; after all, our Christian Action Council supports the lies of omission committed by the Crisis Pregnancy Center in their advertising. For some reason it just surprised me that Christians would be so upset with the concept of honesty.[54]

In another letter, it is argued that I misrepresent Planned Parenthood's mission. "According to Scott, Planned Parenthood exists only to promote abortion and sexual promiscuity," she writes. Funny, I do not quite remember saying any such thing. "He compared the founder of Planned Parenthood to Adolph Hitler in her advocation of birth control," she continues. No, only in her rabid support of eugenics. "Planned Parenthood is not about abortions. It offers gynecological care, education and family planning services. All of these are made available to women regardless of income," she writes. I am accused of being "remiss in seeing the true role of this agency: to provide education and enlightenment to women of all backgrounds and quality, affordable gynecological care. It is unfortunate that an agency which tries to promote a woman's wellness should be maligned by a fanatic trying to peddle morality."[55]

This letter-writer is not the only person to misrepresent what I have said. Jon Kerr, who is rabidly supportive of legal abortion, attended a speech I was giving in Minnesota. He was there with notepad and camera crew. Kerr claimed he had received permission to have the camera crew present by asking the leader of the organization sponsoring the speech. The leader later said the statement was completely false. Kerr told me he was doing a documentary and he is affiliated with a university in Massachusetts. In an article titled "A is for Abstinence," Kerr writes that I compared Planned Parenthood to Nazi Germany.[56] In reality, I compared Sanger, and only Sanger, to Adolf Hitler.

Kerr also writes that the sponsors of the event "attempted to exclude a TV crew" from the site of the speech.[57] He did not note that it was his crew and that he gave what appears to be fallacious information to justify his presence. Kerr may have misrepresented himself in the hope that I thought I was in the presence of supporters only and would, therefore, give one of our big secrets or say what we really think. Unfortunately for him, there are no big secrets and we are always honest about what we think—despite what certain people may like to believe.

The experience with Kerr reminded me of another experience and, between the two of them, I believe I have now learned that not all "journalists" can be accepted at face value. Dave Ransom of the National Committee for Responsive Philanthropy called me to do an interview. He dropped the names of several anti-abortion friends of mine. He asked a few seemingly innocent questions about my friends, acted friendly, and made me believe we agreed on the issues. When the article he wrote was published, I felt mislead. The article was titled, "Special Report: Rightwing Attacks on Corporate Giving."[58] I had been raised with the thought that unless someone gives you reason to distrust them, you should inherently assume the truth is being told—within reason, of course. However, my parents surely were not thinking of the media when they taught me this lesson.

Another letter-writer refers to my statement that Planned Parenthood leaders duck debates with skilled opponents. He cites an example of an anti-abortion speaker who broke the rules a year before my arrival in Normal. "Perhaps the real reason pro-choice people are hesitant to debate the anti-choice folks too often," he theorizes, "is that they cannot be trusted to do what they say they will do, agreeing to rules and then intentionally breaking them to suit their purposes."[59]

Of course, an example could not be given of a debate in which I broke the rules. I *always* adhere to them, regardless of how ridiculous they may be. Is the writer suggesting that only abortion foes have ever broken the rules in a debate on this issue? This is an excuse, not a reason.

My favorite letter uses the old, "Aside from the obvious problems with Scott's facts and documentation . . . "[60] No examples, absolutely none, are given.

Of course, my challenge has always been the same: If anything I say during a speech or anything written by me is a lie, simply prove it. Do not imply I am lying and ignore the real issues. Either way, I am honored to be attacked by these individuals. It lets me know an impact is being made. They must be concerned about something or I would be ignored. Maybe it is the truth they are concerned about.

While criticism is to be expected, some people have a hard time sticking to the issues. They prefer to attack the people instead. Consider this letter received after an anti-abortion group I was working for published a list of corporate contributors to the National Abortion Rights Action League:

> Scott,
>
> your "politics" stink! goddamn your vile, sexist, monomaniad [sic], brain-damagged slime-self to hell!
>
> Your phenominal presumption makes me puke.
>
> Sincerely,
>
> someone you probably know[61]

The letter was sent with a "Love" stamp.[62]

Another anonymous letter-writer considers the publication of the list of corporate supporters of the National Abortion Rights Action League to be "blackmail":

> "A little blackmail" . . . "for SUCH a *good* cause"—Shame on your moral codes. Im [sic] afraid to sign my name—wouldn't want to be blackmailed for disagreeing with you.[63]

A third letter offers suggestions such as "mind your own business" and notes that "Hitler was a 'human life' too" and asks whether I would have wanted to protect him? I am called a "first-rate a—hole non-taxpayer for increasing welfare."[64]

A cartoon showing a woman, barefoot and pregnant, cooking in the kitchen, has a hand-written note underneath it, "your ideal Woman! Then [you] wonder why she's dull and boring."[65]

It has always puzzled me how someone can believe such activity will positively effect the belief system of the target. In order to change someone's views, we must rely on methods which would be effective in changing our own. Would we be convinced by people showing how much they loathe us? Never. The point, of course, is that no one side of the abortion debate has a monopoly on hate mail or other abuse.

THE CHURCH

Attacks launched against Christians and Christianity by Planned Parenthood have been horrendous. Roman Catholics have been under siege more than any other group, with "fundamentalists" coming in a distant second.

A pamphlet called *Facts About Threats to the Supreme Court Decisions on Abortion* devotes the entire text to "attacks" on legal abortion by the abortion foes.

"They have the strong backing of the hierarchy of the Roman Catholic Church," the pamphlet reads, "despite polls which show increasing support for abortion among the Catholic laity."[66]

A Planned Parenthood document states that, "Fanatics, stirred into activity by the bombast of 'churchmen,' are running about with matches."[67] A reason for this alleged activity is provided:

> Because some people, some religious and semi-religious groups dominated by elderly men, simply cannot deal rationally with sex. They can't talk about it rationally, and above all can't give up the power which controlling other people gives them. They control other people through sex.
>
> What groups? The Roman Catholic Church is pouring millions of dollars into the fight against women's freedom to choose abortion. The Mormon church is pouring money into the defeat of the ERA [Equal Rights Amendment]. The John Birch Society, the Ku Klux Klan, and certain fundamentalist churches are fighting against any form of sex education. All of them oppose contraceptive clinics, and the "Right to Life" group (financed by the Catholic Bishops) has announced its intention of getting all birth control funding withdrawn.
>
> All of these groups control people through controlling their sexual activity. All of these groups are totalitarian groups which offer women no freedom of choice in sexual matters. If they advocated their beliefs for their own members, no one would mind.
>
> But, they want to force their beliefs on you, and they are very likely to succeed. . . .[68]

Later in the document, it is suggested that without abortion and birth control, women will "start dying again."[69] Consequently, more hysteria regarding birth control and the Roman Catholic Church is raised:

> They [women] can start dying again because a tiny, vocal minority of religious fanatics, led and financed by the Roman Catholic Church, has decided that American women are to be deprived of abortion *and* birth control. Yes. That is the publicly announced goal of the "Right to Life" group, to remove all financing for birth control . . . so that women can start dying again.[70]

If the text of the Planned Parenthood document were not enough, cartoons are included. Titled "Don't Lose Your Right to Choose," the first depicts a Catholic bishop or pope. His words, divided into six frames, are as follows:

> We lost some of our flock over birth control—but we weren't worried . . .
>
> The faithful remained.
>
> We lost some more of them on the subject of homosexuality—but we weren't worried . . .
>
> The faithful remained.
>
> Now we're losing the flock on the subject of abortion—but we're not worried . . .
>
> We've got the faithful out burning down the clinics.[71]

Another cartoon depicts a general who, in six frames, makes the following statements:

> It's going to be a fight.
>
> I can see it coming . . .
>
> and we can't do it with no frigg'n volunteer army.
>
> It will take millions of men—men we don't have . . .
>
> We gotta stop this birth control, abortion crap . . .
>
> and get those cute little gals busy having babies. Instead of yelling about equal rights.[72]

A third cartoon depicts a woman. Over eight frames, she mal statements:

> The church taught me that birth control was wrong.
>
> So I had five miscarriages and six pregnancies.
>
> The church taught me that I would find the strength to go on.
>
> So I just hit the kids alot [sic] when things got tough.
>
> The church taught me that abortion was wrong.
>
> So I had Buddy when I was forty-two. He's retarded.
>
> Now these tramps are trying to tell me that birth control is OK—that abortion is OK—that sex is OK
>
> [same woman, now angry with a raised fist, holding a sign which reads, "Right to Life"]—over my dead body!![73]

An advertisement placed in the *Dallas Observer* also refers to Catholics:

> Myth: If you're careful about rhythm, it always works.
>
> Fact: Tell that to a Catholic mother of ten kids.[74]

Most Roman Catholics would surely be offended to read the newsletter of the Planned Parenthood League of Massachusetts. The first page covers the keynote speech presented by Daniel Maguire at its 56th annual meeting. Maguire is professor of moral theology at Marquette University:

> The battle has been difficult because religion and politics are "inextricably conjoined." Both are "out to define the 'good' life," and both are "moral authorities that control the thinking, choices, and judgments of people." When we cling to the words of "a magically interpreted Bible, a magically interpreted Pope, a magically interpreted Constitution," Professor Maguire maintains, "we are still hankering for that early security" we found in trusting the authority of our parents. Too often this yearning leads to excessive dependence on various authority figures and has led to fanaticism both in religion and in politics.[75]

Maguire, a member of Catholics for a Free Choice, does not understand why people oppose Planned Parenthood and its agenda. "Why is it that in our kind of work we run into problems convincing people of what seem obvious goods?" The Planned Parenthood newsletter cites contraception and abortion as examples of "obvious goods." Maguire specifically refers to abortion as a "negative good" which "may often be the most life-affirming decision that a woman has to make."[76] He also has specific thoughts regarding why there are unplanned pregnancies:

> Behind this woman's desperate situation, Maguire says, is a sexism that infects us all and contributes to the "hostile inseminator syndrome"—when men consider women inferior and thus make love carelessly. Religion promotes such sexism by supporting and creating male monopolies and hierarchies, at the end of which is a "male" God who gives male supremacy divine sanction. A second reason behind a woman's anguish when she seeks an abortion is poverty, caused in the U.S. by massive overspending on our military budget. Little revenue is left to combat the social chaos that produces the interpersonal chaos that leads to unwanted pregnancies and abortion. A third force driving women to have abortions is ignorance. If better education about sexuality were available, fewer people would have "eruptive," unplanned sex; fewer would fail to realize very early on "that pregnancy . . . [being] with child . . . is a twenty-two-year condition"; fewer would be content with the poor quality of the contraceptives now available; and fewer of us would be deluded by romantic notions of love that deny the need for commitment, spirituality, and caring for one another.[77]

Maguire claims there is not a consensus among Catholic theologians on abortion. He argues that abortion should remain legal in the absence of such a consensus because "to crush respectably debated issues in the name of false and ultimately unenforceable consensus" is to "indulge in the fascist instinct."[78]

Giving some personal thoughts is impossible to resist. Maguire seems to want Catholic leaders to base their interpretation of Scripture on what is popular. This amounts to "Cafeteria Catholicism"—take want you want, leave what you do not want, but you can still call yourself a "Catholic." Are you a Catholic just because you call yourself one? Maguire seems to have a basic misunderstanding about Christianity, particularly Roman Catholicism. It appears he wants to call himself a "Catholic" while wanting to change Catholicism to "Maguirism."

Being a member of Catholics for a Free Choice is like being a member of Palestinians for Israel, or like saying, "I'm a Christian, but I just can't accept that Jesus stuff." Of course, none of Maguire's comments are ever supported by Scripture—including his interpretation of Scripture. This assumes, however, that Maguire views the Bible with any sense of reverence and Divine inspiration.

As noted in chapter 8, Planned Parenthood occasionally uses the "automobile sales technique" in its abortion counseling, particularly when a case involves overcoming religious concerns. *Papers 1975*, a Planned Parenthood publication, gives an example of a teenager who wanted an abortion and her "extremely religious" mother who was against it.[79] The parent and her daughter were referred to a psychiatrist who was a Planned Parenthood volunteer. At the time of the incident, parental consent was required for a minor's abortion:

> The mother of a 15 year old girl came into the [Planned Parenthood] clinic in great distress. After being seen by the counselor, she was referred to me. Her daughter was pregnant and had decided to have an abortion. The mother, an extremely religious woman, considered abortion against all her principles. Her daughter demanded that her mother sign a consent for her abortion and added that if the mother refused, the daughter would get an illegal abortion. The mother's conflict was obvious. She was encouraged to express her feelings and at that point I realized that the mother needed the authority of a minister of her faith to bring about the resolution of this conflict. I referred her for further help to a minister, whom we knew to be empathetic and helpful. The end of the story is that the mother signed the consent form.[80]

Our Bodies, Ourselves, a book which Planned Parenthood recommends to teenagers, includes a comment regarding Catholicism:

> The day I left the Church was the day I had an argument in the confessional with the priest about whether having intercourse with my fiancé was a sin. I maintained it wasn't; he said that I would never be a faithful wife if I had intercourse before marriage. He refused me absolution and I never went back.[81]

Medical History of Contraception, by Norman Himes, was first printed in 1936. It was reprinted by Planned Parenthood in 1965 with an introduction by Alan Guttmacher, M.D., who at the time was president of the Planned Parenthood Federation of America. Himes raises an interesting question:

> Are Catholic stocks in the United States, taken as a whole, genetically inferior to such non-Catholic libertarian stocks as Unitarians and Universalists, Ethical Culturalists, Freethinkers? Inferior to non-Catholic stocks in general? No one really knows. One is entitled to his hunches, however, and my guess is that the answer will some day be made in the affirmative.[82]

Professor Jacqueline Kasun of Humboldt State University, writing in *The Family in America,* notes that Christians have been verbally abused by sexuality educators:

> Traditional religion is . . . [a] favorite whipping boy. The typical Christian "cheats on his income tax each year, but donates all the money . . . to his church." . . . Christians are bigoted, ignorant, and even wear funny shoes. . . . The [sexuality education] programs ask children if they would really want to "go to heaven if it meant playing a harp all day." . . . and "how many of you would be upset if organized religion disappeared?" . . . Religion, according to sex educators, is not only absurd but, worse yet, it causes sexual dysfunction. . . .[83]

Kasun documents all of the quotations in the article.

Faye Wattleton managed to do her fair share of Catholic bashing. In a debate with an advisor to New York's Catholic Archdiocese, the speakers were disagreeing over whether $200 million are being spent on sex education. "Who spends that," Wattleton fired back with a bit of sarcasm, "the Archdiocese to speak about abstinence and 'just say no' as an answer to teenage sexuality." The remark was followed by audience applause.[84]

When not attacking religion or religious people, Planned Parenthood is using both. Planned Parenthood's lists of supporters and board members almost always include clergy from denominations supportive of legal abortion. One example of Planned Parenthood using religion is an advertisement that appears in three newspapers in the Albany, New York, area:

> As clerical leaders of a rich and diverse religious community, we represent a wealth of differing beliefs. But we stand together in our certitude that abortion must remain a personal decision made within a woman's own moral framework. Churches and synagogues, as well as legislatures, should provide compassion and support—not condemnation and barriers—to any woman faced with an unwanted pregnancy.
>
> We are pro-choice advocates and call upon people of conscience everywhere to recognize that the principles of separation of church and state and the right to privacy protect us all. It's time to go public for privacy.[85]

The $2,400 advertisement lists the names of 117 "Jewish" and "Christian" clergy who support legal abortion.[86] As is often the case, because of its controversial nature and because it was done by "religious people," a news article was written about the advertisement in at least one of the Albany area newspapers. This serves to increase the impact of the advertisement.

Planned Parenthood's use of religion and religious leaders is not a new practice. A 1955 *Planned Parenthood News* article is titled, "Family Planning is Moral Duty, Religious Leaders Say." The article quotes Bishop G. Bromley Oxnam of the Methodist Church:

> "Procreation is not the only purpose of sex," he said, "and those who in the name of religion defile a holy and beautiful relationship that has its own intrinsic values do themselves commit sin. *Christian parents are morally obligated to plan for the coming of their children.*
>
> "The proper spacing of children is an expression of love, and therefore is a religious obligation. Those who condemn such planning as sinful commit sin, and cast reflection upon Christian men and women who in love take those wise steps necessary to the spacing of children and the health and happiness of the home."[87]

The article also quotes the Clergymen's Advisory Committee of the Mothers' Health Centers of New York City. "Every child has a right to come into the world, welcomed and loved," the statement reads. Titled, "The Ethics of Planned

Parenthood," the authors assert that, "It is a child's right to come into the world as planned for and wanted. Both of these factors will enhance the high and sacred meanings of family life."[88] The writers go on to endorse Planned Parenthood:

> Every married couple should decide in a sense of vocation under God whether they ought at a given time to increase the size of their family. Mothers should be provided with adequate, healthful, and scientific means to help them have their babies at such times and under such circumstances as will ensure that parenthood is indeed a sacred responsibility and privilege. It is every child's birthright to be reared by parents who feel that parenthood is a voluntary sharing in God's creativity. It is our strong conviction that the service of Planned Parenthood Mothers' Health Centers, in making possible the birth of children under such wholesome and desired circumstances, is a service of religion.[89]

According to the newsletter, the Clergymen's Advisory Committee is composed of "Protestant and Jewish leaders."[90]

A different Planned Parenthood newsletter draws a distinction between religious faiths opposed to legal abortion and those which support it. According to the newsletter, those that oppose abortion are not representative of "mainstream religions."[91]

Planned Parenthood occasionally refers to religion when urging people to participate in its programs. One Planned Parenthood poster depicts Mary and Joseph looking at the baby Jesus in a manger. The caption reads, "God had only one Son . . . [F]ollow HIS example. Visit your local Planned Parenthood."[92]

Another poster depicts God the Father seated amongst the angels. The caption reads, "If God could control how many children you should have . . . We think He would say two. We think He would bless you if you visit your nearest Family Planning Center."[93] If God *could?*

One Margaret Sanger biographer makes several references to religion. Virginia Coigney, author of *Margaret Sanger: Rebel With a Cause,* writes, "Birth control is still a controversial subject. Some religious groups still oppose it." Notice the words "still oppose it," as though they just have not caught up with the times.[94]

"In all but official Catholic circles," Coigney writes, "birth control methods are equally acceptable on moral grounds." It is noted that, "A recent publication of Planned Parenthood Federation included statements of support from spokesmen representing fourteen different religious faiths." Coigney charges that South America is still "held back by the [Catholic] Church."[95]

The German affiliate of the International Planned Parenthood Federation of America even takes on Mother Teresa of Calcutta, India. "This very successful old and withered person, who doesn't look in the least like a woman, especially when she raises her clenched fists in prayer, and who, for us, is a very suspect holder of the Nobel Prize, sees her task as that of reducing the pain and suffering brought about as a result of their having too many children," Planned Parenthood argues.[96] The attacks continue in a way reminiscent of Margaret Sanger:

> We have praised this woman's good deeds: We have respected her celibacy and the fact that she never smiles when facing the camera. Now, however, she has become for us the symbol of all that is bad in motherhood and womanhood—an image with which we do not wish to be associated.
>
> This Mother Teresa, this perfect picture of heavenly salvation, works untiringly and unselfishly to alleviate the suffering of the innocent. She cleans away their excrement, slime and snot; then asks for no reward—other than, of course, to be allowed to sit on God's righthand side (naturally at his feet). She shows us how women should behave; she

> ridicules everywhere and openly the sinfulness and arrogance of modern women; she offers for comparison the picture of herself and the sacrifices she makes, that is, when she can find time between her ideological campaigns.
>
> It's high time we rejected the menial tasks forced upon us by our society in general and by some of the male species in particular; they serve only to create in us a feeling of nausea. We refuse to make any more sacrifices, although even that is difficult to do because our mothers, aunts and nuns have raised us to do just that. We were motivated by the beatings and the false kisses which we received from them. But then, even they were only carrying out orders.
>
> Mother Teresa is the perfect image of a sexless, religious woman. This is, however, not the image of womanhood that we want. Show us instead the mother or daughter who can take delight in the most enjoyable of all worldly pleasures, sexual intimacy.
>
> We want to have the enjoyment of erotic love between men and women. No longer are we going to allow the mothers, aunts and nuns to smack little girls on their knuckles or their bottoms to ensure that they despise their physical attractions instead of being proud of them.[97]

If this does not make Catholics and those who oppose religious bigotry angry, there is much more. However, one could wonder whether the words are inspired by Margaret Sanger or Ebenezer Scrooge:

> Mother Teresa, this personification of Christian virtue, wants to show the world the way. And once more, it's a path which leads the bodies and wombs of women.
>
> Let the children come! Observe their skeleton-like heads and their greedy emaciated arms which reach out to those who may bring them food.
>
> Is it not a source of great joy and comfort to be able to feed them and clothe their nakedness? Imagine the heavenly hours of pleasure one could spend nourishing them back to health and then filling their minds with rules and regulations and then the satisfaction of watching how well they obey.[98]

Planned Parenthood shows that there is enough blame to go around:

> Oh! You poor little nuns who stand at Mother Teresa's right hand. Let us rid ourselves of these old mothers, aunts and nuns who appropriate for themselves the sorrow and suffering of those stillborn babies conceived but delivered by the beautiful bodies of the white, brown, yellow and black women who have been physically and morally destroyed by the exploitation of macho men. These exploiting males also know no better, having received their teaching from these selfsame mothers, aunts and nuns.
>
> Mother Teresa, you can't really expect us to believe that the suffering of women can be identified at one and the same time with the joys of motherhood. You must know better. Is your merciful ear aware of the cries of all these mothers when you are before photographers pictured laying your bony hands on the shorn heads of those who have brought about their own deaths by giving birth?
>
> You, you nightmare of women! You unliberated, enslaved wives, mothers, nuns and aunts, what do you want from us, who have finally decided that we are going to take control of our bodies, our children and our destiny into our own hands. Do you not realize that you are all merely puppets of the devil?[99]

Planned Parenthood officials accept religion and religious people so long as they do not believe strongly enough to act accordingly. If you call yourself a Christian and support legal abortion, you are acceptable to Planned Parenthood. In fact, your Christianity will be flaunted. If you call yourself a Christian and oppose abortion, but you are willing to oppose efforts to "impose this morality on others," you are acceptable. However, if you want to see abortion outlawed because you are "so Christian" that you want to act upon your beliefs, you are an unacceptable, close-minded, bigoted minority, or worse. Planned Parenthood's message to Christians can be summed up this way: Call yourself a Christian if you must, just do not act like one.

There is one step which can be taken that will help the anti-abortion movement more than most others: Protestants must be willing to stand up for Catholics when religious bigotry is demonstrated, such as in the German Planned Parenthood publication. Catholics must be willing to stand up for Protestants when religious bigotry is demonstrated. In 1991, Catholic leaders had come under attack for urging lawmakers who claim to be Catholic, but who support legal abortion, to act appropriately. This most often meant asking the offending lawmaker to refrain from taking communion.

In a press release, I argued that Catholic leaders were right to act against those who claim to be Catholic but who do not act accordingly. After Molly Yard, then-president of the National Organization for Women, criticized the Catholic Church, the following statement was released:

> Why should any Roman Catholic listen to the objections of Molly Yard, an enemy of the Catholic Church? She has no problem defending religious leaders who speak out in support of abortion rights. The problem is what the Catholic leaders are saying, not that they are exercising their right to free speech.[100]

Why should Ted Kennedy or any other person be allowed to call themselves Catholic and be allowed to participate in Catholic Sacraments, unchallenged, when they do not believe what their church teaches?

Yard's criticism really annoys me. This is an internal Catholic matter and Yard, the media, and even Protestants have no business interfering, particularly if they are anti-Catholic in the first place.

Concern had been expressed about the consequences of taking action against Catholics who support legal abortion. This issue was addressed in the press release:

> If the decisions lead to fewer parishioners, this may be for the best. Church leaders need to preach the Gospel, not adjust their actions and teachings in an effort to be popular or to appease critics. The same holds true for Protestant churches. If people do not believe what the Bible teaches, the problem is with the people, not the Church.
>
> We urge the Catholic leadership to decide on a course of action and apply it uniformly—irrespective of a person's status or position.[101]

Regardless of the differences between Catholics and Protestants, speaking against religious bigotry will serve not only the anti-abortion movement, it will do wonders for the protection of religious liberty. These goals are highly important to both groups.

While Planned Parenthood routinely attacks religions which oppose its goals, including personal attacks against religious leaders and followers, as previously noted, there is a place for religion. Planned Parenthood obviously uses religion when it suits its purposes, but it refers to it on other occasions. After all, as Planned Parenthood's Arlene Rosenberg says, "birth control is a religion."[102]

13

A PROJECT OF DAVID

For centuries, large organizations and powerful individuals have battled those of smaller stature. The same is true of those involved in the abortion issue. Economic boycotts, campaigns of disinformation, and other strategies have been used not simply to gain advantage in order to increase one's own position, but to decrease that of one's foe.

One might think that any attack against a Goliath like Planned Parenthood would be futile; a waste of both time and money. On the other hand, a Goliath might think itself so big and powerful that the point of immunity to the attacks of smaller organizations has arrived. Of course, if Goliath is spending a lot of time attacking its enemies, an opportunity could exist for a counterattack. Having enjoyed many years of attacking organizations opposed to abortion, this Goliath was surprised to learn that David was not mortally wounded.

One of the most recent campaigns used by abortion foes to strike at Planned Parenthood is an economic boycott of corporations which support the organization. Such donations have totalled up to $5 million per year. Some of the world's best-known corporations have made contributions to Planned Parenthood. Most grants have been made through the corporate foundation structure.

INITIAL INTEREST

While executive director of HUMAN LIFE, Washington state's largest organization opposed to abortion, I was surprised to learn that the state affiliate of the National Abortion Rights Action League was receiving support from many local businesses. In its newsletter, the League listed the names of businesses which had donated money, goods, or services in support of the group's annual auction. The list was reprinted in *HUMAN LIFE News*.

The reaction in ultra-liberal Seattle was interesting. The *Seattle Times* published an editorial titled, "Taking the Low Road," in which it was argued that launching a boycott is unconscionable.[1] It was insinuated that even alluding to a boycott is tantamount to a threat—extortion, if you will. In reality, a boycott had not been called and, at that time, not even considered.

HUMAN LIFE claimed the people have a right to know. It was also argued that the *Seattle Times* had failed to print an editorial against the animal rights, labor, civil rights, and environmental defense movements for resorting to economic boycotts, which HUMAN LIFE had not done.

Soon after moving to Arizona in 1987, I learned that a national corporation was supporting Planned Parenthood. Recalling the old expression, "Where there's smoke there's fire," it seemed that if one corporation supports Planned Parenthood it is likely that others are doing the same thing—quietly.

When I went to work in Washington, D.C., the effort to expose corporate supporters of Planned Parenthood became of increasing interest to me. Why should corporations be allowed to support the nation's number one abortion provider without being questioned?

CAMPAIGN BEGINS

An outline for a Planned Parenthood Federation of America workshop notes that, "Pharmaceutical companies, and corporate America in general, are afraid of the anti-choice movement."[2] I was determined to encourage corporations to change their philanthropic practices in a proper manner. The Corporate Funding Project began in 1988 with a letter sent to approximately one dozen corporations which simply inquired as to whether the corporations support Planned Parenthood. Of the responses received, almost all were in the affirmative.

Corporate supporters of Planned Parenthood, once confirmed, were sent information about the organization, particularly with regard to its role in the abortion industry. Corporate leaders were asked to stop supporting Planned Parenthood. After a reasonable amount of time, a letter-writing campaign was launched. A few corporate leaders agreed to end support of Planned Parenthood soon after the campaign commenced.

In an article titled, "Planned Parenthood Didn't Plan On This," *Business Week* informs corporate leaders that supporting Planned Parenthood has come under fire from some of the most active groups opposed to abortion.[3] This is not untrue. One of the primary strategies of the Project has always been to convince organizations which oppose abortion to inform their respective supporters of the letter-writing campaign. Focus on the Family, Concerned Women for America, the Ad Hoc Committee in Defense of Life, and the American Life League were the first to assist in the task.

"Inundated by letters and calls from vocal, well-organized abortion foes," *Business Week* reports, "several companies have cut off contributions to Planned Parenthood." One corporate leader is quoted as saying that "as long as Planned Parenthood supports abortion, we won't support them, because the country is too torn up about it right now." Another corporate leader tells the magazine, "No CEO [chief executive officer] is comfortable with letters saying: 'You're murdering babies.'"[4]

Other corporate leaders quoted in the article say they have no intention of ending support of Planned Parenthood. A spokesman for one company says the three Planned Parenthood facilities it supports "meet a vital need in helping to minimize the problem of teen pregnancy through education." A spokesman for another company says Planned Parenthood has "done an excellent job of helping low income women achieve self-sufficiency by controlling their reproductive choices."[5]

Planned Parenthood's vice president for resources, Peter T. Wilderotter, accuses corporate leaders who bend to the pressure of abortion foes of "corporate cowardice." Faye Wattleton, then-president of the Planned Parenthood Federation of America, said she expects most corporations to continue supporting the organization.[6]

Most corporations attempt to justify support of Planned Parenthood by saying the funds are restricted for specific projects, such as "education." This allows unrestricted Planned Parenthood funds to be released for abortion and abortion advocacy. Moreover, Planned Parenthood's brand of "education" has come into serious question.

SUCCESS

Efforts to end corporate funding of Planned Parenthood have seen considerable success. The decision of American Telephone and Telegraph (AT&T) to drop its support was clearly the most impressive victory and, moreover, it convinced others to take the same action.

The decision shocked Planned Parenthood into a counter-attack. Faye Wattleton appeared on NBC's "Today" and the "CBS Morning News," where she accused the Christian Action Council of pressuring American Telephone and Telegraph to end support for her group. Officials of American Telephone and Telegraph, Planned Parenthood, and the Christian Action Council, were interviewed on the "CBS Evening News," "ABC World News Tonight," and the "MacNeil/Lehrer News Hour," along with several radio stations and newspapers. Strangely enough, "NBC Nightly News" interviewed an anti-abortion leader who has resisted the Project. *USA Today* interviewed a person who claims to oppose abortion but who also strongly opposes the Project. Nevertheless, these individuals seem willing to speak to the media when successes occur.

In April 1990, Planned Parenthood attacked the American Telephone and Telegraph decision by placing a full-page advertisement in several of the nation's most prominent newspapers. Headlined, "Caving In to Extremists, AT&T Hangs Up On Planned Parenthood," the advertisement includes two coupons. One was to be sent to American Telephone and Telegraph in protest of its decision. The other was to be sent to Planned Parenthood, along with a donation of cash, American Telephone and Telegraph shares, and/or proxy votes for a stockholders' meeting:

> In March, AT&T announced it was cutting off twenty-five years of philanthropic support to Planned Parenthood.
>
> For the record, AT&T's annual grant was devoted to preventing teen pregnancy.
>
> It did not pay for abortion services.
>
> Nor did it aid Planned Parenthood's efforts to protect the health of women by keeping abortion safe and legal.
>
> In fact, AT&T was helping us avert abortion by teaching teenagers how to avoid unintended pregnancies.
>
> Yet AT&T caved in to anti-choice extremists, just weeks before the annual meeting at which the question was to be openly discussed and voted on by shareholders.
>
> And decided to leave teens at risk.
>
> The free exchange of information is basic to AT&T's communications business.
>
> By catering to a close-minded minority intolerant of differing ideas, AT&T is working against its own best interests.

> It only encourages those who use bullying tactics to stop women of all ages from getting the information they need to make their own personal, private decisions.
>
> The saddest part of this shameful episode is that AT&T's action has only made abortions more likely.
>
> Indeed, in a panic to distance itself from Planned Parenthood, AT&T has sent a message that education and family planning—the only safe and sure ways to reduce abortion—are unworthy of support.
>
> That's precisely what the anti-choice extremists want. To see their threats succeed. To silence discussion. To take away all our choices, one by one.
>
> This time, family planning was the target.
>
> But what's next on their hit list? And who will have the integrity to stand fast?
>
> We urge you to send a message back by mailing the coupons below.
>
> AT&T advertises itself as "the right choice."
>
> It's time to remind the company what the word really means.[7]

American Telephone and Telegraph held firm. Its spokesmen were eloquent in explaining its position.

A response to the advertisement is warranted. Name-calling is not unusual for Planned Parenthood speakers and in advertisements. "Anti-choice extremists," "closed-minded minority," and "intolerant." Margaret Sanger was called a lot of names, too. I once saw a sign which read, "Call me an extremist, but I just don't like killing babies."

While American Telephone and Telegraph grants did not directly support Planned Parenthood's multi-million dollar abortion business, they did release unrestricted funds which could be used for abortion-related activities. The company also supported Planned Parenthood programs related to the "prevention" of teen pregnancy, yet the problem continues to get worse. Furthermore, the grants legitimize Planned Parenthood by saying, in effect, that American Telephone and Telegraph supports the organization and its mission.

A commentary appearing in the *Milwaukee Journal* notes that the $50,000 per year American Telephone and Telegraph grant "is small potatoes." It suggests that the true reason for Planned Parenthood's massive campaign was merely to get "propaganda mileage."[8]

Faye Wattleton defended Planned Parenthood's decision to bite the hand that had fed it:

> There was no other option to take—and let me explain to you why. We had been in conversations with AT&T for a number of months—as a matter of fact, more than a year, about the concerns they had about the opposition . . . We urged them to let us work together to generate expressions of support, the likes of which you saw in Dayton Hudson [which announced an end to funding and then resumed it] from people who would gladly step up and say, "Absolutely not, do not give in."
>
> AT&T refused to accept that offer of partnership in confronting this problem. We said to them, "you can't avoid this by de-funding. This is an issue that will not go away—it will only give life and strength to people who think that they can push you around when you don't reach out into the broad reservoir of public goodwill for what you are doing."[9]

Wattleton said she could not think of "any situation in which corporations want to be involved in what they see as controversy." However, she believed the manner in which American Telephone and Telegraph "handled this particular situation is evidence of their lack of ability to even understand controversy, let alone handle controversy."[10]

Members of Congress entered the fray with those supporting Planned Parenthood urging American Telephone and Telegraph to reverse its decision, and those opposing Planned Parenthood thanking the company. Congresswoman Barbara Boxer, D-California, led the fight among members of Congress urging American Telephone and Telegraph to restore funding to Planned Parenthood. Congressman Robert K. Dornan, R-California, led the opposing side.

In April 1990, American Telephone and Telegraph shareholders considered the issue of funding abortion advocacy organizations. Many shareholders left the meeting when the issue came up. The shareholder resolution under consideration asked that the company no longer fund groups involved in the abortion issue. I urged that the resolution be withdrawn, victory declared, and thanks be given to American Telephone and Telegraph. The sponsor of the resolution refused to do so, but my suggestion was based on a strategy idea which would have undercut the plans of legal abortion proponents.

While the resolution received only about 5 percent of the vote, it needed only 3 percent to automatically qualify for the next year's ballot. The defeat of the resolution was painted by advocates of legal abortion as a loss for abortion foes and left some people believing that American Telephone and Telegraph funding of Planned Parenthood would be resumed. The fact is that getting more than 10 percent of the vote on a resolution opposed by corporate leaders is almost impossible and funding was not resumed.

In 1991, American Telephone and Telegraph shareholders had two opposing resolutions to consider on the abortion issue. One was the anti-abortion resolution which had qualified to reappear on the 1991 ballot. The other was sponsored by Planned Parenthood supporters who urged that the March 1990 decision to end funding be reversed. The anti-abortion resolution failed to garner enough votes to qualify for the 1992 ballot. Like the anti-Planned Parenthood measure, the pro-Planned Parenthood resolution was opposed by American Telephone and Telegraph management. While the anti-Planned Parenthood funding resolution is dead, the pro-Planned Parenthood resolution received about 8 percent of the vote and consequently qualified to appear on the 1992 ballot. However, at the 1992 meeting, shareholders refused to require the company to restore its contribution to Planned Parenthood, but it qualified for the 1993 ballot.

Shareholders at several other corporations are expected to see similar resolutions at their respective shareholder meetings. Corporations such as Bristol-Myers Squibb have already faced such issues.

The successful effort has led several writers not associated with anti-abortion groups to mention the Project. Alan J. Miller, author of *Socially Responsible Investing*, writes about the success in dealing with the American Telephone and Telegraph Company:

> Through it all, the company held firm. Robert E. Allen, chairman and chief executive officer, explained the company's position as follows: "Much to our regret, Planned Parenthood has raised the level of their political advocacy with respect to abortion. . . . Our contribution to a specific segment of Planned Parenthood has become tainted and tarnished with a number of our constituencies because their actions were interpreted as being in favor of a pro-abortion stance. This is not an issue on which this corporation ought to come down either one way or another."

> What all of this means is that if you truly do see yourself as a socially responsible investor and you believe that generous charitable contributions by corporations are desirable, you still shouldn't just settle for investing in the stocks of those companies that contribute a lot and let it go at that. It really is incumbent upon you to try to determine *what* it is that they are contributing to, so that you can be sure that the charities being supported are ones that you want to support too.[11]

While the principle is generally true, it is particularly so for Christians. Paul McGuire, author of *Who Will Rule the Future,* writes that success can be achieved:

> Many people look at the mega-corporations and big business and throw up their hands in resignation. Some of these corporate giants are unwittingly helping to establish a New World Order. However, as the Bible tells us "giants can be slain." Christians, like their spiritual predecessor King David, can slay the "Goliaths" of our day. One person or a small group of people can change the direction of massive conglomerates.[12]

McGuire cites the Corporate Funding Project as an example.[13]

The success involving American Telephone and Telegraph was followed by several others. More importantly, state and local anti-abortion organizations began using the Project. Smaller companies have been identified and targeted on local and regional levels. Wisconsin Right to Life is one group which has taken on business donors to Planned Parenthood of Wisconsin. It has been reported that the effort has seen some success. As with the international Project, Planned Parenthood has accused Wisconsin Right to Life of using an unfair and illegitimate tactic.[14]

Local efforts are critical to the success of the Corporate Funding Project. It is not enough to end support to Planned Parenthood provided by major corporations when smaller companies are doing so. While the scope of the Project has been limited to corporations which cross state lines, a local, state, and regional attack is essential and should be a part of all groups which seek to limit Planned Parenthood's influence.

Canadian anti-abortion groups can be helpful here. Canadian divisions of corporate supporters of Planned Parenthood are claiming to be completely independent of their American counterparts. While this is doubtful—very doubtful—Canadian abortion foes can still say, "Well, that's fine, but until you convince your American counterpart to stop supporting Planned Parenthood, we cannot support you." Unfortunately, many Canadian groups have been reluctant to do so.

OFFICIAL INTERNATIONAL BOYCOTT

In August 1990, virtually every nationwide organization opposed to Planned Parenthood agreed to participate in a Washington, D.C., press conference during which the groups urged corporations to end funding of Planned Parenthood. All identified corporations had been informed that an official boycott would be announced at the press conference. On the same day, I appeared on "CBS This Morning" where the list of corporate supporters of Planned Parenthood was announced to the public. A Planned Parenthood spokesman refused to appear opposite me.

Due to efforts to end corporate support of its organization, Planned Parenthood published an article in its newspaper titled, "Public Affairs Special Report on the Opposition: Christian Action Council." The article is riddled with inaccurate information:

> Founded specifically as a counterpart to the National Right to Life Committee and the American Life League, both of which were originally Catholic organizations, the Christian Action Council is predominantly a Protestant anti-choice group. It lobbies not only against the right to abortion but also against Title X, the national family planning program.
>
> The council has about 148 state groups and a network of more than 300 crisis pregnancy centers in the United States and Canada that are now its main occupation. The first crisis pregnancy center was started in November 1980. Such centers lure unsuspecting women into their facilities by offering free pregnancy tests, counseling, and services. Once women are inside the centers, their staff members show films like "The Silent Scream," [sic] give inaccurate information about abortion procedures and services, and try to intimidate women into carrying their pregnancies to term.
>
> "Operation Nehemiah" is the network of administrators who operate the crisis pregnancy centers.[15]

The Christian Action Council was not founded "specifically as a counterpart" to any organization. In addition, in early 1992 it had approximately 100 local chapters. Additionally, the Christian Action Council has approximately 425 affiliated pregnancy counseling centers. Operation Nehemiah is its network of local chapters, not affiliated pregnancy counseling centers.

Specific mention is made of the Corporate Funding Project. "In 1988 the Christian Action Council began its campaign to boycott corporations it believes support Planned Parenthood," the newsletter reads. "It issued 'A Brief on Public Policy,' on corporate support of Planned Parenthood . . . "[16]

The boycott actually did not begin until August 1990. Furthermore, the Christian Action Council did not publish the names of corporations "it believes support Planned Parenthood." Support must be confirmed before a corporate name is published. Additional points are made in the newsletter:

> Among the council's targets was the American Telephone and Telegraph Co. (AT&T), whose foundation has provided support since 1984 to PPFA's teen pregnancy prevention program. Bowing to pressure from the CAC [Christian Action Council], Jane Redfern, senior vice president of the AT&T Foundation, sent a letter to CAC on March 13, 1990, announcing its decision to end support for Planned Parenthood.[17]

American Telephone and Telegraph had been supporting Planned Parenthood for 25 years, not simply since 1984 as the article implies. The company was never the "target" of a boycott because it changed its philanthropic practice five months before a boycott was instituted. The media helped Planned Parenthood spread this inaccuracy by writing that American Telephone and Telegraph ended support of Planned Parenthood because the company was "facing a threatened boycott."[18]

The press conference announcing the boycott is mentioned in the Planned Parenthood newsletter:

> On Aug. 8, 1990, CAC held a press conference to announce a listing of corporations it believes support Planned Parenthood and to target another major international corporation, American Express, for increased attention. At the press conference, other national anti-choice organization leaders announced support of the CAC campaign.[19]

The Planned Parenthood article also lists the old address of the Christian Action Council, out-of-print publications, and some projects of the organization are listed as "Affiliated Groups."[20] The National Abortion Rights Action League and several other groups supporting the Planned Parenthood agenda also published articles regarding the boycott.

Planned Parenthood adopted an interesting strategy which consisted of getting an unchallenged point of view in front of the public. In April 1990, Faye Wattleton of Planned Parenthood and Marilyn Laurie of the American Telephone and Telegraph Foundation had to be interviewed separately on a network morning news program. In late 1990, WWOR, a television station based in New York City and carried by many cable companies nationwide, attempted to set up a debate between me and a Planned Parenthood spokesman. WWOR asked Planned Parenthood officials at the national and affiliate levels to appear but they all refused. Not wanting to feature the anti-Planned Parenthood side alone, the plans were scrapped. Planned Parenthood officials agreed to be interviewed on the matter, but not with someone from the opposing side present.

The Dayton Hudson Corporation, which announced it would end support of Planned Parenthood, soon reversed its decision. The reversal came because the leadership consists of strong supporters of Planned Parenthood, though they claimed public pressure was involved. It is believed the decision to end funding may have been a ruse in an effort to convince some corporations which had ended funding to reverse their decisions as well. Like Dayton Hudson officials, Faye Wattleton claimed the reversal was based on large numbers of people who had protested the decision:

> Well, I think there was just overwhelming public outrage. People were returning merchandise, I understand, they were cutting up their credit cards—it was an economic decision. . . . And I think that they came to see that there was much broader and greater support that was willing to express rage for the work that Planned Parenthood has been doing than against what we are doing.[21]

The *Wall Street Journal* reports that a favorite cause of the "upper-class" spouses of corporate leaders is Planned Parenthood. "It's amazing how few of them are conservatives," says George Gilder, who wrote an introductory essay to 1991's "Forbes 400" list.[22] This has led to great support for Planned Parenthood through the corporate structure.

BOYCOTT HIGHLIGHT

It was announced at the press conference that all corporations listed would be boycotted. However, the American Express Company was highlighted due to its consistent giving pattern.

This action, too, was addressed on the floor of the United States House of Representatives. Congressman Robert K. Dornan, R-California, said, "Mr. Speaker, my American Express card grows radioactive in my pocket as it does every time I read that they give money to Planned Parenthood."[23] American Express has expressed some concern. The company is responding:

> Amex [American Express], which admits to receiving "several thousand letters from concerned card members and clients," is worried about CAC's [Christian Action Council's] efforts, which included getting "Christian owned-and-operating companies" to *refuse to honor the Amex credit card* (and those of other financial powers which fund Planned Parenthood.) The company's managers and "800" phone operators have been briefed on how to answer [pro-lifers and "downplay"] CAC-generated complaints about the Planned Parenthood funding policy.[24]

DIFFERING STRATEGIES

While the Christian Action Council had been the recognized leader in fighting corporate support of Planned Parenthood, the American Telephone and Telegraph success led other anti-Planned Parenthood groups, some of which had called the Project a "waste of time," to take an interest, particularly when it made headlines. *Newsday* printed an article titled, "Companies in Abortion Crossfire." The article points to differences in strategy emerging from the various groups.[25]

With the number of groups involved in the Corporate Funding Project rapidly expanding, disagreements have emerged regarding how to proceed. Some want to extend boycotts to those corporations which advertise on abortion-related television programs. Some want to target one or two particular corporations for a major boycott. Some believe the economic boycott can be an effective tool used against offending corporations. Others believe it will have limited economic impact and, therefore, is more of a symbolic and moral action. In an effort to avoid problems which would arise from changing its approach, the Christian Action Council continued to exercise control over the Project while accepting the suggestions of other groups. Nevertheless, some groups decided to go their own way.

One large anti-abortion group was hesitant to endorse the Corporate Funding Project. Its leader at the time argued that one product of one subsidiary of one corporate supporter of Planned Parenthood should be selected for a boycott. He contended that this approach would allow other corporations to see what could be done by abortion foes who boycott a product. This approach was given serious consideration, but rejected for three reasons: 1) Why should the other offending corporations be left unchallenged?; 2) What if the "wrong" corporation were selected and the company never changed its philanthropic practices? How would that look to the other corporations?; and 3) How could anyone argue with success?

The organization's leader eventually agreed to endorse a boycott of American Express, but not the entire list. The group's newsletter called for a boycott of American Express but ignored, and continues to ignore, the rest of the Project. After being forced to leave the group, the anti-abortion leader met with me to discuss the Project in greater detail, asking for the first time how the effort had been managed. He inquired as to the steps used in identifying corporate supporters of Planned Parenthood and suggested that his new organization would be good for expanding and managing the boycott. He continues, however, to cling to the different strategy. In addition, he wishes to take what seems to be a "we were just kidding about that anti-boycott stuff before, but now we're serious" approach. Ordinarily, this alternate approach would not have potentially serious consequences, but another anti-abortion leader, in an attempt to get control over the Project, could severely weaken its impact.

At the other extreme, the Saint Antoninus Institute insists that offending corporate chief executive officers sign its "Pro-Life Principles of Corporate Conduct" before dropping a company from the boycott list. The principle includes one provision with which I could not agree:

> Should the corporation, or the corporation-sponsored foundation, have funded such organizations in the past, whether knowingly or not, its chief administrator will donate corporate funds, in the amount of the total sum of the different previous donations to pro-abortion organizations (in constant dollars), to any legitimate pro-life organizations of his choice. A pro-life organization is to be construed as an organization whose prime objective is the furtherance of the pro-life cause, the abolition of abortions and the assistance to victims and potential victims of abortions.[26]

This "principle" is to be in addition to a requirement that the chief executive officer not fund abortion advocacy organizations in the future and that current commitment to these organizations cease. The chief executive officer is required to sign the "pro-life principles of corporate conduct."

It seems that a corporate chief executive officer will *never* agree to sign such a statement and will absolutely *never* agree to pay reparations for past philanthropic practices. To do so would, in some cases, amount to more than one million dollars—a high price to pay. Moreover, requiring restitution could be seen as a form of extortion. It may not constitute extortion from a legal perspective, but it may from a moral one. It is more important to get corporations to stop doing evil. Getting them to make up for it might be a little too much to expect chief executive officers to swallow.

BOYCOTT EFFICACY

Do boycotts really work? Is an economic boycott an appropriate way to impact philanthropic policy? The answers depend on whom you ask. Call for a boycott against something we care about and you are a terrorist. Call for a boycott against something we loathe and you are behaving in the tradition of Martin Luther King, Jr., and Caesar Chavez.

The economic boycott has been utilized by many kinds of groups, most of which have been on the left of the political spectrum. Recent use by groups such as the American Life League, the American Family Association, and Christian Leaders for Responsible Television have demonstrated a willingness by those considered to be on the right to take a page out of the "how to impact policy" strategy of those considered to be on the left.

The Green Consumer Supermarket Guide, which endorses purchasing products which are environmentally friendly, takes a strong position on the question of the effectiveness of economic boycotts:

> Let's start with the basics: Every time you open your wallet, you cast a vote "for" or "against" the environment.
>
> This is more powerful than you might imagine. First and foremost, the marketplace—whether the supermarket, hardware store, or appliance showroom—is not a democracy. It doesn't take 51 percent of people "voting" in any one direction to affect environmental

change. Far from it. In fact, a relative handful of shoppers can send shock waves through an industry simply by making good, "green" choices.[27]

The author of the *Guide* notes that consumer pressure was the primary factor convincing three major corporations to sell only "dolphin-safe" tuna. When tuna company executives announced the policy shift in April 1990, they did not say it was being done because of a concern for the environment or dolphins. They attributed the decision to "consumer pressure":

> What's amazing about this is that it was a relatively small number of consumers who were "pressuring" the tuna companies—probably less than a million active individuals, according to some reports. That's less than 1 percent of the American marketplace. In fact, during the twelve months preceding the tuna companies' announcement, tuna sales had barely changed. As so the "votes" of a very small number of individuals revolutionized an entire industry.[28]

According to the *Guide*, consumer pressure also convinced McDonald's to use paper rather than polystyrene foam hamburger boxes. In fact, sales of McDonald's products had been rising before the announcement was made. The president of McDonald's did not say the company's decision was made because there was something wrong with using the boxes, but because McDonald's customers just did not "feel good" about using them.[29]

The *NonProfit Times* cites a public opinion poll conducted by the Barna Research Group of Glendale, California. According to the survey, 67 percent of the American people *disagree* with the statement that boycotts "don't really accomplish anything." Only 30 percent believe boycotts are ineffective while 3 percent are not sure. Barna Research Group estimates that 25 million Americans had boycotted something in the month preceding the survey.[30]

Even the rabid National Abortion Rights Action League refers to the Corporate Funding Project as "marginally successful."[31] This is actually a telling statement when one considers its source. *NARAL News* printed the list of corporations and asked its supporters to do what they can to counter the Project.[32]

It is clear that the Corporate Funding Project will have a limited impact on Planned Parenthood's nearly $400 million annual budget. However, it is not just about money. It is about moral involvement with the abortion industry. Every time a company ends its support for Planned Parenthood, it represents a relatively small loss of dollars to the group but a big slap in the pubic image. When Pioneer Hi-Bred International withdrew its funding from Planned Parenthood, Jill June, director of Planned Parenthood of Greater Iowa, demonstrated her understanding of the real impact the Project can have on her group. "It's beyond monetary value," June said, "it's much greater than that."[33]

EXTORTION?

Other corporate officials desire to end support of Planned Parenthood, but they have expressed fear of retaliation by Planned Parenthood. The *Chronicle of Philanthropy* reports that, "Some grant makers who are anxious to end their long-time support for Planned Parenthood say they fear reprisals if they do so."[34] The newspaper quotes a corporate leader:

For us to publicly withdraw our support from Planned Parenthood at this point would be suicide. If we make a mistake, we're going to rise into the sights of Faye's [Wattleton's] 48-inch guns. She will use AT&T mercilessly. We can't be next. We'd be in a worse position.[35]

Another grant-maker told the newspaper:

None of us can afford what Planned Parenthood is going to do to us [if funding is withdrawn]. The worst of all things is to antagonize them. I don't know how much heat our business people can take. Faye [Wattleton] has maneuvered beautifully to take advantage of our moral cowardice.[36]

The National Organization for Women launched a boycott against a national pizza chain because the company's chief executive donated to an anti-abortion-funding campaign in Michigan.[37] Some of the groups opposing Planned Parenthood funding have cried foul because the donated funds were not pizza company dollars. Companies cited by those groups opposed to Planned Parenthood are only targeted if corporate funds are donated.

A CHANGE IN MANAGEMENT

The Christian Action Council expressed a desire to "wind down" the Corporate Funding Project. This essentially means the organization no longer wants to make it a primary project. The Project is now managed by Life Decisions International, based in Amherst, New York.

The primary goal of Life Decisions International is to decrease the influence Planned Parenthood now enjoys throughout the world. This includes not only opposing its funding but also its controversial programs. The organization has developed brochures and other helpful literature on Planned Parenthood.

Life Decisions International has several seasoned and well-respected board members including George Grant, Jim Sedlak, Joseph R. Stanton, M.D., Michael Schwartz, Thomas L. Jipping, J.D., Molly Kelly, Cindi LoForti, and Robert McFadden. More importantly, board members also include individuals whose names are not as widely known but whose work is making a difference.

SUPPORT V. OPPOSITION

While the vast majority of dedicated and far-thinking anti-abortion activists see the wisdom and strategic importance of the Corporate Funding Project, there are a few who not only do not support it, but are doing what they can to undermine it. While I believe these attacks to be more personally motivated than reflective of philosophical or strategic concerns, the fact remains that such efforts and statements could seriously harm the Project.

One individual, who works for an anti-abortion organization that publicly endorses the Project, went so far as to avoid using one boycotted item while having lunch with an important avid supporter of the Project. On other occasions, when not in the presence of such an individual, he routinely ignores the boycott. In addition, he has attacked the Project both in written and oral communications.

Such actions, I believe, are driven by ego or animosity rather than good judgment and godly wisdom. Whatever their basis, they could seriously harm the Project. Only Planned Parenthood would be served in the long run. Naturally, when criticism is not based on an effort to protect those not yet born, they can only be called ungodly.

One of the most difficult parts of the Corporate Funding Project has been convincing some Christian radio stations to participate. Christian radio station owners had never been asked to refuse advertising of corporations which support Planned Parenthood. However, when an internationally popular weight loss program was added to the boycott list, a problem developed. Christian radio personalities had personally endorsed the weight loss program. The company relies heavily on such personal endorsements.

Several Christian radio personalities, including Neil Boron then-of WDCX in Buffalo, New York, and Al Krestsa of WMUZ in Detroit, among others, refused to endorse the company's weight loss program. Many people urged owners of Christian radio stations to refuse to accept the advertisements but they met considerable resistance. One radio station simply asked employees with weaker or no opinions on abortion to do the advertisements.

The greatest problem was with Donald Crawford of Crawford Broadcasting Company. Crawford claims to be anti-abortion but he refused to cooperate. Project organizers were left with the impression that the stations are businesses first and ministry-oriented second.

While a handful of people are doing what they can to draw attention to their *personal* projects, apparently believing it is necessary to diminish fervor for the Project in order to be personally successful, virtually all others have come out strongly in favor of it. George Grant, who arguably knows more about Planned Parenthood than any man alive, outside of those in the organization, writes, "I am an enthusiastic supporter of the boycott . . ."[38]

When asked to endorse the Project, the Rev. Olga Fairfax, Ph.D., leader of Methodists for Life, wrote, "Absolutely! Thank-you!"[39] American Family Association's president, the Rev. Donald E. Wildmon, writes, "Keep fighting!"[40]

Earl W. Essex, Esq., executive director of Defenders of Life, writes, "Planned Parenthood is a 'kingpin' in the 'evil empire' of Satan functioning in our world today. . . . We will gladly use our resources and contacts to promote the boycott . . ."[41] Ralph Reed, Jr., executive director of the Christian Coalition, writes, "Best of luck on the ongoing boycott effort . . . "[42]

Gregg Cunningham, leader of the Center for Bio-Ethical Reform and maker of the pro-life seminar/videos titled *No More Excuses*, mentions the Project in his video series:

> There have been books written aplenty about the sorts of activities you can become involved with—letter-writing activities and all that sort of stuff. One thing that hasn't been discussed very much that I think is going to play an ever more important role is the economic boycott and I'd like to talk about economic boycotts in a couple of ways that you're not likely to hear other people discussing. . . . *Every* church should be distributing that [boycott] list and encouraging people in the church to not patronize the companies that support Planned Parenthood. This list is readily available and it's a wonderful activity. It's passive, it's non-threatening and it's very good.[43]

Judie Brown of the American Life League has also enthusiastically endorsed the Project and has been helpful in spreading information about it.

The following is a partial list of nationwide or international Canadian and American organizations that have endorsed the boycott of all corporate supporters of Planned Parenthood: Ad Hoc Committee in Defense of Life, Advocates for Life Ministries, Alliance for Life (Canada), American Coalition for Life, American Collegians for Life, American Family Association, American Life League, Americans United for Life, Bernadell, Brokers for Life, Campaign Life (Canada), Catholic League, Center for Bio-Ethical Reform, Christian Action Council, Christian Coalition, Christians for Life (Canada), Coalitions for America (associated with the Free Congress Foundation), Concerned Women for America, Defenders of Life, Eagle Forum, Family Research Council (associated with Focus on the Family), Feminists for Life, Human Life International, Legacy Communications, LifeNet International, Lutherans for Life, Methodists for Life, National Association of Evangelicals, National Conservative Political Action Committee, Pro-Life Action League, Public Advocate, Saint Antoninus Institute, Stop Planned Parenthood, and the Traditional Values Coalition.

Teaching Home, a magazine for parents who operate home schools, has been extremely helpful in spreading the word about the Project. It published a card listing the corporations and included it in the magazine. The response has been tremendous. I have always suspected that home schoolers are pro-family, but I had no idea they were so activist-oriented.

COMMITMENT

The pro-life movement will succeed only to the extent that pro-life people are willing to be inconvenienced. In fact, I have not even considered the Project to be much of an inconvenience. It is a matter of the heart and the will. I believe excuses for ignoring the Project are either based on ignorance of economic boycotts or reflective of the degree of commitment of the person using the excuse.

In a September/October 1990 newsletter, the Christian Action Council writes:

> We believe the boycott should last as long as corporations are supporting PP [Planned Parenthood]. If this takes until Judgment Day, so be it. Corporate leaders are hoping we will eventually get tired, bored and give up. They are wrong. Even if no other corporations change their policies and they continue to support PP, at least they will do so without pro-lifers contributing to it.[44]

One editorial on the issue was printed in the newsletter of a local anti-abortion organization:

> I do not think it unreasonable to expect pro-life Christians to educate themselves and to deny themselves products and/or services whose purchase aids in financial contribution to Planned Parenthood. Patronage (buying the products or services) of corporations that support Planned Parenthood enables them to continue their support. Planned Parenthood's programs are anti-family and anti-child. They serve to disrupt parent-child relationships.[45]

Patricia Bainbridge, author of the commentary, refers to specific types of products:

Are you willing to be inconvenienced by finding substitute services and p *are* other ketchups . . . but even if there weren't, do you want to help . . . su Parenthood? Are you willing to deny yourself and/or your family members ce services, and/or restaurants that you "like," or "have a coupon for" or "are ju corner" or "are the only cereals or *(fill in the product)* that my kids like?" . . . [hamburger] is, in my husband's opinion, the "*best!*" But . . . we refuse to eat . . . [the] establishment until the parent company . . . stops contributing to Planned Parenthood.[46]

The author suggests that those opposed to abortion must compare this position with their lifestyle:

Do the excuses you offer for not familiarizing yourself with the boycott list and not purchasing the products/services listed, accurately reflect your pro-life stance?

James 4:17 says: "Anyone, then, who knows the good he ought to do and doesn't do it, sins." I pray that you will give serious prayer and thoughtful consideration to what I have shared. God Bless You![47]

It seems as though I have received hundreds of letters regarding the Corporate Funding Project. Most request additional information and seek advice on how to do a better job urging corporations to stop supporting Planned Parenthood. While many people seem to have a different opinion as to how the Project should be managed and while some believe it is their duty to tell me what a waste of time they believe the effort is, I occasionally receive letters that make the criticism and destructive comments diminish in their importance:

[R]egarding the writing of my second letter to each corporation, I handwrote the first letter, having been advised that a handwritten letter gets prompt attention and is often seen by the CEO [chief executive officer] of the company rather than being handled by a less significant department. However, I have sustained nerve damage in my right hand and it takes me two hours to handwrite a two page letter. Based on your vast experience in dealing with these corporations . . . , do you feel a second letter from me, typed, might get less attention and have less of an impact on the company? If a typed letter will have little effect on the company, I will handwrite them. I feel I could send letters on a more regular basis . . . if I could type them . . . I am at present writing to 10 corporations asking them to reconsider contributing to PP [Planned Parenthood].[48]

Another letter also shows great dedication:

I have not found it easy [to boycott the products] . . . I personally love . . . [two restaurants on the list]. However, I love children more.

Thank you for this opportunity to make a difference.[49]

One word comes to mind when I read these letters: commitment.

In August 1990, David J. Andrews, executive vice president of the Planned Parenthood Federation of America, said he did not believe many corporations would end support of his organization.[50] Despite Andrews' prediction, 22 major corporations had permanently ended support of Planned Parenthood as of March 1992. This number does not account for those which have ended support without announcing that Planned Parenthood will receive no future funding, nor does it include corporations which will never start supporting the group because of the controversy. Life Decisions International has agreed to keep the list of 22 corporations confidential so they will not become targets of a Planned Parenthood advertising campaign or boycott.

Consider the commitment of those who are involved in boycotts for other causes. Queer Nation, a militant homosexual rights organization, has organized a boycott against Cracker Barrel restaurants because of their policy against hiring ıomosexuals. Barbara Walters, of ABC's, "20/20" said of the effort, "I, however, think I might be able to find another restaurant to go to if I were in that area." Tom Jarriel, a "20/20" correspondent, responded, "As a consumer that is certainly your right."[51] If abortion foes were as committed to their cause as other groups, things would change even more rapidly.

The Corporate Funding Project should continue as long as it takes to achieve the goal: ending corporate involvement with Planned Parenthood. Leaders of Planned Parenthood predict their opponents will eventually grow weary of the boycott and call it off. They must be shown that abortion foes are committed to do what it takes to end abortion and Planned Parenthood's role in it.

There is one other aspect of this Project which opponents of abortion should consider. No corporate leader wants picketers outside his or her place of business with signs reading, "This establishment supports abortion providers so please don't support it!" If picketing is used along with the boycott and the introduction of stockholder resolutions, it is just a matter of time before the battle will be won.

While this Project has seen considerable success, there are still many active abortion foes who really do not care what they buy. As dedicated as they seem to be, many who are involved in civil disobedience are among the biggest patronizers of corporate supporters of Planned Parenthood. This Project calls for a private, moral witness against abortion. Acts of civil disobedience call for a public witness and for all the burden such activity brings, it also brings praise from others. Boycotting corporations does not do so. It requires everyone to do so because it is the right thing to do, not because it will make the evening news or participants will be given recognition or thanked by others. Food for thought.

14

A PROJECT OF GOLIATH

The boycott of corporate supporters of Planned Parenthood followed a project initiated by the Planned Parenthood Federation of America to discredit pregnancy counseling centers. Joined by several other organizations which support legal abortion, the effort is designed to "expose" the "bogus abortion clinics."

Planned Parenthood charges that pregnancy counseling centers, which offer free services to women facing an untimely pregnancy, masquerade as abortion clinics in order to lure women into their centers. Once inside, women are allegedly verbally and emotionally abused, threatened, and even physically restrained.

The campaign to "expose" pregnancy counseling centers did not begin by accident. It was not the result of "investigative journalism." It was not the result of law enforcement efforts.

MAKINGS OF A CONTROVERSY

A January 22, 1987, Planned Parenthood Federation of America news release created a new front in the abortion battle as it issued a statement made by Faye Wattleton, then-president of the organization:

> On this day, 14 years ago, the right of every American woman to receive a safe and legal abortion was resoundingly confirmed by the U.S. Supreme Court's 7-2 vote.
>
> Although, throughout the past 14 years, we have seen extremists who have tried to construct barriers to that right or eradicate it completely, they have failed dismally because the right to privacy is one which Americans hold as inalienable.
>
> In their frustration, however, these extremists have sunk to new depths in an effort to harass and punish women who seek abortion services. They have resorted to intimidation and even violence to inflict their own views on an unwilling America. The latest effort in their campaign of deception is the creation of anti-abortion counseling centers, many of which appear to offer abortion services, but actually lure unsuspecting pregnant women into their clutches under false pretenses. . . .
>
> These centers, for the most part, exist only to inflict upon very vulnerable women their own views of morality and religion and to harass women who seek abortion as their legal alternative.[1]

In conjunction with the National Abortion Federation, the Planned Parenthood Federation of America published a document (and now a brochure) titled, "A Consumer's Alert to Deception, Harassment and Medical Malpractice":

> In their zeal to stop women from having abortions, anti-abortion activists have set up "counseling centers" in hundreds of communities around the country. Far from true coun-

> seling, these centers are designed to misinform and intimidate women—some will go to any lengths necessary to dissuade women from ending their pregnancies.
>
> Increasingly, women complain about their unwitting encounters with anti-abortion centers. Women describe being harassed, intimidated, and given blatantly false information. They complain that confidential information they provided was used against them. In some cases, they describe instances of medical malpractice which threatened their lives.[2]

Included in the document is a section called, "How to Recognize Anti-Abortion Counseling Centers." Characteristics of such centers allegedly include: 1) falsely suggesting or promising a full range of reproductive health services; 2) offering free pregnancy tests but giving ambiguous answers about the results; 3) showing shocking and deceptive films or slide shows; 4) attempting to induce guilt by engaging women in discussions about their religious views and beliefs; 5) refusing or failing to provide contraceptive information; and 6) making exaggerated promises.[3]

A warning is given to the reader of the document:

> Caution: if you find that the facility from which you have sought help is actually an anti-abortion facility, protect yourself from further harassment. Leave the premises immediately and do not return. When you do locate a professional clinic or counseling center that offers all available alternatives, you may find it helpful to share those experiences with your new counselor so that whatever distortions and misinformation you may have received can be corrected.[4]

Guidelines are offered for finding "professional pregnancy counseling centers." They include: 1) selecting clinics and pregnancy counseling centers that have clearly established reputations; 2) selecting clinics that provide a full range of contraceptive alternatives; and 3) selecting clinics that have or are supervised by physicians, nurse practitioners, or other licensed health professionals.[5]

The campaign against pregnancy counseling centers, which educate women about abortion and fetal development, provide support, free clothing, baby products, referrals for medical care and other services, was kicked off by Faye Wattleton at a January 1987 press conference. A list of pregnancy counseling centers from around the country was published. In order to avoid a lawsuit, a disclaimer is included:

> The facilities on this list have been reported to us as providing anti-abortion counseling and failing to provide counseling or information as to where and how abortions may be obtained. Inclusion on this list is not a representation that a facility has engaged in any particular deceptive practice. This is not a complete list and the fact that any facility is not mentioned should not be regarded as an indication of approval.[6]

LOCAL ATTACKS

One of the primary aspects of Planned Parenthood's project has been to concentrate on a local approach. Its affiliates and other local groups supportive of legal abortion have been urged to generate press by attacking pregnancy counseling centers at the local level. One victim of the Planned Parenthood effort was the Crisis Pregnancy Center of King County (Washington). Participating in the Planned Parenthood Federation of America campaign was its Seattle-King County affiliate.

The public broadcasting television station in Seattle, KCTS, aired a program on January 22, 1987, called "NightSight." The program is a live news magazine which includes some pre-recorded material. The lead story was introduced as relating to the anniversary of *Roe v. Wade*. However, a story on *Roe* is not what followed.

"NightSight" was hosted by Leila Gorbman and Victoria Fong. Consider the opening statements of the program:

Gorbman: "Today marks the anniversary of *Roe v. Wade*, the historic Supreme Court decision that legalized abortion 14 years ago. Despite the passage of time, the clash over the issue of abortion is still as heated as ever."[7]

Fong: "The newest wrinkle in the conflict is the growing number of so-called fake abortion clinics. In their advertising these clinics appear to offer abortion services, but critics say they do just the opposite. They pressure women to decide against abortion."[8]

Gorbman: "Last October, one such clinic in Texas was fined $39,000 for deceptive trade practices. Because of that decision and because of lawsuits filed against clinics in other states, local anti-abortion clinics have toned down their approach. But as Victoria reports, the pro-life clinics are still stirring up controversy."[9]

The program switched to a pre-recorded report prepared by Fong. Interviewed for the report were the directors of two pregnancy counseling centers; Ric Woodrow, executive director of the now defunct Life Amendment Political Action Committee; Marcy Bloom, an activist with the National Abortion Rights Action League; and Jennifer Carl, M.D., an abortionist.[10]

The pre-recorded segment was followed by a live debate between Lee Minto, then-executive director of Planned Parenthood for Seattle-King County, and myself, then-executive director of HUMAN LIFE, Washington state's largest anti-abortion organization. The first question was to addressed to me. "Doug, the right to lie. Is that really what's at issue here?"[11]

Crisis Pregnancy Center leaders attacked the program as biased, especially the pre-recorded segment. KCTS defended the program and called it fair despite several problems that were brought to the attention of station executives:

1. Ric Woodrow is not an authorized spokesman for the Crisis Pregnancy Centers targeted in the report. A statement made in the program that the Centers are partially funded by the Life Amendment Political Action Committee is completely untrue.[12] This information was gathered with little research. KCTS said it relied on Woodrow's word. Crisis Pregnancy Center leaders were not told that Woodrow was interviewed. Consequently, Center officials could not inquire as to why Woodrow was interviewed and what he had said. Some accuse Woodrow of misrepresenting himself and blame KCTS for not checking into this more deeply. Some Crisis Pregnancy Center supporters believe KCTS kept the Woodrow interview a secret because of the kinds of statements he made—most of which would not be supported by the Center leaders.
2. The activist roles Marcy Bloom and Jennifer Carl play in the pro-legal abortion movement were never clearly outlined. KCTS portrayed them as neutral rather than avid supporters of legal abortion. Bloom was identified in the report as an "abortion counselor." Carl was identified as a "pro-choice

physician."[13] In addition, nothing was said of their financial interest in abortion.

3. Some crisis pregnancy centers nationwide are listed under "Abortion Services" or "Birth Control." While one Crisis Pregnancy Center in Thurston County, Washington, had apparently been listed in the yellow pages under "Abortion Services," KCTS failed to research the reason(s) for the listing. The telephone company placed the Crisis Pregnancy Center under "Abortion Services" without consulting the Center. The yellow pages did not carry a category appropriate to crisis pregnancy centers so the advertisement was placed where yellow pages officials thought most appropriate. Some telephone book companies now list "Abortion Alternatives" as a separate category.

   The same issue became a problem for Arizona Right to Life, which is not a crisis pregnancy center. Arizona Right to Life was listed under "Birth Control." Having had the experience in Seattle, I specifically asked that we not be listed under that category. We were listed there anyway because, as the telephone company employee explained, it was the "most appropriate" category available.

4. Crisis Pregnancy Center officials informed KCTS executives that the entire nature of the Fong report was biased. This was true in the editing as well as the comments made by Fong. Fong was clearly taking a side. After a Crisis Pregnancy Center official said the centers were neutral, Fong made the statement, "Most anti-abortion clinics can hardly be called neutral . . ."[14] This is simply editorializing. Similar comments were made throughout the report.

5. Victoria Fong interviewed Les Newton, M.D., an opponent of abortion. Crisis Pregnancy Center officials agreed to participate in the program only after they learned Newton had been interviewed. However, his interview was not used in the report. Instead the Woodrow interview was aired.

Despite these clearly documentable facts, KCTS avidly defended its reporters and the job they had done.

MEDIA/ABORTION-PROVIDER CONSPIRACY?

Media participation in the campaign against pregnancy counseling centers is evident nationwide. A study by Marvin N. Olasky, Ph.D., journalism professor at the University of Texas at Austin, documents that this campaign is no coincidence. The Olasky study documents the conspiracy between Planned Parenthood, the Religious Coalition for Abortion Rights, and the Reproductive Freedom Project of the American Civil Liberties Union.[15]

The American Civil Liberties Union Foundation's Reproductive Freedom Project publishes a booklet called *Women's Legal Guide to Reproductive Rights*. It is noted that the booklet will appear as a chapter in the American Civil Liberties

Union's handbook called *The Rights of Women*. The printing of the booklet was donated by the Playboy Foundation.[16] Do American Civil Liberties Union officials consider Playboy to be a strong supporter of the rights of women?

Olasky notes that Amy Sutnick, public information associate for Planned Parenthood of New York City, spent about 1,000 hours with a single purpose—creating a negative image of pregnancy counseling centers. To do this, she convinced a *New York Daily News* reporter who supports legal abortion to run a story based on information provided by Sutnick. Once the story appeared, Sutnick sent the article to other reporters, along with a media packet, to prompt the writing of more articles.[17]

Evidence has mounted which indicates that the attacks on pregnancy counseling centers are based on the actions of those operated by the Pearson Foundation, a Missouri-based anti-abortion group now believed to be effectively defunct.[18] Centers associated with the Pearson Foundation do not oppose the use of deception if it results in saving the life of an unborn human being. Officials of the group have been almost unanimously shunned as an illegitimate organization by other anti-abortion leaders, both Christian and non-Christian alike. They represent less than 5 percent of all pregnancy counseling centers nationwide. Nevertheless, all centers are lumped together by the media, even though most had issued statements saying women should always be told the truth.

USA Today writer Marlene Perrin contacted leaders of pregnancy counseling centers opposed to deception. However, when she heard from women who claim to have been clients at one pregnancy counseling center, Perrin decided she did not believe center leaders were telling the truth. Consequently, Perrin refused to include comments of center leaders in the story. The women who claim to have gone to pregnancy counseling centers were supplied by Planned Parenthood.[19]

It soon became clear that the unwarranted attacks on pregnancy counseling centers would pay off. Many centers reported a temporary drop in clientele and financial resources. Even some strong Christians who had supported pregnancy counseling center efforts ended their backing because they believed media reports.[20]

It has been shown that the media attacks on pregnancy counseling centers are a well-planned, well-coordinated effort. Several groups supportive of legal abortion simply conspired with many legal abortion supporters in the media to do a slash job on pregnancy counseling centers.[21] Why? Pregnancy counseling centers take business (profits) away from these groups.

Olasky points out the unethical practices in what took place. He also notes that the pregnancy counseling centers, which operate largely with volunteer staffs and on low budgets, were assailed by groups that can afford to put millions of dollars into a campaign to discredit them. Against such odds, fighting back is difficult.[22] This is especially true when the media, the self-described "investigative reporters," choose to narrow the investigation and report only what they want the public to know.

ADVERTISING CAMPAIGN

Planned Parenthood has stepped up its attacks on abortion opponents as well as centers assisting women faced with untimely pregnancies. As part of their, "Don't

Wait Until Women Are Dying Again," advertising series, Planned Parenthood again lumps all pregnancy counseling centers together. The full-page advertisement is headlined, "Would You Lie to a Pregnant Teenager?" It attacks center counseling by claiming women are shown frightening and untruthful films.[23] (See Appendix C for an analysis of selected Planned Parenthood *Time* advertisements.)

Centers that assist women come under many names, including Crisis Pregnancy Center, Problem Pregnancy Center, Aid to Women, Birthright, Alternatives to Abortion, Pregnancy Counseling Center, and so on. Many are independent organizations with standards of operation varying from center to center. Others are affiliated with national organizations such as Alternatives to Abortion International, the Christian Action Council, Birthright International, and Save-A-Life. The standards applied to local pregnancy counseling centers by national organizations also vary.

Birthright International has more than 650 centers worldwide. It reports it has never put a girl into a room to watch anything more than a film on fetal development which is a film produced by scientists, not abortion foes.

Denise Cocciolone, former national director of Birthright USA, says Planned Parenthood takes the actions of one individual, as noted in the advertisement, and tries to argue that all pregnancy counseling centers are the same. "All we do is tell them the truth. No audio visuals or pictures are used except for *Window to the Womb*," Cocciolone states.[24]

Birthright offers women information on fetal development, a place to stay, medical care, legal assistance, professional psychological counseling, clothing, materials for the baby, and referrals to agencies of the woman's choosing if she decided on adoption. Some services are provided by the Birthright staff while others are referred out. "We're here to show the woman that somebody cares," Cocciolone says. "We're giving them a real choice. If she chooses abortion, we give her literature on abortion and fetal development and we ask her to read the literature before making a final decision." Photographs of aborted human beings are given only to the women who say they are going to have an abortion and are leaving the center. "It is given as a last resort," Cocciolone states.[25]

Alternatives to Abortion International has hundreds of loosely affiliated centers, none of which use "graphic" films. The international organization serves more as a clearinghouse of what almost amounts to independent pregnancy counseling centers.[26]

The Christian Action Council has approximately 425 affiliated pregnancy counseling centers in the United States and Canada. It has standards for honesty and care as detailed in its "Crisis Pregnancy Center Statement of Principle":

> The CPC [Crisis Pregnancy Center] is committed to providing its clients with accurate and complete information about both prenatal development and abortion. The CPC is committed to integrity in dealing with clients earning their trust and providing promised information and services. The CPC denounces any form of deception in its corporate advertising or individual conversations with its clients.
>
> The CPC is committed to assisting women to carry to term by providing emotional support and practical assistance . . . The CPC does not discriminate in providing services because of race, creed, color, national origin, age, or marital status of its clients . . . The CPC offers assistance free of charge at all times . . .
>
> The CPC recognizes the validity of adoption as one alternative to abortion, but is not biased toward adoption when compared to the other life-saving alternatives. Centers are

> independent of adoption agencies, relating to them in the same manner as to other helpful referral sources. CPCs receive no payment of any kind from these agencies, do not enter into contractual relationships with them, and do not share combined office space. CPCs neither initiate nor facilitate independent adoptions, though they may refer for independent adoptions in states where it is legal.[27]

Despite the attempts of the vast majority of pregnancy counseling centers to remain honest and professional, Planned Parenthood attacks have only increased. It seems the attacks are really based on the fact that such centers are taking business away from Planned Parenthood.

"Honesty is more than the best policy," says Harriet R. T. Lewis, vice president for pregnancy counseling center ministries at the Christian Action Council. "By being honest with our clients from the beginning we demonstrate that we are trustworthy. The relationship between the crisis pregnancy center volunteer counselor and client must be founded on trust if it is to be effective." Lewis argues that those who practice deception "under the guise of rendering helpful services" are, in reality, "deceiving themselves."[28]

The tie between pregnancy counseling centers is often in name only. In some cases, those belonging to a parent organization have nothing more than a clearinghouse for information with no policy-making powers. Planned Parenthood, on the other hand, is a closely knit group with strong ties which are based on specific national and international standards.

Lewis argues it is the pregnancy counseling center movement that is offering women a real choice and that it is not the centers which are the true deceivers:

> Abortionists, who have never provided the breadth of services available to clients through crisis pregnancy centers, have consistently tried to distance themselves from the most radical wings of their industry. Yet many find it acceptable to stereotype those who give abortion alternative services. The use of broad generalizations in publicly expressed rhetoric has the potential of being financially advantageous. By creating popular distrust of those who render abortion alternatives without cost, the abortion industry promotes itself as the only "safe" refuge for those in need. How much more deceptive can you get?[29]

One argument used against pregnancy counseling centers affiliated with the Christian Action Council is that counselors are encouraged to share the Gospel with clients. It is true that evangelism is encouraged, but only when the woman allows the counselor to do so. Christian Action Council officials feel that while their primary and immediate role is to assist the woman facing an untimely pregnancy, it would be a shame not to share the Word of God which leads to a change in lifestyle and, most importantly, acceptance into the Kingdom of God.

While Planned Parenthood officials approve of the activities of religious people who will help further their agenda, they apparently oppose those who actually put biblical principles into practice. To some Planned Parenthood leaders, it appears that evangelism is the worst thing happening at the centers. Lee Minto, former executive director of Planned Parenthood of Seattle-King County, said she takes "great exception to the fact that the primary purpose of this is, and it's not in front of the public at all, is that it's a Christian ministry." She asserts that women are not allowed to leave a pregnancy counseling center without hearing the Gospel.[30]

NEW COMMAND

After Planned Parenthood fired its initial shot at abortion alternative centers, the project was picked up by others in the movement for legal abortion. People for the American Way launched a campaign against pregnancy counseling centers in mid-1991. The effort was intensified in the fall of 1991 when Congressman Ron Wyden, D-Oregon, chairman of the Subcommittee on Regulation, Business Opportunities and Energy, held a public hearing on allegations made against pregnancy counseling centers. Wyden has a 100 percent pro-legal abortion voting record and has been a vocal and active supporter of legal abortion. He asked the staff of the subcommittee to "investigate" the allegations.

The subcommittee staff issued a report and memorandum titled, "Investigation and Hearing on Bogus Abortion Clinics: The Role of False, Deceptive and Misleading Telephone Directory Advertisements and Listings; State Enforcement Efforts and the Extent of Federal Consumer Protection Jurisdiction." In the report, several charges are made against pregnancy counseling centers.

Early in the report, the staff notes how the investigation began:

> At your direction, subcommittee staff beginning earlier this year initiated an extensive inquiry of unfair competition issues, and consumer protection complaints, stemming from the emergence of "bogus" abortion or abortion referral clinics.[31]

A June 20, 1991, memorandum from Ron Fitzsimmons, executive director of the National Coalition of Abortion Providers (NCAP), to "NCAP Members and Interested Parties," points to the organization's involvement in the congressional hearing:

> I recently met with Congressman Ron Wyden to discuss the format of his hearing on phony clinics. We now expect the hearing to occur sometime in September. We want to have a panel of women who have had bad experiences in phony clinics, a panel of state Attorneys General who can testify to the need for a national solution to the problem, the Federal Trade Commissiona [sic] and a panel of telephone company executives who can discuss why they are not as cooperative as we would like. I could use your help with two things: we need women are [sic] willing to testify about their experience (we could guarantee anonymity) and a tape recorded conversation with a phony clinic. Please call me if you think you can help.[32]

A September 4, 1991, memo from Fitzsimmons to "All Abortion Providers" states, "While this issue may not be a high priority item for some providers, I still thought the issue deserved attention so I approached the Chairman of the Subcommittee, Rep. Ron Wyden (D-OR), approximately seven months ago and suggested he hold a hearing to help publicize the issue. My thinking was that the resulting publicity would at least make some women more aware of the problem."[33]

It is incredible that Wyden, using taxpayer money, would hold a hearing at the request of Fitzsimmons, lobbyist for the multi-million dollar abortion industry. It is an attempt to attack and regulate all pregnancy counseling centers even though only a handful are using the methods in question. Why? As previously noted, the centers are depriving the abortion industry of millions of dollars. Moreover, abortion providers do not advertise as "abortion clinics." Their purpose is diffused by a name such as "Women's Choice Clinic."

In short, this entire controversy has been raised by people intimately involved in the abortion industry. When Subcommittee staff write, "At your direction . . . ," it should really be writing, "At your direction, which is at the direction of the abortion industry . . . "

One part of the staff report provides a definition of a "bogus abortion clinic":

> For the purposes of this investigation, and a hearing on these issues scheduled for September 20, 1991, a "bogus clinic" is a facility which typically is not staffed by professional health care providers. Abortion and abortion referral services are neither given nor contemplated by the operator. Instead, these facilities are by design venues for hard-sell, and often abusive anti-abortion arguments and tactics aimed at unsuspecting and vulnerable consumers.[34]

While it is interesting that those who seek an abortion are viewed as "consumers," the point is that a "bogus clinic" is being defined in a "bogus" way. A pregnancy counseling center does not need to be staffed by "professional health care providers" (read, supporters of legal abortion) in order to be free of deception. The reverse is also true. Even if "professional health care providers" are hired, this does not mean deception cannot take place. There is no reason why volunteers, who care about women and who wish to assist them, must be "professional health care providers" unless they are practicing medicine, which is not the case at pregnancy counseling centers. It is also interesting to note that Planned Parenthood sites are not exactly riddled with "professional health care providers." In fact, a small minority of its employees could be described as such.

It is inferred that, unless abortion and abortion referrals are offered, the center is automatically to be considered deceptive and bogus. This would be true only if the center implies it is an abortion clinic which is the situation in a handful of cases.

Arguing that the centers are designed as "hard-sell" and that they use "often abusive anti-abortion arguments and tactics" against "unsuspecting and vulnerable consumers" is a clever use of rhetoric, but lacking in truth. Pregnancy counseling centers affiliated with any reputable group certainly do not fit into this category.

The broad definition provided in the Subcommittee staff report would include virtually every pregnancy counseling center in North America, except that they are not involved in hard-sell, abusive practices. Not offering abortion services or referrals does not make a center "bogus," except to the abortion industry. Not being staffed by "professional health care providers," when medicine is not being practiced does not make a center "bogus," except to the abortion industry. The use of hard-sell (undefined) or abusive arguments and tactics (unspecified) have been condemned by most pregnancy counseling center leaders. It seems, however, that anything which may encourage a woman to give birth is considered hard-sell and abusive to abortion providers, including a discussion of fetal development.

Subcommittee staff seeks to provide specific examples of inappropriate conduct on the part of pregnancy counseling centers:

> These "clinics" tend to mislead the most socially vulnerable women seeking an abortion. Those most likely to be duped are women who because of economic status, age or cultural background have no personal physician, and who rely on telephone directory advertising as their principal means of selecting a pregnancy termination service.
>
> In many cases, these women are deceived by a misleading ad designed by a "clinic" operator with no intention of providing a legal, medical service.[35]

Pregnancy counseling centers are most often listed under "Abortion Alternatives." However, in some areas it is the telephone company which places a center under the category of the company's choosing—without regard to the wishes of the center. Women who call or go to a pregnancy counseling center for an abortion need only ask if abortions are provided. The answer given is straight-forward and honest—"no." Once again, it is implied that by refusing to provide a "legal, medical service" which destroys human life, the centers are somehow deceptive. Women are capable of reading the telephone directory and making a telephone call to learn more about any business or organization listed in the yellow pages.

It is assumed that the term "clinic" implies medical service. In fact, the terms "clinic," "center," and "medical clinic" have been used synonymously and loosely by those attacking pregnancy counseling centers throughout this ordeal. *The Random House College Dictionary* offers several definitions of clinic, including this one: "any class or group convening for instruction, advice, remedial work, etc., in a special field: a marriage clinic; a speech clinic."[36] Nevertheless, pregnancy counseling centers are urged to advertise under "Abortion Alternatives." Those which have advertised under "Clinic" are urged to include a statement that the center is not a licensed medical facility.

Unfortunately and quite unfairly, Subcommittee staff seeks to paint almost all pregnancy counseling centers as being exactly alike:

> An extensive survey by subcommittee staff of yellow page directory listings in all fifty states tends to support earlier claims that there may be as many as 2,000 *of these deceptively promoted facilities, nationwide*.[37]

The 2,000 figure represents virtually every pregnancy counseling center in the country. Unfortunately, this is the number which has been quoted by the media.

The crafty language used by the Subcommittee staff is interesting, yet it curses the entire pregnancy counseling center movement. The staff writes that there *may* be "as many as 2,000 *of these deceptively promoted facilities, nationwide.*" True, or there could be as many as two. The truth is that if some pregnancy counseling centers purposefully use deceptive tactics, they are the exception, not the rule. The point of the hearing, however, was to infer that all pregnancy counseling centers wish to abuse women in an effort to discourage them from seeking alternatives. After all, who knows what might happen to these women once in an "anti-choice" chamber? Another point is to establish a congressional record for efforts to pass federal, state, and local legislation.

Had pregnancy counseling center representatives been allowed to testify, an opportunity denied by Wyden, the Subcommittee and its staff would have learned that a small minority of them use deceptive tactics, although using the definition of deception provided by the staff, it seems most every group is doing so. The fact is that the definition is ludicrous.

The Subcommittee staff is not unwilling to draw conclusions from its so-called investigation:

> Staff surveyed more than 200 yellow page directories encompassing all fifty states, with specific attention to the character and quantity of bogus clinic listings. In staff's view, given this random sampling, previous estimates that there may be 2,000 "clinics" nationwide, seem entirely reasonable.[38]

Judging the "character" of yellow pages listings, especially given the broad definition of what encompasses a "bogus clinic," is subjective. It seems the Subcommittee staff has a political agenda similar to that of Wyden. This is further evidenced by the nature of the rhetoric used throughout the report.

The Subcommittee staff continues:

> Staff heard personal stories, and collected affidavits, from a number of individuals who had been deceived and abused in such clinics. The abuse ranged from personal recriminations from clinic staff toward persons seeking abortions to attempted physical restraint of those persons. Some of these incidents were repeated in instances where subcommittee staff visited bogus clinics to verify implied offerings of abortion or abortion referral services.[39]

Once again, pregnancy counseling centers receive few complaints from real clients. They are consistently seeking ways to improve. Most complaints come from "plants" who represent news agencies, congressional offices, and/or those who are sent by pro-legal abortion groups. In other words, people who come looking for a controversy may be able to create one, but those truly in need are pleased with the services.

Planned Parenthood and similar groups actively solicit people to file complaints against pregnancy counseling centers. Centers have served hundreds of thousands of Americans and they are pleased with the services. Consequently, personal stories and affidavits which attack pregnancy counseling centers are likely from "plants," not from individuals who are really in need or those seeking information without organizational backing.

Note the use of rhetoric once again. Words like "abused" and "deceived" are pejorative and subjective. Unfortunately, Subcommittee staff apparently feel that discussion of the abortion procedure or the showing of fetal slides are "abusive" and the equivalent of "terrorism."

Subcommittee staff take yellow pages publishers to task:

> In its survey of yellow page directories, subcommittee staff found a wide degree of variance in use of disclaimers, restriction of advertising placement, and policing of claims or implications in the substance of display ads . . . Some yellow page publishers, for example, require disclaimers that precede abortion alternative listings *specifying* that those advertisers *will not* provide abortion or abortion referral services, but most directories do not. In many cases, directory publishers allow bogus operators to list themselves under the "clinics" heading, even though no professional services are provided.[40]

The Subcommittee staff wants to place yellow pages officials in the position of determining what is and what is not a "bogus abortion clinic." Once again, using the definition provided by the staff, this would include virtually every organization which does not perform or refer for abortions. Moreover, there is nothing inherently wrong with advertising under "clinics," so long as false or misleading statements are not made about services offered. It is the abortion industry which seeks to write the definitions and set the standards in order to support itself.

Some wish to use a definition of "clinic" derived from what the majority of people think of when they read or see the word. A "clinic," it is argued, treats people for a medical problem. This argument essentially says we should ignore the actual definition(s) of words in favor of public ignorance. In addition, using this standard would make it difficult to refer to facilities which only perform abortions as "clinics."

The Subcommittee staff addresses the corporate structure of pregnancy counseling centers:

> These bogus clinics often are operated as individual, mom-and-pop facilities, with little or no corporate structure, and no direct ties to a national organization. However, subcommittee staff have identified at least two informational and assistance organizations with an aggressive anti-abortion agenda, which provide clinics with various how-to manuals and other organizational and promotional aids. The prevalence of these organizational materials appears to account for, in part, generic name similarities (i.e., Women's Choice, Crisis Pregnancy Center, AAA Center for Women's Choice, etc.).[41]

It is argued that abortion foes have "robbed the vernacular of the pro-choice movement." Of course, those who support legal abortion do not have a lock and key on certain words in the English language.

It is not true that "bogus clinics" often are operated without structure or ties to a national organization. Most of those pregnancy counseling centers identified as deceptive *are* affiliated with a national organization. Such affiliation does not necessarily mean deceptive practices are not being used. This depends on the national organization and its standards for affiliation.

The Christian Action Council standards are clear when they state:

> The CPC [Crisis Pregnancy Center] is committed to providing clients with accurate and complete information about both prenatal development and abortion. The CPC is committed to integrity in dealing with clients, earning their trust and providing promised information and services. The CPC denounces any form of deception in its corporate advertising or individual conversations with its clients.[42]

In addition, the Christian Action Council's *Crisis Pregnancy Center Volunteer Training Manual* states:

> The caller should never be lied to or deceived in any way. Everyone at the crisis pregnancy center must be completely honest with the public at all times. As representatives of Jesus Christ, all of the activities of the CPC must be above reproach.
>
> There are three pragmatic reasons for this policy: 1) God will not honor the efforts of anyone who is deceitful. Scripture makes it clear that God hates lying (Proverbs 6:16, 12:2). The CPC ministry will be effective only to the degree that God blesses it; 2) Deceitfulness is self-defeating. A woman who has been deceived into coming into the CPC will justifiably react with anger when she discovers the truth. Once that happens, she will not be open to anything the CPC has to share, and the opportunity to minister will have been lost; 3) Lying to or deceiving the public can give the opposition an opportunity to sue the CPC. Pro-abortionists will not be successful in their opposition as long as the CPC remains above reproach in every aspect of the ministry. . . .
>
> Always be truthful. The client should never be lied to or misled. Responses such as, "The crisis pregnancy center will meet all your needs," when the client asks "Do you do abortions?", are misleading.[43]

The two organizations specifically identified later in the Subcommittee staff report are the Pearson Foundation and the Christian Action Council. This is grossly negligent on the part of the staff. The former organization has defended practices the latter considers to be deceptive. Christian Action Council standards are clear. Any Christian Action Council-affiliated pregnancy counseling center found to be in violation of the letter or spirit of the standards regarding the use of deceptive practices is required to immediately change its practice(s) or be dropped as an affiliate.

What is meant by "an aggressive anti-abortion agenda" is unclear, though pregnancy counseling centers are indeed opposed to abortion. The staff, once again, refers to its definition of deception.

Subcommittee staff believe that yellow pages advertising is a problem, primarily because of the fact that abortion alternative organizations are placed so close to abortion providers:

> These operators often advertise under "clinic" listings in yellow page directories. In those directories which also offer both "abortion services" and "abortion alternative" listings, these operators generally are correctly listed under "alternatives." However, often these deceptive facilities *share* display advertising space, usually on the same page, with legitimate abortion providers. This proximity problem has been the cause of confusion and consumer abuse, according to persons interviewed by the subcommittee staff.[44]

Pregnancy counseling centers are generally and appropriately listed under "Abortion Alternatives" in telephone directories where a distinction is made. This is clearly not deceptive and shows a desire to be up-front. The fact remains that in many areas it is the yellow pages publisher who determines the most appropriate category for a pregnancy counseling center. Unfortunately, expressed desires of pregnancy counseling center leaders regarding their placement in the yellow pages are often ignored.

One main objection is that groups offering abortion alternatives are often listed on the same page as abortion providers with regard to display advertising. This is nitpicking. As previously mentioned, an intelligent person can easily look at the regular yellow pages listing to determine the appropriate category for the display advertisement. We are not dealing with illiterate people and the yellow pages publisher should not have to adjust their practice on such a basis. However, every yellow pages publisher should offer the listing category of "Abortion Alternatives."

The "proximity problem," as it is called, is not the cause of "consumer abuse." There is no link here. If confusion is caused, it is because the reader of the yellow pages does not know how to use the directory.

It seems the agenda of abortion providers is to remove the "Abortion Alternatives" category altogether. Since "Abortion Alternatives" appears before "Abortion Services," as does "Abortion Information," some women may contact one of the alternative groups because they did not originally know alternatives are available. This impacts the income of abortion providers. In addition, women who seek counseling at a pregnancy counseling center are given accurate information which is not made available by abortionists, such as fetal development, possible abortion-related complications and abortion procedures.

According to Subcommittee staff, law enforcement officers are reluctant to prosecute cases of "consumer abuse." This assumes that law enforcement officers, who are not politically motivated, have a case to prosecute:

> As previously stated, legal authorities contacted by subcommittee staff said that most states *have* consumer protection statutes to address false or deceptive advertising. However, it appears that only a handful of state attorneys general and local district attorneys have enforced protective statutes in this area. This leaves us to conclude that either (1) state statutes generally are inadequate to deal with the problem of such "clinics," or (2) there is a lack of political will by individual state agencies to prosecute.[45]

Consumer protection laws should be enforced, but this is not a consumer issue as no money changes hands. Such laws should not be abused by the abortion industry or its apologists. Law enforcement agencies should enforce the law in a fair manner, regardless of the potential political consequences. Anti-abortion law enforcement officials, and law enforcement officials who work in anti-abortion communities, should always equitably enforce the law when sufficient evidence has been presented. It should not be assumed, however, that lack of enforcement is based on a lack of will. Law enforcement officials may understand that in many cases the complaints are coming from people with a political axe to grind.

The Subcommittee suggests solutions to the problem:

> At best, the federal jurisdiction in this area is cloudy. The Chairman has written to Janet Steiger, chairman of the Federal Trade Commission, requesting information on FTC jurisdiction and activities in this area . . . Subcommittee staff asked the American Law Division of the Library of Congress to study the Federal Trade Commission's authority. Its findings . . . cited the current prohibition against pursuit of cases involving nonprofit corporations—an apt description of most if not all of the bogus clinics.
>
> However, in legal terms the lack of jurisdiction could be easily remedied by removing the nonprofit exemption within section 4 of the Federal Trade Commission Act, according to the Division.
>
> A less wholesome alternative, according to the Division, would be to an amendment [sic] removing the nonprofit exemption "only to those nonprofits which advertise concerning abortion or pregnancy-related services." The Division points out that the FTC statutes in general have been kept non-industry specific, and that little precedent exists for this alternative remedy.[46]

Such action would clearly be politically motivated. The reason there is no move to exclude other groups from the enforcement exemption is because there is no politically charged issue involved. Consequently, it is not surprising that there is little precedent for doing so.

It would not be surprising if an advocate for legal abortion in Congress moves to sneak language into a bill to accomplish that which is outlined as a "remedy" or "less wholesome alternative" to the abortion industry-caused problem. Abortion foes in Congress and members of their staffs should track and carefully watch any legislation through which this might be attempted.

The Subcommittee staff gives its version of the history of pregnancy counseling centers and the problems caused by them:

> The bogus abortion clinic phenomenon emerged in the early 1970s, spurred initially by the work of the St. Louis, Missouri-based Pearson Foundation, an aggressive anti-abortion organization. The Foundation provides training manuals, urine tests, videos such as the anti-abortion staple "Silent Scream," [sic] and detailed training for operators of bogus clinics.[47]

These comments attack the Pearson Foundation, yet they are meant to be extrapolated to the entire pregnancy counseling center movement. The staff report continues:

> Pearson's formula for clinic operation is recounted in a 93-page manual, "How to Start and Operate Your Own Pro-Life Outreach Crisis Pregnancy Center." The Foundation's methods were later adopted, replicated and/or refined by other groups, including the Falls Church, Va.-based Christian Action Council, which publishes "How to Start a Crisis Pregnancy Center."[48]

The Christian Action Council's *How to Start a Crisis Pregnancy Center* is in no way related to the Pearson Foundation or any of its publications. The manual was not "adopted, replicated and/or refined" from the Pearson manual. Such a statement is thoroughly false and reflects more negligence on the part of the Subcommittee staff.

Additional information is provided as to the history of pregnancy counseling centers:

> Although the source of the advice may change, the basic suggestions and direction remains consistent:
>
> 1. Name. Choose a neutral name which does not indicate you have no intention of providing an abortion service.
>   "The woman who wants an abortion may not come to the center if the center appears to be pro-life." *Pearson Manual.*
> 2. Location. Choose an address near a legitimate abortion clinic, in the same building if possible. Assume a business name similar to the nearby legitimate clinic.
>   "The whole idea for this . . . is if the girl who would be going to the abortion chamber sees our office first with a similar name, she will probably come into your center." *Pearson Manual.*
> 3. Decor. The bogus clinic's interior should have a medical flair.
>   "You want your office to look like an abortion clinic." *Pearson Manual.*
> 4. Telephone procedures. When a potential client telephones the clinic, do not disclose that you will not provide an abortion.
>   "Do not indicate you are pro-life. If she is seeking an abortion and indicates she won't come in because she knows we are pro-life, assure her we can still help her by giving her all the information on abortion." *Pearson Manual.*
> 5. Telephone listings. List your office in the yellow pages.
>   "Make sure your center is listed in the yellow pages of the telephone directory with abortion clinics—under 'Clinics, Medical.'" *Pearson Manual.*[49]

Once again, due to the above statement regarding manuals, it is implied that the Christian Action Council concurs with deceptive strategies and with the statements in the Pearson Manual. This is totally false. Notice that only the Pearson Manual is quoted. I challenge the Subcommittee staff to find a quotation in any Christian Action Council publication even remotely similar.

Toward the end of the Subcommittee staff report on pregnancy counseling centers, an attempt is made to claim that not all centers are guilty of deception:

> These bogus operators do not necessarily represent the majority of the anti-abortion counseling movement. Recognized groups such as Birthright have gone on record as opposing the deceptive practices of the bogus clinics. But the sharpest criticism, naturally, has come from pro-choice groups.[50]

The Subcommittee staff concedes that "bogus operators do not necessarily represent a majority of the anti-abortion counseling movement," though virtually every other statement made throughout the report and during the oral testimony (note the 2,000 figure) imply otherwise. The media reported such figures as "gospel truth" without mention of the above quotation.

Birthright is the only organization listed as having condemned deceptive practices. The Subcommittee staff has not done its homework. The Christian Action Council condemned deceptive practices many years ago and has repeatedly done so. Had the staff checked with Christian Action Council leaders, this could have been made clear. Recall the Standards of Affiliation previously quoted.

Birthright has denounced deceptive practices, but surely not on the basis of definitions provided by the Subcommittee staff. Like the Christian Action Council, Birthright opposes deceptive practices. However, what the Subcommittee staff determines to be a deceptive practice is not what pregnancy counseling center leaders believe to be a deceptive practice.

People for the American Way, which has recently become involved in pushing the attack against pregnancy counseling centers, is described in glowing terms by Subcommittee staff:

> People for the American Way, a non-profit, constitutional rights organization, recently demanded that the Maryland state attorney general conduct an investigation of a chain of "Crisis Pregnancy Centers" in that state. The group said the centers "through ads and conversations with callers . . . deliberately mislead women to believe they provide abortion services and give false information about abortion and birth control."
>
> "The centers disseminate false information regarding the risks and effects of abortion," reads the complaint. "The centers provide anti-abortion information and engage in scare tactics with the intent that women will rely on the false information and decide not to seek the services of a legitimate abortion clinic."[51]

People for the American Way is identified as a "non-profit, constitutional rights organization." Founded by Norman Lear, the organization is staunchly supportive of legal abortion and the abortion industry. It has even filed *amicus* briefs on abortion-related cases before the judicial branch of government, including the *Webster* case. People for the American Way is simply not a neutral organization.

It is alleged that pregnancy counseling centers have disseminated "false information regarding the risks and effects of abortion" and they "engage in scare tactics." If it is assumed that only those statistics released by pro-abortion organizations, such as the Alan Guttmacher Institute, are acceptable, I beg to differ. The "scare tactics" referred to concern the showing of fetal development slides or abortion procedure information. While these may be surprising and even disconcerting to some clients, such information is nevertheless scientifically sound and accurate. Women who know the whole truth are likely to decide against abortion for very real, practical reasons.

After claiming that there has been little ligation against pregnancy counseling centers, Subcommittee staff reference some cases:

> An attorney general's action in Maryland would be unusual, but not unique. Attorneys general or district attorneys in at least three states—California, New York and Texas—have sued bogus abortion clinics for deceptive or misleading promotional tactics. In each case, the foundation for action was the state's consumer protection law.
>
> In the New York case, clinics settled out-of-court with the state, agreeing to amend counseling and advertising methods.
>
> The Texas suit resulted in an injunction against the offending clinic, followed by a jury verdict which resulted in a large cash award to plaintiffs. The decision has been sustained in lower court appeals, and the U.S. Supreme Court has declined to review.
>
> In California, courts enjoined a clinic requiring that it only advertise that it provides abortion alternatives.[52]

Assuming that politics does not play a role in enforcement, and definitions such as those offered by the Subcommittee staff are not being used, these actions may be appropriate. This was clearly not the case with all three, however. For example, Gloria Allred, a radical feminist and activist for legal abortion, was the lead attorney in the California action. Political motivation cannot always be ruled out. The report continues:

> Some state attorneys general have declined to act against bogus clinics based on interpretations of state consumer protection laws. In Washington state, for example, the state AG

argues that since no money changed hands at a bogus clinic which was the subject of a complaint, no "commerce" took place which places the activity under the consumer protection statute's authority . . .[53]

This is a legitimate decision on the part of Washington's attorney general. The fact is that consumer fraud is not taking place because pregnancy counseling centers do not exist to sell commodities or services to the consuming public. They are nonprofit, charitable organizations providing welcomed services free of charge. Pregnancy counseling center personnel are most often volunteers. They are people helping people. Women are being offered a real choice and abortion providers do not like it.

CONGRESSIONAL "HEARING"

After the Subcommittee staff prepared its report, Congressman Ron Wyden held a hearing on pregnancy counseling centers. There were three panels established for testimony given at the hearing. Panel one included Shannon Lock, identified as "a victim of bogus clinic practices"; Jennifer Kraeger, identified as "a victim of bogus clinic practices"; Lynn Taliento, subcommittee staff investigator; and Ron Fitzsimmons.

Panel two included Robert Abrams, attorney general for the State of New York (who actively supports legal abortion); Arlo Smith, district attorney in San Francisco (who supports legal abortion); Stephen Salo, assistant attorney general for the State of Texas (who supports legal abortion); Mark Salo, executive director of Planned Parenthood of San Diego and Riverside Counties; Marcia Greenberger, co-president of the National Women's Law Center (which litigates for legal abortion); and Deanna R. Duby, deputy legal director of People for the American Way.

The third panel consisted of representatives from various telephone companies. Wyden chose to use these gentlemen for his grandstanding by grilling them on their practices. This grandstanding and grilling was not unexpected.

Despite repeated requests for an opportunity to testify, crisis pregnancy leaders were not allowed to do so. Wyden appeared on NBC's "Today Show" the morning of the hearing during which he said that representatives of the "bogus abortion clinics" had *refused* to testify and that he would have loved the chance to hear from them. Given that the staff report clearly accuses the Christian Action Council, Wyden must decide whether he does not consider Christian Action Council-affiliated centers to be "bogus," which conflicts with the staff report, or whether he lied to the American people.

Media coverage of the Subcommittee hearing was extensive and largely unfair. Statements made by those testifying and accusations made in the Subcommittee staff report were often reported as fact, not opinion.

"PRIMETIME LIVE" EXPOSÉ

The September 4, 1991, memorandum from Ron Fitzsimmons shows the connection between the abortion industry and the media:

> To publicize this issue as much as possible, I went to the ABC program "Prime Time" several weeks ago and they immediately agreed to do an "expose" [sic] on the issue. I have directed them to bogus clinics around the country and to several "victims." Their producers tell me that they have some terrific footage using undercover cameras. At this time, they hope to air the program sometime in mid-September [airing was actually on October 31, 1991]. This show airs at 10:00 EST on Thursdays. I will alert all providers with fax machines once I hear when the show is going to air. . . .[54]

In the same memo, Fitzsimmons urged members of his group and others to stage a media event outside of a pregnancy counseling center. This led to many local stories on the issue.

"PrimeTime Live" producers, two camera crews, and correspondent Chris Wallace visited the Christian Action Council's international headquarters on October 11, 1991, to interview Harriet R. T. Lewis. "PrimeTime" had sent an employee into at least two Christian Action Council-affiliated pregnancy counseling centers posing as a pregnant woman. She carried a hidden camera.

During the interview, Wallace alleged that advertising under "Clinic" in the yellow pages is deceptive. There were two primary reasons for this statement: 1) pregnancy counseling center display advertising is sometimes placed on the same page (even next to) display advertising for abortion clinics. Wallace implied that the advertising was placed in that location on purpose to mislead women; and 2) pregnancy counseling centers do not write in the display advertising, "Don't want to get an abortion? Come see us." In other words, a specific statement, according to Wallace, should be included in the display advertising which expresses the pregnancy counseling center philosophy about abortion. According to Wallace, opposing abortion is what the centers do and offering services are really a peripheral purpose. Wallace also stated that he believes pregnancy counseling center operators really do not care if a woman erroneously goes to a pregnancy counseling center believing she can get an abortion.

One of the specific display advertisements referred to by Wallace states, "offering . . . Free Pregnancy Tests, results while you wait, Lay Counseling, Post Abortion Counseling, Abortion Information and Alternatives, Temporary Housing, 24 Hr. Hotline. All services confidential, all services free."[55] The advertisement is placed in the "Clinic" category. While clarification is advisable, the sentence "Abortion Information and Alternatives" does show that alternatives are offered. The advertisement does not state, nor does it imply, that abortions are done.

Another advertisement used by Wallace reads, "We Care . . . We Want to Help! Free Pregnancy Testing, Confidential Counseling, Referrals, 24 Hr. Phone Service."[56] It is placed in the "Abortion-Alternative Organizations" category. Given the category, I see no problem with this advertisement.

Wallace has a basic misunderstanding about the reasons why pregnancy counseling centers were established in the first place. They were established to provide alternative services and care to women and to present them with information about abortion that is being given by abortionists. Pregnancy counseling centers are unashamedly anti-abortion, but the purpose is to offer alternatives to abortion. Offering alternatives and support lead women to decide against abortion. This is a natural by-product of providing positive answers to the problems facing women.

Wallace wants pregnancy counseling centers to blatantly state a philosophical position. Unfortunately, he does not believe abortion providers should place in their advertisements a statement like, "Abortion alternatives and prenatal care are not offered here." A woman could just as easily make the mistake of believing an abortion provider will offer non-directive counseling (which is not the case) and alternatives. Writing "abortions up to 24 weeks" in an abortion clinic display advertisement does not necessarily mean no alternatives are offered.

What is the harm done if a woman erroneously goes to an abortion clinic when she has decided to keep her baby? She need only be directed elsewhere. What is the harm done if a woman goes to a pregnancy counseling center when she wants to have an abortion? She not only may learn that alternatives are available, but she may also learn that she has not been told everything there is to know about abortion. No harm could come to her. Nevertheless, such a mistake would be based on a misunderstanding, not deception (overt or covert), and it is easily cleared up.

Wallace questioned the description of an abortion given by one Christian Action Council-affiliated pregnancy counseling center director. A second trimester abortion was described, but the phony client was in her first trimester. The director says she explained abortion procedures at all stages. "PrimeTime Live" says the center employee described a second trimester procedure for a first trimester pregnancy. Wallace said the part of the taped interview which clearly shows that the description given by the center employee was for a second-trimester abortion would be aired as part of the report. It was not.

Wallace questioned references to possible abortion complications. He said the Centers for Disease Control claims there were *only* six deaths attributed to abortion last year. What Wallace does not say is that abortion-related deaths are under-reported. Abortion providers have nothing to gain by listing a death as relating to abortion. Most often, a more specific cause is listed, such as "heart failure." In addition, abortion-related deaths which occur after the procedure are usually listed as being due to other reasons.

The Centers for Disease Control tells me that no public data must be reported. It acknowledges that states have different reporting requirements (some have none for complications, but deaths must be reported—in some way). Simply put, reporting is a state matter. When asked about under-reporting and attributing abortion-related deaths to other causes, the response was, "That happens, I'm sure."

The American Cancer Society, according to Wallace, said there is no increase in the possibility of breast cancer due to an early first trimester abortion. Wallace also said that, according to the Centers for Disease Control, there is no increase in the possibility of spontaneous abortion following an induced abortion. Once again, I checked with the Centers for Disease Control.

The Centers for Disease Control says there are conflicting studies on both issues, though there is not an increased risk of spontaneous abortion following a *first trimester* (suction aspiration) abortion. With this in mind, telling women that some studies have shown a potential problem is advisable, as this is the case. The issue is how the information is presented. It should not be presented as fact, but as a possibility. Telling women there is a chance of these problems is not inaccurate. There is, indeed, such a chance.

Wallace presented his statements as Centers for Disease Control facts. They are not.

At the urging of the National Coalition of Abortion Providers, several similar reports on pregnancy counseling centers by the media have been done and more are expected. The "PrimeTime Live" report generated extensive local media. KVEN radio in Ventura, California, featured a report done by Phil Hendrie, one of those radio show hosts who apparently believes controversy is necessary to get listeners. In one program aired on September 20, 1991, Hendrie said he "found out about the Ventura County Crisis Pregnancy Center and, ah, I'm a little bit troubled . . ." He went on to imply that the Ventura County Crisis Pregnancy Center is deceptive.[57]

Hendrie was not satisfied with implying that the Center engages in deception. In a conversation with a woman identified as a member of Hendrie's staff, another issue of concern is raised. The woman, who apparently did some "investigation" work on the issue, said of the Ventura center, "They do offer, ah, medical treatment should you decide to, to keep your pregnancy, but pretty much if you decide to terminate [the pregnancy] they won't have anything to do with you."[58]

Hendrie asked the woman, who has never been involved in a post-abortion counseling program at the center, what it is like:

Hendrie: And what does that mean? They'll save your soul from eternal damnation?

Woman: Yea, probably.

Hendrie: They'll save you from burning in Hell?

Woman: Probably. They'll probably make you see the light.

Hendrie: Either that or they'll make you feel even more guilty than you, than you might already feel walking in the door there.

Woman: Yea, I think so, because I remember they have a lot of paraphernalia and films and propaganda that they show you before hand. . . . I think what it is, basically, is, ah, they used, ah, the scare tactic type thing. Most of them do, when you think about it. You know, they don't counsel you as far as decisions, they show you only a one-sided thing. . . .[59]

Amazingly, Hendrie backed off of his strident position after his station manager received a six-page letter detailing the unfair treatment and suggesting that legal action was being considered. Radio program hosts of his ilk, however, often seem to do so given similar circumstances. In other words, they are good at opening their mouths, but weak at backing up their words with facts. Nevertheless, many seem to think, in their own minds, that they are Sherlock Holmes.

It seems one can logically reach the following conclusions with regard to the attacks launched against pregnancy counseling centers:

1. The charges against pregnancy counseling centers, even if true, only concern the operations of a few. Nevertheless, they are used as a broad way to attack all.
2. Most pregnancy counseling centers have strict standards relating to integrity. This fact has been ignored.
3. Representatives of the pregnancy counseling centers were not allowed to testify before the Subcommittee because a one-sided, blanket attack on the centers was intended.
4. Wyden, at the urging of the abortion industry, has used taxpayer dollars to wage a personal war against pregnancy counseling centers. (Wyden was the

only member of Congress to attend the hearing.) This was also done to generate unfavorable publicity against all pregnancy counseling centers and to create a congressional record for future legislation at all levels of government.

5. The attack against pregnancy counseling centers is part of a long, organized effort started by Planned Parenthood, the nation's largest abortion provider.
6. The definition of terms provided by the Subcommittee staff are flawed and serves the abortion industry.
7. Allegations of abuse are fabricated or exaggerated and most often come from "plants" encouraged by the abortion industry.
8. Like certain members of Congress, the media will do its best to present a tainted view of the pregnancy counseling center movement at the urging of the abortion industry.

Wyden's hearing itself seems to have intimidated yellow pages publishers into doing what the abortion industry and its cohorts in Congress want. Yellow pages publishers are now printing "clarifications" under "Abortion Alternatives" which reads, "Advertisers under this heading provide assistance, and/or information on abortion alternatives. They do not provide abortion services, nor do they provide counseling or information on abortions."[60]

Do the publishers consider this some sort of compromise, even though it is at least partly inaccurate? Advertisers under the heading *do* provide counseling and information on abortions, just not that approved by the abortion industry and the easily intimidated yellow pages publishers. Unfortunately, some of the nation's largest national and international pregnancy counseling center organizations appear unconcerned about this action.

It is interesting to note that Planned Parenthood has nothing negative to say about a person who goes into a center under false pretenses. This has not always been the case. In 1985, a parent went into a Planned Parenthood clinic with the specific purpose of finding some of the organization's indecent literature. "I frankly don't know what to think about people who come to an agency under false pretenses and hunt around and try to find evidence for their charges," the Planned Parenthood spokesman said. The parent found what she had been seeking.[61]

15

THE THREAT TO *ROE*

Planned Parenthood's abortion advocacy significantly increased following the United States Supreme Court decision in *Webster v. Reproductive Health Services*. Planned Parenthood submitted an *amicus* ("friend of the court") brief on behalf of Reproductive Health Services. (See Appendix F for a partial list of organizations submitting briefs in *Webster*.)

In *Webster*, the Supreme Court upholds a Missouri law restricting public (state) participation in abortion. Moreover, the decision virtually invites state legislatures to pass laws on abortion. The Court does not reverse *Roe v. Wade*.

WAITING FOR THE DECISION

Like groups opposed to abortion, Planned Parenthood and its allies had no idea what the Supreme Court would do in *Webster*. There were essentially three likely scenarios. First, the Court could have upheld the Missouri law in full or in part without specifically reaffirming *Roe*, which the Court did. Second, the Court could have explicitly reaffirmed *Roe* and declared the Missouri law unconstitutional. Third, the Court could have overturned its 1973 decision in *Roe v. Wade*, which would have said there is no constitutional right to abortion. This latter action would have allowed lawmakers to determine abortion policy.

Planned Parenthood, the National Organization for Women, and the National Abortion Rights Action League used the fact that the Missouri law was going to be considered by the Supreme Court as a major fund-raising campaign. This campaign was highly successful. Claims that legal abortion is in serious jeopardy assisted the organizations in adding thousands of names to their respective mailing lists to be used for later fund-raising and political action.

Advocates of legal abortion predicted the Supreme Court would issue a decision that would have a negative impact on *Roe*, if it were not overturned outright. Abortion foes had heard rumors that the Court was going to reverse *Roe* on a five to four vote. Another rumor said the Court would reverse *Roe* by a six to three vote. As the day for the decision approached, Justice Sandra Day O'Connor appeared to be the swing vote.

Public comments made by Planned Parenthood, the National Organization for Women, and the National Abortion Rights Action League served to arouse great public interest in *Webster*. Abortion opponents took a wait-and-see posture, knowing that a total reversal of *Roe* would mean a battlefield in each of the 50 states, Washington, D.C., and the American territories.

RESPONSE TO THE DECISION

Faye Wattleton, then-president of Planned Parenthood Federation of America, was quick to attack the decision in *Webster*. Wattleton spoke to reporters on the steps of the Supreme Court building immediately following the decision:

> "This Supreme Court decision once more slaps poor women in the face and says you do not have constitutional protections if your state sees fit to restrict them and you do not have the resources to circumvent those restrictions," Wattleton said. "The Court says certain fundamental protections that are part of your human dignity and part of being a respected and decent human being are not yours."[1]

Wattleton did not limit her remarks to the Supreme Court's decision. While speaking to reporters, Wattleton was moved aside by John C. "Jack" Willke, M.D., who at the time was president of the National Right to Life Committee. Willke wanted to speak to the press. The *New York Times Magazine* reports that while Wattleton was still answering a reporter's question, "he [Willke] strode up to the microphones and shoved her [Wattleton] aside. . . ." According to the magazine, Wattleton "stood firm against Wilke's [sic] incursion."[2] Following her statement on *Webster*, Wattleton commented on the incident:

> "I was so stunned at the outrageous rudeness of it that my mind did not function as quickly as it should have. I didn't say that this is just symbolic of the way that men push women around. He is ready for me to go, so he comes along and tries to push me away, and I did not permit him to do it. And we will not permit women to face the possibility of illegal abortion any more than I permitted Jack Wilke [sic] to push me away from the microphones."[3]

A videotape shows that the incident, as reported by the *New York Times Magazine*, is largely accurate, though the term "shoved" seems strong. Unfortunately, one can likely expect similar incidents to occur as the verbal battle, as well as the fight for the attention of the media, heat up.

ADVERTISING

Soon after the *Webster* decision was announced, both Planned Parenthood and the National Abortion Rights Action League placed full-page advertisements in major newspapers across the country. One Planned Parenthood advertisement pictures the five members of the Supreme Court who voted in the majority in *Webster* with a headline reading, "Five U.S. Supreme Court Justices Just Had Their Say On Abortion. Now It's Your Turn."[4]

Coupons are addressed to President George Bush, Speaker of the House Thomas Foley, and Senate Majority Leader George Mitchell. The coupon for President

Bush begins, "You swore to uphold the Constitution, not undermine it." It reminds the President that he is supposed to "represent all Americans, not just an extremist few." The support given by the White House to the movement against abortion and in opposition to what Planned Parenthood refers to as "responsible family planning" is called "a betrayal of American women." The coupon ends with, "Stop trying to punish women for unwanted pregnancies and start doing more to help prevent them."[5]

A fourth coupon appears at the end of the advertisement. It was to be used to send a "tax-deductible contribution to Planned Parenthood's Campaign to Keep Abortion Safe and Legal."[6]

The remainder of the advertisement includes many paragraphs attacking the decision in *Webster,* the White House, and abortion opponents. Familiar arguments, such as "back-alley" abortions, are repeated:

> WOMEN will always have the final word on abortion. No legislator, Supreme Court Justice or President can change that. All they can do is make it illegal or harder to obtain, drive it into dirty back alleys and endanger the lives of women. . . .
>
> Abortion is still legal. But the Supreme Court—aided and abetted by the White House—has opened the door for anti-abortion extremists to impose limits on abortion in each state. . . .
>
> This is more than a theoretical injustice. It could lead to the death and maiming of thousands of desperate women in back-alley butchery and horrifying self-induced abortions. And all women would suffer the indignity of hurdling barriers designed solely to harass them.
>
> We can't let that happen. Planned Parenthood is committed to fighting in every state to keep abortion safe, legal and available for all women. But to take this battle to fifty state legislatures, your active support is essential.
>
> Elected representatives can no longer be allowed to remain equivocal on abortion. They can't permit themselves to be bullied or intimidated by a few vocal and violent anti-abortion extremists. . . .
>
> This is still a democracy. And when an intolerant, fanatical few seek to impose their will on the rest of us, we can and must fight back.[7]

The advertisement ends with, "Send a message they can't ignore. Don't wait until women are dying again."[8]

In November 1989, one day after the Supreme Court heard arguments in two parental consent cases, a full-page advertisement was printed in *USA Today*. Part of Planned Parenthood's "Don't wait until women are dying again" campaign, the advertisement is headlined, "What Extremists Couldn't Do With 100 Firebombs, the Supreme Court Might Do With One Decision."[9]

The advertisement includes the usual coupons. One is addressed to President Bush. It centers on his veto of three bills. Two of the bills would have expanded the Hyde Amendment, which bans federal funding of abortion except when necessary to save the mother's life, to include rape and incest. The third bill would have restored funding to the United Nations Population Fund, a group that has poured more than $157 million into supporting China's forced abortion policy. It is expected that the same legislation will resurface in the future. The coupon to President Bush reads as follows:

> Mr. President:
>
> Your vetoes of federal legislation protecting the right of the disadvantaged to make responsible, safe decisions about abortion were cruel and unjust. Don't you realize you are accountable to the majority of Americans who want the health and privacy of women pro-

tected? Reject narrow extremism and take a responsible position on abortion and family planning.[10]

Of course Americans support protecting "the health and privacy of women," but they do not consider abortion to have anything to do with either "health" or "privacy."

Thomas Foley and George Mitchell were to receive coupons:

> The White House's aggressive intervention in personal and private decisions about abortion calls for decisive leadership in Congress. Millions of women have been targeted, their rights and their lives threatened. I strongly urge you to take whatever action is necessary to correct the Supreme Court's errors and protect the health and privacy of every American woman.[11]

Naturally, one coupon is to be sent to Planned Parenthood—along with a tax-deductible contribution. The rest of the advertisement is divided into three parts:

> Frustrated because they haven't been able to outlaw abortion for everyone, extremists are using desperate maneuvers to stop specific groups of women from being able to obtain safe, legal abortions.
>
> On July 3, in the *Webster* case, the Supreme Court gave states more power to restrict access to abortion, touching off a legislative and political firestorm.
>
> And anti-choice zealots are pushing for states to use their power against the young and the poor.
>
> Right now, in two cases before the Supreme Court . . . , anti-choice forces are attempting to strip young women who seek safe, legal abortion of their privacy and protection against harassment and physical abuse.
>
> Another measure headed for Supreme Court review might have shut *three out of four* clinics offering family planning and abortion services.
>
> Confronted with public outrage at such threats to women's health, the state attorney general in that case backed away, but medically unnecessary "clinic standards" . . . are a favorite extremist weapon and will doubtless appear on the Supreme Court's docket again.
>
> A bad Supreme Court decision in any of these cases would do more to deny women access to safe, legal abortion than a decade of firebombings and clinic blockades.
>
> President Bush has continued the attack started by President Reagan. Allied with anti-choice extremists, his administration has again asked the court to reverse *Roe v. Wade*, the historic decision that legalized abortion nationwide and ended the back-alley carnage sixteen years ago.
>
> He has overruled Congress three times and vetoed the right of poverty-stricken rape and incest victims to terminate their pregnancies.
>
> The White House must take responsibility for the chaos in abortion laws and the growing danger to women.
>
> When voters get the chance to reject extremism, they do so, as the races in Virginia, New York and New Jersey made clear.
>
> America stands for choice.
>
> And it's time for our elected officials to respect the views of the majority, undo the damage done by the Reagan-packed court, and act to preserve the safety and privacy of *all* women—including the millions who happen to be young or poor.
>
> Please mail the coupons immediately.
>
> Don't wait until women are dying again.[12]

A second section of the advertisement is titled, "What's Wrong With 'Parental Consent'?":

> The *Hodgson* case before the court challenges a Minnesota requirement that a woman under 18 notify both parents before an abortion. Most teens already consult a parent, without such laws. Almost half don't live with both parents. One in four teens seeking a judicial "bypass" of the law is accompanied by the parent who has custody, pleading not to have to involve the other parent. Most Americans agree a teen who can't talk with her parents should be able to consult another responsible adult. Indeed, after hearing evidence

of family conflict and brutal violence, an appeals judge wrote "compelling parental notice . . . is almost always disastrous." We're also contesting an Ohio law with a similar destructive impact.[13]

The third section is titled, "Clinic Marauders Raise 'Safety' Concerns?":

> Abortion is practically risk-free . . . one hundred times safer than an appendectomy. Yet extremists now call for every clinic to be equipped and staffed like a major hospital. Net effect? To padlock 75 percent of women's health centers. Outrage against such extremist tactics forced Illinois Attorney General to settle the *Ragsdale* case just days before the Supreme Court was to hear it. But similar assaults are proposed in other states. Catastrophe is still only five Supreme Court votes away.[14]

Some comment is appropriate. Planned Parenthood has intensified its name-calling campaign. Using terms such as "anti-choice," "extremists," and "zealots," when Planned Parenthood knows those opposed to its agenda do not have the funds for counter-advertising, evokes the desired response.

Planned Parenthood raises the issue of mandating parental involvement in the abortion decision of a minor. A June 1990 *New York Times*/CBS News poll shows that 76 percent of Americans support parental notification laws.[15] An NBC News/*Wall Street Journal* poll released one month later shows that 75 percent of Americans support mandated parental notification.[16] One of the most compelling reasons for such laws is that if complications arise, it is the parents who must pay for it—both financially and emotionally. In addition, such laws lead to reductions in both the teen pregnancy and abortion rate. Why? Teens change their behavior when they learn abortion cannot be obtained without parental notification. Planned Parenthood officials have conceded that such laws reduce the teen pregnancy and abortion rate, yet they still oppose such legislation.[17]

Planned Parenthood refers to the poor. The issue here is not the poor, especially when Planned Parenthood bills the government to pay for the services of those it claims are "poor." Planned Parenthood wants the government to pay for its services so it can have more money. If abortion and its other services are not paid for by the government, Planned Parenthood will lose many customers. Planned Parenthood is certainly not interested in providing these services unless either the government (preferred) or customers pay for them. The bottom line is that Planned Parenthood officials believe every person should receive its services free of charge and, therefore, the government should pay for them. In the eyes of Planned Parenthood officials, these services are equivalent to Medicare or Social Security.

"Safe, legal abortion" is the common theme. It is a phrase Planned Parenthood desires to bury in the minds of the American public.

The most amazing attack is that Planned Parenthood claims the Illinois attorney general, Neil Hartigan, backed away from the Supreme Court case due to "public outrage." Justice Department officials told some leaders of the anti-abortion movement that the case would be settled out of court long before it came to the attention of the public.

Why did Hartigan settle the *Ragsdale* case, as though he has the right to thwart the will of the Illinois legislature? Hartigan became a Democratic candidate for Governor. He believed abortion foes would have no better choice as the Republican candidate had always been radically supportive of legal abortion. Therefore, at the urging of pro-legal abortion leaders, Hartigan settled to prevent the Supreme Court from using the case to reverse *Roe v. Wade*. Hartigan apparently believed he could get the votes of both sides in the abortion debate. Most observers would probably say Hartigan managed to lose the support of abortion foes while his Republican opponent, always a friend of the legal abortion cause, retained his support. Hartigan lost the election.

The advertisement refers to the victories of candidates who support legal abortion in New Jersey, Virginia, and New York City. It is not mentioned that the "pro-life" candidates in these races never made abortion a positive issue. Instead, the candidates either ignored the issue or softened their anti-abortion positions. Winning candidates in other races put on the gloves and made abortion a central issue, showing that most candidates who support Planned Parenthood's position on abortion are radically out of step with the American people.

The advertisement fails to mention the victories of candidates opposed to legal abortion in other areas where abortion was an equally volatile issue. The moral for politicians is simple. Do not stick by your principles (be a traitor to your cause) and you can expect to lose. There are few exceptions.

Supporters of unrestricted abortion have succeeded in convincing many candidates for public office that being opposed to abortion is a losing position. This has been accomplished by consistently referencing the gubernatorial races in New Jersey and Virginia and the mayoral race in New York City. Even local races have been effected. In a race for the state senate in a northern Virginia district, the Democratic candidate, Jim Tso, made abortion an issue by claiming his opponent, Warren Barry, is anti-abortion. Barry's response was to mail a circular to voters addressing the issue. Examine the rhetoric used by the Republican candidate:

> *On abortion:* Using abortion as a political tool is wrong. While Mr. Tso is for abortion on demand, Warren's more moderate position is that abortion is a personal moral matter which should be decided by the woman in concert with her Family, Doctor and Clergy—*not the politicians in Richmond.*[18]

Reading the circular, some abortion foes could come to the conclusion that the candidates have the same position. However, Barry said during a telephone call that he opposes second and third trimester abortions and he supports requiring parental consent.

It became clear that Barry's support for first trimester abortions is based largely on political considerations, not moral ones. The candidate wanted to win the election and he was convinced that being against abortion, given what happened in the race for governor one year earlier, this would not be possible. Barry was informed that if he were trained on how to make the abortion issue work for him, such worthless rhetoric and an alteration of his political views could have been avoided. Barry won by a lopsided margin.

The state senate election points to another problem facing abortion foes. Supporters of legal abortion recruit, train, and "educate" candidates for public office. Abortion foes rarely do any of these.

It should not be assumed that only frightened abortion foes make use of rhetoric to mask their positions. In early 1990, Leslie L. Byrne, a Virginia state legislator, wrote to her constituents asking them to answer several survey questions. A zealous supporter of unrestricted abortion, Byrne asked one question about abortion:

"Should Virginia's current abortion laws remain unchanged?" According to Byrne, 68 percent said "yes," 16 percent said "no," and 16 percent were undecided.[19]

Some important questions come to mind: How many people answering the survey know the abortion law in Virginia? How many people understand that unless the law allows abortion for any or no reason and at any time in the pregnancy, it is worthless due to *Roe v. Wade* and *Doe v. Bolton?* It would not be unreasonable to assume that most survey respondents know little about the issue, yet Byrne could use the "survey of the ignorant" to claim her position on abortion is consistent with that of her constituents. Byrne surely knows this to be the case and the question was surely written in a way to generate the desired response, not the true feelings of voters in her district.

It must be noted that every election, whether won by a supporter or opponent of legal abortion, has a tremendous impact on public policy in both the short and long terms. In March 1992, Governor Ann Richards, D-Texas, appointed Susan Larsen to the Eighth Supreme District Appeals Court. Larsen is actively involved with El Paso Planned Parenthood.[20]

EFFECT ON PRO-LEGAL ABORTION GROUPS

Planned Parenthood's effort called the "Campaign to Keep Abortion Safe and Legal" has succeeded in improving fund-raising for Planned Parenthood and other pro-legal abortion groups. It has also succeeded in boosting membership in groups dedicated to legal abortion.

As previously noted, fund-raising and support for pro-legal abortion groups increased at the very threat of the *Webster* case. Once the decision was actually handed down on July 3, 1989, the fund-raising and memberships increased even more. For example, *Time* reports that the National Organization for Women and the National Abortion Rights Action League each signed up 50,000 new members shortly after *Webster*. As for money, "NARAL [National Abortion Rights Action League] added $1 million to its coffers in July [1989] alone."[21]

A story appearing on the Associated Press wire reports that the political action committees of groups that support legal abortion have "built up a political war-chest . . . nearly seven times as large as the funds held by the chief anti-abortion organization . . . "[22] Political action committee funds are used to support candidates for public office.

The point the Associated Press story fails to raise is from where the money is coming. According to Federal Election Commission reports for the first quarter of 1992, organizations opposed to legal abortion had raised $629,099. Groups supporting legal abortion had raised $7,026,052. Opposing abortion is costly. Performing abortions is highly profitable. For abortion foes, contributing to a political action committee is a sacrifice. For performers of abortion, it is an investment.

DIRECT MAIL CAMPAIGN

Many of those who write to Planned Parenthood about its Campaign to Keep Abortion Safe and Legal are sent a brochure picturing televangelist Jimmy Swaggart, a "Statement of Affirmation" supporting Planned Parenthood's goals, and a fund-raising letter. The fund-raising letter attacks anti-abortion leaders and generally outlines Planned Parenthood's agenda:

> When we've received one million or more signed statements, we will use them as a lobbying tool before Congress and state legislatures and as a tool to show the media the overwhelming number of Americans who support the right to choose.
>
> Next, you can return the signed statement to Planned Parenthood with as generous a contribution as you can afford today.
>
> Your tax-deductible contribution will help Planned Parenthood to . . .
>
> - expand a massive public information campaign to get the facts about the right to choose to as many Americans as possible, and to expose the leaders of the anti-choice movement for the ruthless fanatics they are.
> - mobilize the vast majority in America who support the right to choose and show these concerned citizens how to make their will known to our elected representatives.
> - convince the policy makers in every state that it is politically foolish to pander to the anti-choice extremists.
> - enact mandated sexuality education programs to teach teenagers about the risks of unintended pregnancy and the spread of sexually transmitted diseases, including AIDS.
> - convince Congress to reauthorize Title X, our nation's family planning program, which has been under siege by anti-choice zealots since 1985.
> - begin a major offensive to increase funding for badly needed new contraceptive research. This will also force the opposition to reveal their true position on contraception.
>
> President Bush has worked against abortion rights since his first day in office. But if he truly wishes to reduce the number of abortions, he should not pander to the zealots who cry for punishment over prevention. Rather he should join with Planned Parenthood and use the power of his office to foster the development, testing and distribution of more effective new birth control methods.
>
> For 73 years, Planned Parenthood has been working to ensure that every child is a wanted child. And now it appears that everything that we have worked for may be reversed. *We must not let a minority of anti-choice fanatics turn back the clock.*
>
> Please join us in our Campaign to Keep Abortion Safe and Legal. Don't wait until women are dying again.
>
> Reaffirm your belief in the American values of self-determination and personal freedom by supporting Planned Parenthood today.[23]

READY FOR A FIGHT

While abortion foes fight to determine the best strategy for when *Roe* is reversed, supporters of legal abortion are facing the same struggle, but to a lesser degree. Abortion supporters must decide how far they wish to go in defending such rights.

While still president of the National Organization for Women, Molly Yard called for the formation of a new political party dedicated to reproductive rights, the environment, and other issues. Yard believes the Democratic party, which has enjoyed the vast majority of the votes of those who support the goals of the National Organization for Women, has abandoned that agenda. The organization also has called for an expansion of the Bill of Rights in the Constitution. One amendment would guarantee abortion as a constitutional right while another would protect all sexual orientations. Patricia Ireland, current president of the National Organization for Women, not only supports the call for a new political party, she has announced that the organization now officially calls for civil disobedience.

Faye Wattleton supported the idea of a constitutional amendment protecting abortion. However, she did not endorse the idea of working outside of the two-party structure.

Planned Parenthood continues to prepare to have a key impact on legislation and political races. A coalition has been formed including all major pro-legal abortion groups. The leaders of the coalition have formed several task forces to assist in achieving their goals. Planned Parenthood heads the State Task Force which is charged with doing "intensive research on existing state laws pertaining to abortion," monitoring "any attempts to pass new" state laws, and following "state political races."[24]

Since Planned Parenthood is a nonprofit organization and receives tax-deductible donations, it cannot be directly involved in political campaigns. Planned Parenthood will, however, work to get its message to the public through its affiliates.[25]

That is not all. Planned Parenthood has conducted a massive public opinion poll designed to assist in the development of a campaign to reach the millions of Americans who do not have strong feelings about abortion. While Planned Parenthood cannot be directly involved in political campaigns (through endorsement and donations), it can assist in other substantial ways, including releasing mailing lists, "educating" its supporters as to which candidates support Planned Parenthood's agenda, and providing thousands of volunteers to work on political campaigns. All of these activities are legal under Internal Revenue Service guidelines.

Faye Wattleton realizes the most important lesson of all. "The reality has set in," she says, "that more effort and resources will have to be invested in the electoral process. In the end it's going to have to be the people, and I go even further to say it's going to have to be women . . ." According to Wattleton, "If women determined to settle the abortion issue, it would be settled. The power is within ourselves."[26]

MEDIA BLITZ

On May 15, 1989, almost two months before the decision in *Webster* was handed down, NBC aired a made-for-television movie based on *Roe v. Wade*. Following the movie, after local news, NBC ran a special program titled, "The Abortion Dilemma: Rights and Lives."

The NBC special featured a panel discussion consisting of Faye Wattleton, then-president of the Planned Parenthood Federation of America; Anna Quindlen, an author; Congressman Christopher Smith, R-New Jersey; and Olivia Gans, head of American Victims of Abortion. The program was moderated by NBC's Tom Brokaw. (See Appendix D for excerpts and commentary from "The Abortion Dilemma: Rights and Lives.")

Roe vs. Wade was just one abortion-related program to be aired on television following the decision of the Supreme Court to hear the *Webster* case. Other television films and programs (mostly news-related programs) that addressed the abortion issue were aired. For the first time since 1973, most in the media saw the Supreme Court decision in *Webster* to be crucial to the future of legal abortion.

As noted in chapter 6, Planned Parenthood has teamed up with the Better World Society, headed by R. E. "Ted" Turner, founder, president, and chief executive officer of the Turner Broadcasting System. This relationship has proved invaluable to Planned Parenthood.

Following the decision in *Webster*, WTBS aired a film called, *Abortion: For Survival*. Produced by the Fund for the Feminist Majority, a pro-legal abortion group headed by the former president of the National Organization for Women, Eleanor Smeal, the film is a strong attack on the movement opposed to legal abortion, as well as a strongly pro-legal abortion piece.[27]

When aired on WTBS, *Abortion: For Survival* opened with the statement, "The views presented are not necessarily those of the TBS [Turner Broadcasting System] Network."[28] While the views may not represent Turner's company, they certainly represent Turner. The *Chattanooga News-Free Press* quotes Turner as saying that anti-abortion activists are "bozos." Turner, speaking to television critics and writers at the National Cable Forum, does not care whether anyone likes *Abortion: For Survival*:

> "You bet you're bippy we're taking a position," Turner said. . . .
>
> Turner, his language weaving in and out of what's allowed in a family newspaper, criticized anti-abortion activists, saying they try to impose their views on others.
>
> "I don't want anybody else telling me what my daughter's got to have, or my wife, or my girlfriend . . . We live in a free country. There is absolutely no way that that's anybody's business but the person that's involved. That's my opinion."
>
> Despite his convictions, Turner will broadcast a panel discussion after "Abortion for [sic] Survival," with people on both sides of the issue. Just don't expect him to listen.
>
> "We'll give the other Bozos a chance to talk back," Turner said. "They look like idiots anyway."
>
> And that's not all, he said.
>
> "The pro-lifers say we don't want people to have sex for fun, only to have babies. It's sinful. Sex is sinful," Turner said. "Well, that's fine if those people don't want to ever have sex. Swell. I happen to enjoy it. I don't get near as much as I want to."[29]

Abortion: For Survival is riddled with ludicrous and surprising content. One of the most shocking sections is the acknowledgment of World Vision at the end of the program. Why would World Vision, one of the most respected Christian relief and development organizations in the world, assist groups like the Fund for the Feminist Majority and the Better World Society?

It appears that the Fund for the Feminist Majority used an independent company, On the Screen Productions Incorporated, to obtain World Vision film footage of the 1984-1985 Ethiopian famine. According to World Vision officials, the company acquired the footage by misrepresenting the purpose of the program in which it was to be included. World Vision was told that the subject of the program was "overpopulation" and that the organization would have an opportunity to clear the program before it was aired in its final form. World Vision was given no other information about the program.[30]

In May 1989, when World Vision learned the actual circumstances in which its Ethiopian film footage was to be used, the relief organization demanded that the footage and its name be removed from *Abortion: For Survival.* World Vision threatened legal action to seek damages for fraud and deceit if the Fund for the Feminist Majority included the World Vision footage in its program.[31]

On June 2, 1989, an attorney for On the Scene Productions Incorporated denied any wrongdoing but agreed to World Vision's demands. Nevertheless, the World Vision acknowledgement was not deleted from the program.[32] World Vision's president, Robert A. Seiple, issued a strongly worded statement on the issue:

> This program misrepresents World Vision on an emotional and divisive issue. We inexorably oppose the use of abortion for population control in the third world. For World Vision to be identified in any way as supporting or encouraging abortion runs contrary to everything we stand for. All of World Vision's efforts seek to save, extend and enhance life.[33]

Following *Abortion: For Survival,* a one-hour "panel discussion" was held between the two factions. Congressman Robert K. Dornan, R-California, and Nellie Gray, president of March for Life, represented those opposed to abortion. Faye Wattleton and Eleanor Smeal represented those supportive of legal abortion. This part of the program was called "Abortion: An Issue Forum" and was hosted by Martin Agronsky.

Agronsky, while billed as the moderator, actually participated by commenting on statements made by Gray and Dornan. While Agronsky had a difficult job, given constant interruptions, his participation with regard to arguments made by the abortion opponents was unwarranted. For example, Dornan noted Turner's comments that opponents of abortion are "bozos" and that the format was unfair since Turner refused to air an anti-abortion film (such as *The Silent Scream* or *Eclipse of Reason*) along with *Abortion: For Survival.* Dornan argues that a panel discussion following the showing of both films would have been fair.[34]

Following Dornan's comments, Agronsky says, "Let me say to you that this whole business of dragging Turner into it doesn't make a hell of a lot of sense." Dornan replies by pointing out that Turner had commented on the program publicly and, more importantly, Turner was paying for the program since no advertising was sought given its nature. Agronsky replies:

> Well, sure, he's paying for it, but, but, you know, Turner is giving you an opportunity to set forth whatever your point of view may be and you may do it at great length if you wish. Nellie's already done it, despite what she calls the stacked nature of the program. But I do think, I do think that it's only fair, that instead of doing this kind of name-calling, we address the issue.[35]

A thorough check of the transcript shows that the only name-calling with regard to the exchange came from Dornan's quotation of Turner's widely reported "bozos" comment.

Another exchange regards Dornan's assertion that the government of the People's Republic of China uses infanticide. Dornan asserts that China "has an infanticide program to back up its abortion program and the Better World Society gave Zhou Boping an award." (More accurately, the Better World Society gave the award to the China Family Planning Association. The award was accepted by Wang Wei, vice president of the Association. Zhou Boping serves on the board of directors of the Better World Society.) Agronsky, billed as the debate moderator, not as a participant, counters with, "An infanticide [interruption] . . . You mean the Chinese government is committed to killing babies?" When Dornan responds by saying the Chinese "kill the babies after they're born if they don't get them before," Agronsky says, "Oh, that's nonsense."[36]

There were other examples of bias on the part of Agronsky. In his first question to Gray, referring to the Fund for the Feminist Majority program, Agronsky says, "That was really a powerful 30 minutes, I thought, evaluating why so many people all over the world are in favor of women having access, free access, to legal abortion."[37]

Agronsky chastises Gray saying, "I raise questions, you don't address them. You go off into a completely opposite direction." When Agronsky tries to discredit Gray's knowledge of law by saying, "Nellie, don't . . . get off into an area where there are different areas of competence and I don't think you are really competent in dealing with the judicial or legal problems," he learns that Gray is an attorney and World War II veteran.[38]

Most of Agronsky's other degrading and hostile comments are also directed at Gray. They clearly show bias. For example, Agronsky says, "Oh, Nellie, you're setting forth all these phony propositions," and, "Nellie, . . . you, you just, you know, go completely off the course here," and, "You get completely disoriented and all of a sudden you're talking about murdering babies."[39]

It is clear that Agronsky did not want Gray to talk about the preborn. Agronsky makes comments such as, "We're not trying to talk about murdering babies," and, "I don't want to talk about killing babies. Can't we, can't we address other questions that are of equal significance?"[40] Of equal significance to killing babies, Mr. Agronsky? Like what?

Agronsky interrupts one of Gray's first comments with, "You keep saying innocent people. Why?" Gray responds, "Because a child is innocent in the womb. It has not done anything at all . . ." Agronsky interrupts again with, "No, people and children is what you said."[41]

A check of the transcript shows that Gray refers to "innocent preborn children." At no time was the word "people," which seemed to bother Agronsky, used.

One question must be asked. Why do abortion opponents agree to go on programs that are clearly stacked against them? Turner knew exactly which people he wanted on the program. Turner knew they would agree to participate. Turner knew he could then say he had been fair to the "bozos." Had abortion foes refused to participate, Turner would have simply announced that time was offered and refused, which could have been better than allowing Turner to *appear* fair. (See Appendix E for excerpts and commentary from *Abortion: For Survival* and "Abortion: An Issue Forum.")

ANOTHER IMPORTANT EVENT

On April 5, 1992, the National Organization for Women sponsored a pro-legal abortion march in Washington, D.C. Some media estimates said 500,000 people attended. The park police reported 250,000 in attendance.

Many people believe the large crowd is comparable to the March for Life, which takes place every January 22, and the Rally for Life held in April 1990. The events are not comparable. Supporters of legal abortion held a march in 1989 and 1992. They concentrated on getting virtually every advocate of legal abortion in the country to attend the infrequent events. Since abortion foes march every year, in what is often terrible weather, the make-up of the crowd significantly changes from year-to-year.

The day following the pro-legal abortion march, the *Washington Post,* a newspaper which admittedly supports legal abortion, included an article titled, "Rally Draws Movement Veterans: Poll Suggests Abortion-Rights March Failed to Attract Diverse Crowd." The article notes that those who marched were "mostly veterans of previous abortion-rights rallies . . . "[42] Consider the results of the poll conducted by the newspaper:

- 78 percent of the marchers were female;
- 3 percent were between the ages of 13 and 17, 47 percent were 18–29, 31 percent were between 30 and 44, and 19 percent were 45 or over;
- 30 percent were married;
- 26 percent were parents;
- 25 percent were students;
- 59 percent held full-time jobs;
- 15 percent called themselves Catholic, 25 percent called themselves Protestant, and 21 percent said they were Jewish;
- 59 percent said they were Democrats, 5 percent were Republican;
- 30 percent categorized themselves as very liberal, 49 percent called themselves liberal, 16 percent said they were moderates, 3 percent labeled themselves as conservative, while 1 percent said they were very conservative.
- 82 percent say they have had a close friend or relative who has had an abortion;
- 99 percent said abortion should be legal if the mother's life is in danger (compared to a national figure of 87 percent), 97 percent said abortion should be legal if there is a chance the baby will be born deformed (compared to 63 percent nationally), 100 percent said abortion should be legal if the pregnancy is the result of rape or incest (compared to 79 percent nationally), 96 percent said it should be legal if the family cannot afford another child (compared to 39 percent nationally), and 95 percent believed abortion should be legal if the parent(s) simply do not want another child (compared to 32 percent nationally);
- 93 percent believed the law should not require parental notification for a minor wishing to have an abortion (compared to 18 percent nationally); and
- 96 percent of the marchers said a woman should not be required by law to get the permission of her husband before getting an abortion (compared to 33 percent nationally).[43]

The march not only included the most rabid advocates of legal abortion, it is clear that these women and men are not representative of the population. The idea that lawmakers would cower by seeing the large crowd is simply laughable.

Moreover, the idea that the decisions of the Supreme Court would be influenced by such a spectacle is ridiculous.

The Court is likely to make sweeping changes in *Roe v. Wade*. If the 1973 decision is not overturned outright in *Planned Parenthood of Southeastern Pennsylvania v. Casey*, it is only a matter of time. On this point, both sides of the abortion debate agree.

In *Planned Parenthood v. Casey*, virtually all leaders in the abortion debate, on both sides, expected the Supreme Court to uphold all of the Pennsylvania law, including spousal notification which had been struck down by a lower court. Many leaders expected the Court to reverse *Roe v. Wade* while others believed the Court would wait for an even more direct challenge to *Roe* posed by the Guam and Louisiana laws. Both sides were shocked to see what the Court had done.

The Supreme Court upheld the parental consent, 24-hour waiting period, informed consent, definition of "medical emergency," and clinic reporting requirements of the Pennsylvania law. They found spousal notification to be unconstitutional. However, the Court *reaffirmed Roe v. Wade*. The Pennsylvania laws do not, the Court decided, impose an undue burden on women seeking an abortion, but the basic holding in *Roe* still stands, although the Court toned down its "abortion is a fundamental right" rhetoric.

The decision was a great surprise because Justices Sandra Day O'Connor, Anthony Kennedy, and David Souter joined in reaffirming *Roe v. Wade*. The three use precedence and a desire to protect the court's "integrity" to justify their decision, despite the fact that they virtually admit *Roe* was wrongly decided. Prior decisions led virtually everyone to believe that at least Kennedy would vote in favor of reversing *Roe*. Chief Justice William Rehnquist and Justices Antonin Scalia, Byron White, and Clarence Thomas argued for reversal. Justices Harry Blackmun and John Paul Stevens had always been supporters of *Roe v. Wade*.

Predictably, supporters of legal abortion slammed the *Casey* decision because the Supreme Court upheld most of the Pennsylvania law. This shows their unwavering dedication to completely unregulated abortion. Moreover, it helps to galvanize support. After all, if everyone can be convinced the abortion sky is falling, even though *Roe v. Wade* was explicitly reaffirmed, maybe they will give more money and time to pro-legal abortion groups.

Surprisingly, some abortion foes sought to paint the decision as good for their movement. Granted, the Supreme Court did uphold most of the Pennsylvania law, but to claim these provisions are, in the long-run, meaningful restrictions is preposterous. They are, at best, regulations not restrictions. Moreover, the reaffirmation of *Roe* is a stunning set-back, and no positive thinking will change this fact. With the present Supreme Court, one can expect meaningful restrictions on abortion, such as those found in the Guam and Louisiana laws, to be found unconstitutional.

One excuse for putting the *Casey* decision in a good light is that abortion foes will become discouraged if the truth is told. Hogwash!

If the people cannot hear and deal with the reality of the situation, they are not up for the real fight ahead, and a fight will come whether *Roe* is reversed or not. If those opposed to abortion are that weak, they may deserve to lose, but those they seek to protect do not. The question is simple: Are abortion foes more dedicated to protect strangers, those least among us, more than supporters of legal abortion are dedicated to protecting the "right" to destroy the lives of others without interference?

16

PUTTING UP A LOCAL FIGHT

As powerful as Planned Parenthood is (which is largely due to its financial base), the organization can be challenged. This has been proven on both the local and national levels. Such a challenge takes time, determination, hard work, and cooperation, but it can be done.

Planned Parenthood's foes must have the determination of Margaret Sanger, minus the unethical baggage. Strategies aside, it is important to learn from those who have fought the battle before us. There is no reason to make the same mistakes.

TACTICS

There are several strategies which can be used to effectively thwart Planned Parenthood at the local level. If Planned Parenthood is to be stopped, those seeking to employ these strategies should have these goals in mind: education of those in the community, motivation of those in the community so effective action will be taken, and challenging Planned Parenthood at *every* step.

The most common tactic used by citizens opposed to Planned Parenthood is picketing. While some view picketing as a radical action, it has always been viewed as a legitimate form of protest in any free society, particularly in North America. The most common misconception about picketing as it relates to Planned Parenthood is that it is intended to close the facility. This is naive in that picketing itself will almost never close a Planned Parenthood office. This is erroneous in that the purpose of picketing is to inform and educate the surrounding community.

Picketing should not be limited to Planned Parenthood. Picketing at the offices of corporate supporters of Planned Parenthood is an excellent way to convince corporate leaders to change their philanthropic practices. No corporate official likes to see pickets set up outside his or her office, plant, or other work site.

Picketing is effective only when done consistently. Do not set up just one day of picketing. Your commitment, or lack thereof, will be noticed. Do not set up picketing only on Tuesdays. You do not want Planned Parenthood or corporate officials to say, "There are the picketers; it must be Tuesday." Picketing should be done as often as possible.

Numbers are not important. In fact, if you have too many people on a picket line it becomes more of a rally with little room for walking. Even one or two picketers are better than none.

Picketers should not be yelling or harassing passersby. They are there to educate the public in a kind way. Picketers should answer questions when asked but should not get into arguments.

If the police are called, one person should serve as the leader. If the police give instructions, they should be obeyed, but an attorney should be consulted to be sure constitutional rights are not being violated.

Distribution of leaflets is an effective way to spread your message. The leaflets should look good and include only factual, easy-to-read material. The purpose should be stated logically and without emotional rhetoric. Communication should have the receiver in mind, not the sender. Keep the use of religious rhetoric to a minimum as it may give people an excuse to oppose the anti-Planned Parenthood position because of a prejudice toward religion or religious people.

Showing films and inviting public speakers is an impressive way to educate the community, provided that the films selected and the speakers invited are of high caliber. The key in employing this strategy is to use churches, civic groups, newspapers, local media, and other devises to encourage attendance at your meeting. Never hold a public meeting without setting up a system to contact those who wish to get more information and/or become involved.

LOCAL GOVERNMENT FUNDING

In Mecklenburg County, North Carolina, a coalition of groups opposed to legal abortion had been working for years to end funding of Planned Parenthood by the County Commission. Mecklenburg County had funded Planned Parenthood programs for 13 years and Planned Parenthood was requesting funding of $115,000 for 1988. Planned Parenthood had received $110,000 from the county one year earlier.

Led by Barrett Mosbacker, the group opposed to Planned Parenthood funding called itself "The Ad Hoc Committee to Oppose Public Funding of Planned Parenthood." The committee operated professionally but aggressively. Most work was done behind the scenes—rallying support and meeting with lawmakers. Citizens became familiar with the political process on the county level and leaders of the ad hoc committee were often attacked in the local media.

Barrett Mosbacker received most of the media harassment. The *Charlotte Observer* provideed the bulk of the criticism. This is not surprising since in 1985 the newspaper's publisher received the Margaret Sanger Award from the local Planned Parenthood affiliate. The publisher is even quoted as saying he would "personally make up the difference in the budget" if the County Commission refused to fund Planned Parenthood.[1]

Polly Paddock, a columnist for the *Observer*, writes in support of the Planned Parenthood funding:

> We can rant and rave about how teenage sex is immoral, risky, socially destructive—all of which is true.
>
> We may feel exhilarated by our moralism, smug in our self-righteousness.
>
> But does that stop one young couple from experimenting with sex? . . .
>
> If you feel as I do, let your county commissioners know *now*.
>
> Otherwise, the big losers will be our children—and the children they are now producing.[2]

The official newspaper editorials are also in support of funding.[3]

Planned Parenthood officials sent out 3,100 letters urging supporters of Planned Parenthood funding to show up at the meeting of the county commission. On the other side, the Ad Hoc Committee mailed 4,000 flyers.[4] About 150 people opposed to Planned Parenthood funding attended the meeting. About 40 supporters of Planned Parenthood funding attended.[5]

Two county commissioners who had previously supported Planned Parenthood changed sides. By a vote of four to three, Planned Parenthood funding was cut off. In response, Planned Parenthood placed a full-page advertisement in the *Charlotte Observer* attacking, by name, the four commissioners who had opposed its funding.[6] In short, anyone who opposes funding Planned Parenthood is identified, labeled, and maligned.

Barrett Mosbacker believes the success can be duplicated in other areas. He does warn, however, not to expect immediate victory. It is a long-term battle. (See Appendix B for tips on opposing Planned Parenthood at the local level.)

UNITED WAY

Planned Parenthood of Seattle-King County, Washington, had received $430,000 per year in support from the United Way of King County. In December 1987, the Seattle-King County chapter of Planned Parenthood announced it would begin doing abortions in 1989. It had previously referred women for abortions after doing the counseling.

United Way had been criticized for many years by state and local groups opposed to abortion because Planned Parenthood was receiving funding. United Way has always claimed such criticism was unwarranted because Planned Parenthood of Seattle-King County was not doing abortions. However, with the announcement that Planned Parenthood of Seattle-King County would begin doing abortions, the effort to defund Planned Parenthood intensified.

The fight against United Way funding of Planned Parenthood was led by a coalition involving Washington state's two largest groups that oppose abortion, HUMAN LIFE and the local Christian Action Council chapter. The Catholic Church, which had previously done little more than speak negatively about such funding, also assumed an active role in opposing continued United Way support of Planned Parenthood.

United Way of King County has always had an unwritten policy against supporting groups that offer abortion services. On June 20, 1988, the policy was formalized.

The coalition opposed to continued Planned Parenthood funding published a brochure urging people to boycott the United Way campaign and to give to the charities of their choice on an individual basis. A petition drive was used as well.

On the last day of September 1988, the Seattle-King County chapter of Planned Parenthood was told it could continue to receive funding for its services, including counseling and referral for abortion, if it would agree to place its abortion practice under a separate corporation. This would generally involve little more than keeping separate books. The corporation not performing abortions could receive United Way funding. In response, the Seattle-King County chapter of Planned Parenthood decided to completely withdraw as a United Way agency.

The controversy has not ended with the withdrawal of Planned Parenthood. The local media blames a significant decrease in contributions to United Way on the controversy. Some argue that the Seattle-King County chapter of Planned Parenthood should be readmitted as a United Way agency even if it does abortions. Others suggest that individuals be allowed to designate funding for Planned Parenthood through United Way, using the "donor choice" procedure, even if Planned Parenthood of Seattle-King County is not a recognized United Way agency.

LEASE AGREEMENTS

Rocky Mountain Planned Parenthood, one of Planned Parenthood's most controversial affiliates, lost a battle to concerned citizens in Trinidad, Colorado. Planned Parenthood sought to renew its lease but, due to significant public opposition, the Huerfano-Las Animas Counties District Health Board voted not to renew it.

The *Pueblo Chieftain* quotes a spokesman from Life Alternatives, a group opposed to Planned Parenthood, as saying, "We have prayed for months this would be the outcome." The group centers its argument around what it considers to be an inappropriate relationship between the taxpayer-supported facility and Planned Parenthood, a private agency. However, many commented on Planned Parenthood's role in abortion. Planned Parenthood does not yet do abortions in Trinidad, but the organization is the primary provider of abortion referrals.[7]

Planned Parenthood officials attempt to downplay their role in abortion:

> Sylvia M. Clark, Executive Director of Planned Parenthood of the Rocky Mountains, began her remarks with a review of the health services that the organization has made available to Las Animas County residents over the past 18 years . . . She said that as well as providing contraceptives and abortion counseling to clients who request it, Planned Parenthood offers screening tests and referral for breast and reproductive system cancers, diabetes, high blood pressure, blood cholesterol, and sexually transmitted diseases. Staff members refer clients for mental health and addiction programs when these problems are detected.[8]

Life Alternatives organized a postcard mailing to the chairman of the District Health Board. It is estimated that 1,000 postcards were received from opponents to renewing the Planned Parenthood lease.[9] Life Alternatives also presented the board with newspaper clippings outlining the tremendous public opposition to Planned Parenthood.[10]

Planned Parenthood officials claim the failure of the board to renew the lease could mean that Planned Parenthood will not be able to service the residents of the county. Others dispute this claim, saying Planned Parenthood has moved many times before and another will have little impact.[11]

Planned Parenthood officials claim abortion is not at issue, but access to contraceptive services should be discussed. Failure to provide contraceptive services would amount to "medical malpractice," according to Clark, since state and federal law require that such services be made available, including abortion counseling.[12] Nevertheless, the organized and active concerned citizens triumphed.

EXPANSION

Planned Parenthood is working to expand into many more communities in 1992 and 1993. Several areas have been targeted, some of which have low populations. Planned Parenthood is seeking to reach more people with its programs, particularly in schools, and expand its influence.

One of the most interesting battles is taking place in Dubuque, Iowa, where the Coalition for Parental Rights has formed to fight on the same side as the Respect Life Office of the Archdiocese of Dubuque to prevent Planned Parenthood of East Central Iowa from opening a satellite office in its community. The Archdiocese of Dubuque became actively involved in the battle when Planned Parenthood announced it was moving into the city.

Several leaders have emerged in the Dubuque area in opposition to Planned Parenthood, including Jim Giese, Betty Frommelt, Tim Walsh, Carolyn McGloughlin, and James Yeast. Giese, Frommelt, Walsh, and McGloughlin are working with the Coalition while Yeast is working for the Archdiocese. Both groups have developed excellent brochures designed to educate Dubuque area residents about Planned Parenthood.

Frances Hansen, executive director of Planned Parenthood of East Central Iowa, writes that Planned Parenthood "simply won't listen to anyone who screams 'baby killers'" in its face because it is "an organization whose sole purpose is to prevent unplanned pregnancy."[13]

Frommelt, who along with Giese is co-chairman of the Coalition, argues that "Planned Parenthood's philosophy undermines the morality of a community and traditional family values." Walsh states that "Planned Parenthood programs can be compared to throwing gasoline onto a fire through their flawed philosophy . . . Independent studies show they [sic] have actually increased teenage pregnancy and abortion rates."[14]

Giese states that the Coalition is focusing on Planned Parenthood's disregard for the rights of parents when it makes minors part of its programs without parental knowledge. "I would not characterize us as anti-abortion," Giese insists. Instead, Giese suggests Planned Parenthood's school programs are ineffective and make problems worse.[15]

Planned Parenthood leaders have recently claimed that abortions will not be performed if and when a Dubuque clinic is opened.[16] Shortly after the formation of the Coalition, however, a newspaper reported that Hansen said "it remains to be seen" whether abortions will ever be done in Dubuque.[17]

Walsh asserts that claims of no abortion services is a smokescreen. "When Planned Parenthood moves into a community, it starts out as a partial service clinic," Walsh explains. "But it eventually becomes a full service clinic. It also refers people for abortions." Hansen concedes that a Dubuque affiliate will refer women for abortions in Iowa City or Des Moines.[18]

Planned Parenthood was quick to respond to the formation of the Coalition:

> "Planned Parenthood is a convenient place to draw attention" to the Dubuque group's cause, she [Hansen] said. "We don't operate any differently than many organizations and medical facilities, but they're already in existence. This seems kind of like misplaced zealousness. . . ."
>
> Jill June, executive director of Planned Parenthood of Mid-Iowa, said the organization's philosophy is to encourage family communication but to provide an outlet for young people who are unable to turn to parents for help.[19]

Hansen claims she is not sure what the Coalition is opposing. "Are they against health care for disadvantaged women?" she asks.[20] Hansen writes in a newspaper column that the groups stand for the same kind of things:

> Both groups . . . are composed of people who adore children, promote the strength of the families, support education, work for justice, favor health care for the poor and have an abiding respect for life. What makes one of these groups different enough for the other to be "real bad news" ? . . .
>
> Necessarily we are against teenage pregnancy. Who could be in favor of it? Unfortunately, more teens than ever are giving birth in Dubuque, some at the age of 14 or 15. Even more unnerving is the thought that they became pregnant at 13 or 14. . . .
>
> Education is always the best prevention method, and Planned Parenthood empowers parents to be the primary sexuality educators of their children. . . . But what parent is entirely competent or comfortable in delivering such a curriculum? . . .
>
> Pregnancy is not an option for a young teen, no matter what. No one among us believes a child should have a child.[21]

Planned Parenthood apologists suggest that Coalition members should be open-minded. Giese suggests that it is those who adamantly support Planned Parenthood who are not open-minded:

> Having a permissive attitude is not the same as being open-minded. Open-mindedness is being "receptive to arguments or ideas." Those who simply accept Planned Parenthood's rhetoric can hardly be considered open-minded.[22]

Hillcrest Family Services, which provides family planning services in Dubuque, also opposes the Planned Parenthood facility. While several reasons are given, competition seems to be a major factor.

Another part of Planned Parenthood's Iowa expansion includes putting an abortion clinic in Iowa City where the Emma Goldman Clinic for Women already exists. The expansion announcement has left officials of the Emma Goldman Clinic angry, as reported by the *Des Moines Register*. "Anti-abortion forces are gleefully watching from the sidelines as the Emma Goldman Clinic for Women and Planned Parenthood of Mid-Iowa, longtime allies in the fight for legalized abortion, are positioning themselves for an abortion-rights turf war in Iowa City."[23]

The newspaper reports that Planned Parenthood of Mid-Iowa and the Emma Goldman Clinic "have made Iowa City among the largest per-capita providers of abortions in the United States."[24] It further reports that Planned Parenthood also plans to open a clinic in the Quad Cities (Davenport, Iowa, area), which will divert even more business from the Goldman Clinic:

> "My only disagreement with Planned Parenthood is they are not using their resources as wisely as they should," said [Diane] Finnerty [an associate director at the Goldman Clinic]. She denies her argument is based on a fear or resentment of Planned Parenthood, but she acknowledges the Goldman clinic will feel the competition.

> "It will affect us somehow," Finnerty said. "We don't know exactly how much. We do know we have been a thriving business in this community for 17 years, and we plan to continue to be a thriving business. . . ."
>
> Both sides deny there will be an "abortion war" in Iowa City. But they are less than complimentary about each other's services.[25]

Jill June claims that one reason for opening a Planned Parenthood clinic in Iowa City is that there is so much business that people have to travel great distances, from Iowa and surrounding states, to get to her clinic in Des Moines. "We want to take our services to these women," June states. "It's not fair to expect them to travel halfway across the state to find us." Finnerty, however, responds by saying there are cars in the Goldman Clinic parking lot from Des Moines, so, "What does that prove? . . . We are just wondering why in the world we need another one [abortion clinic] here."[26]

Interestingly enough, Emma Goldman and Margaret Sanger were not exactly friends when they were working to spread their "new morality":

> One woman strongly influenced by Goldman was Margaret Sanger. Sanger later tried to hide that influence. Always needing recognition and fearing rivals for power and importance, Sanger underestimated Goldman's contribution to birth control in her later writings.[27]

Sounds like the Hatfields and McCoys. Some things seem to last forever.

The Coalition for Parental Rights has prepared radio commercials and made use of billboards. There are, however, sometimes consequences of taking a bold stand. Jim Giese received a letter in the mail:

> Jim,
>
> Your definition of planned parenthood [sic] is ignorant, uninformed, narrow minded, and pious!
>
> I'm fed up with corn-fed, barley weaned, bucket heads spouting off about what is good for everyone else.
>
> From your letter I can say I know you. Your [sic] a true blue Dubuquer. You believe all non-Catholics are wrong and doomed to hell.
>
> I'll bet you are a bigot, too. . . . . [sic] I guess I don't only know you, but thousands of other people around here who suffer the same afflictions you do.
>
> If you don't want an abortion, I sure won't tell you, you have to have one!
>
> If you want to be a baby factory which produces sexually ignorant and vulnerable children I certainly won't try to say you can't!
>
> You and all the people around here like you are sheeplike and incapable of independent thought. Brainwashed even.
>
> I've met you personally and ideologically, I'm sorry for that![28]

Needless to say, the letter is unsigned.[29]

Of all groups I have witnessed working against Planned Parenthood, and I have seen many, the Coalition has one of the most innovative and far-reaching approaches. Planned Parenthood claimed its Dubuque clinic would be open by the end of 1991. It has not opened.

NO PLACE TO PICKET

Ann Polka is a mother who became involved in the abortion issue when her daughter had an abortion at a Planned Parenthood clinic—without her knowledge. With the support of her husband, Bill Polka, there are few people in North America who have been able to give Planned Parenthood more of a headache. Moreover, there are few more motivated and full of more energy to get the job done.

Polka has organized many events to educate people who live in the Belleville, Illinois, area about Planned Parenthood, but the project which has received the most attention in the community was her fight to acquire a suitable surface upon which they can picket. Picketers at Planned Parenthood's Belleville area clinic have been both committed and persistent. Every fall and winter, however, the area where picketers would walk became an excellent domain for mud wrestlers. Polka decided that a sidewalk had to be laid on the city property in front of the Planned Parenthood facility. It is no easy task.

The 180-foot sidewalk had to be approved by leaders of Fairview Heights and Swansea Village. Fairview Heights had plans to build a sidewalk along the same street, but picketers did not want to wait, so the city allocated $1,000 to cover the cost of materials needed for the 180-foot section.[30]

Polka, a leader of the Citizens Coalition Against Planned Parenthood, won approval to have the sidewalk built. Her greatest feat, however, was in convincing six area contractors to donate the labor and equipment. "Here are six contractors who bid against each other for jobs in the same communities who are working together for this," Polka told the *Belleville News-Democrat*. "It's pretty astounding."[31]

The effort was coordinated by Jack Cunningham, a vice president of highway construction at Keely Brothers. He says the contractors did the work because they believe it was a worthwhile cause:

> "Everybody supplied something. Some supplied labor, some supplied equipment," Cunningham said. "It was a joint effort. We were asked, and we decided it was a good cause."[32]

The response from Planned Parenthood is that the picketers have the right to be there and that they have been "above reproach," but they are wrong in suggesting that this particular Planned Parenthood facility performs abortions. Noncontroversial services, such as cancer screening, are emphasized, but the executive director of the Planned Parenthood affiliate admits that abortion referrals are made.[33]

Leaders at the Planned Parenthood affiliate announced that they hoped to have a free-standing building constructed in another part of the area in 1992. Planned Parenthood announced the site for the new facility. Ann Polka and friends worked to keep the facility where it stands. They managed to convince the man who owns the land on which the new facility would be built to decide against selling or leasing the property.

A MISINFORMED PUBLIC

Planned Parenthood provides strategy education to those who work to turn its agenda into public policy. For example, Lynn Baird of Planned Parenthood of Central and Northern Arizona writes that those seeking to put sex education programs into schools should know the opposition:

> Intimidation is the most powerful weapon anti-sex education extremists have. Intensive letter campaigns, repeated phone calls—sometimes threatening ones—are combined with letters to the editor, and mass appearances at public hearings.[34]

Planned Parenthood even urges its forces to be "wary" of those groups with names that sound patriotic:

> Be wary of groups or committees with very patriotic, moral-sounding names—Concerned Women of [sic] America, the Coalition for Family Values and the Eagle Forum are examples. These may be extremists masquerading as protectors of "American family values," when what they really want is to impose their own narrow religious views on everyone else.
>
> *Don't be surprised if they distort the truth and lie outright* about sex education programs, Planned Parenthood, or school health programs at public hearings and in letters to the editor.
>
> *Don't get sidetracked by their proposals to substitute "Sex Respect"* or other non-informational, doctrinaire curricula for a valid sex education program.[35]

Planned Parenthood urges its supporters to be prepared by getting valuable support prior to attending a public meeting on a sex education program. "[I]t is critical to get support from the highest level of authority you can—school district administrators, principals, school board members, as well as parent groups like the PTA [Parent Teacher Association]."[36] Planned Parenthood foes can learn from these suggestions.

Perhaps the single most powerful barrier to stopping Planned Parenthood is that the average citizen believes the organization is caring, professional, and credible. Naturally, the vast financial resources of Planned Parenthood, which allow for massive advertising campaigns, make it more likely that the public will view Planned Parenthood in a favorable light.

Most people do not know what Planned Parenthood really stands for, especially with regard to its abortion advocacy. If this is to change, it is essential that such information reach as many hands as possible.

History shows that great political power can be wielded by very few. Therefore, even small groups, if well-organized, professional, and caring, can have significant impact on public policy. Adequate education is critical to success.

A CALL TO ACTION

Planned Parenthood can be stopped. Many organizations are working to expose Planned Parenthood by educating policy-makers and the public concerning its real agenda. You can help.

Work to defund Planned Parenthood in your local community. Find out if Planned Parenthood is receiving city, county, or state funds. If it is, work to end this funding. Beginning at the city or county level is best. Success there will serve as a springboard for success at the state level.

Find out which groups are providing health education materials in your public schools. If Planned Parenthood is involved, work to keep its materials out. Even allowing Planned Parenthood's "innocent" material allows it free advertising and legitimacy with policy-makers, teachers, and young people.

Make sure Planned Parenthood is not involved in providing health care to young people through school-based clinics. If Planned Parenthood speakers are allowed in schools, insist that those with an opposite point of view be invited to speak.

It is crucial that young people be taught, by their parents, about the true nature of Planned Parenthood. Parents should explain why they oppose Planned Parenthood. Young people should be given enough information to remain strong when Planned Parenthood philosophies are taught in schools and even if philosophy is taught by official Planned Parenthood spokesmen.

Educate others about Planned Parenthood as often as is appropriate. Encourage those who have a positive view of Planned Parenthood to become educated on its entire organization and philosophy.

Provide literature for your friends to read. Your friends may have a positive view of Planned Parenthood based entirely on its excellent public relations campaigns. What you have to say and teach about Planned Parenthood may not only be surprising to your friends, but also a welcomed education.

Be sure that your civic and church leaders are educated about Planned Parenthood. Receive Planned Parenthood literature so you can keep updated on Planned Parenthood's activities.

Write to corporate contributors of Planned Parenthood. Think twice before you purchase their products or services. Every dollar of profit made by these corporations can be used for Planned Parenthood. Urge the corporate leaders to cease their support of this controversial organization. Making such contributions is simply bad business.

Christians who are involved in the abortion battle should not forget the most important part of the quest for an abortion-free America—prayer. While often the most overlooked weapon, it is the most potent in the arsenal. This is something that must be remembered.

The evidence is clear. Planned Parenthood, despite its huge financial resources, can be defeated by a group of committed citizens. You could be one of those citizens.

APPENDIX A

SUPPORTERS OF BETTER WORLD SOCIETY AWARDS PROGRAMS

At the end of the 1988 Better World Society awards program aired on WTBS on December 10, 1988, the following list of benefactors, patrons, sponsors, and staff was presented:

BENEFACTORS

Adelphia Cable Communications; American Film Technologies; American Express Travel Related Services; Archer-Daniels-Midland; Crawford Post Production; Peggy Dulaney; GE American Communications; Home Box Office; IDG Communications; National Basketball Association; Ogilvy and Mather; Radio City Music Hall Productions; Tempo Enterprises; Time, Inc.; Trump Organization; Turner Network Television; United Artists Communications, Inc.; and von Zerneck/Sertner Films.

PATRONS

1 Percent for Peace; A1 Bacio Restaurant; Joy Bogen; Craver, Mathews, Smith and Company; Lloyd Cunningham; Kay Delaney; William A. Delano; Patrick and Mary Ann Donaghy; Dorothy Rice; Dwire Carol and Joel Glick; Dr. and Mrs. Alexander Gralnick; David Groth; Greenpeace International; Planned Parenthood Federation-WHR; Jim Henson Productions; Brian Lacey; Kathleen Lacey; Markham-Novell Communications, Ltd.; National Audubon Society; National Geographic Society; Miriam and Albert Ornstein; Maurice and Jacqueline Paprin; Sandy Randel; Daniel L. Ritchie; William Samuels; Bernard and Irene Schwartz Foundation, Inc.; Miranda Smith; Maurice and Hanne Strong; The Tobin Group; United Nations Office for Disarmament Affairs; United Nations Population Fund; Steve Vorillas; and Dian Woodner.

SPONSORS

Bank of America; Robert L. Bernstein; Brunswick Construction Company; Coca-Cola; Interamerica Corporation; Arthur Cody; Conair Corporation; Gloria Chu-Feng; Hon. Seymour Halpern; David and Susan Horowitz; Karon Kiss; Joyce Lewis; Joshua Mailman; James R. McManus; Mr. and Mrs. Kenneth F. Mountcastle, Jr.; Mr. and Mrs. Ray Murray; Alan Press; Reiss Media Enterprises; Robert and Betsy Stang; Nina Streich Troutman; Sanders, Lockerman and Ashmore; Laura Utley; Gordon A. Walker; Robert and Gordon Wallace; Yale Wexler; and Stanley Yotes.

STAFF

Thomas S. Belford, executive director; J.J. Ebaugh, associate director; Victoria G. Morkell, associate director; Elaine L. Jones, director of program development; Lori Henry, special donor coordinator; Mark S. Greenberg, associate producer; Hortense T. Hall, program development; Caprice O. Anderson, executive assistant; and Randy M. Shulman, membership.

Artist Peter Maxx was recognized for a gift made to the Better World Society. Maurice Strong, president of the Society, commented, "Peter is absolutely dedicated to the Better World agenda."

At the end of the 1989 Better World Society awards program aired on WTBS in November 1989, the following list of underwriters, benefactors, patrons, sponsors and staff is presented:

UNDERWRITERS

Anheuser-Busch Foundation; American Film Technologies, Inc.; Drexel Burnham Lambert, Inc.; Merrill Lynch; and Turner Broadcasting System, Inc.

BENEFACTORS

Adelphia Cable Communications; Aeroflot Soviet Airlines; American Express Travel Related Services; American Television and Communications Corporation; Bank of America; Crawford Post Production; Dr. and Mrs. Alexander Gralnick; Patrick and Mary Ann Donaghy; Hughes Communications; Home Box Office; Merck and Company; MGM Grand Air; National Audubon Society; National Basketball Association; National Geographic Society; Occidental Petroleum Corporation; PepsiCo, Inc.; Planned Parenthood Federation of America; Time Warner, Inc.; Trump Organization; United Artists Communications; United Artists Corporation; and von Zerneck/Sertner Films.

PATRONS

Craver, Mathews, Smith and Company; Jane Dimmock; Greenpeace; David and Susan Horowitz; International Planned Parenthood Federation-WHR, Inc.; John W. Jordan II; Names in the News; Maurice and Hanne Strong; Triplex Direct Marketing Corporation; United Nations Population Fund; United Nations Office for Disarmament Affairs; and Laura Utley.

SPONSORS

Bear, Stearns and Company, Inc.; Albert Bildner; Cablevision Systems Corporation; Philippe Caland; Clive Duvall III; Gary Ferdman; Sidney Gilbert; Frank B. Hall and Company, Inc.; Ry Hay; Brian and Kathy Lacey; Joshua Mailman; George Martin; Kenneth and Katherine Mountcastle; Albert and Miriam Ornstein; Reiss Media Enterprises, Inc.; Laurance Rockefeller; David Shatz; Robert and Betsy Stang; The Tobin Group; Troutman, Sanders, Lockerman and Ashmore; Fatima Whitaker; and Stanley Yake.

STAFF

Glenn A. Olds, president and chief executive officer; Thomas S. Belford, executive director; Victoria G. Markall, associate director; Norma Davidoff, senior producer; Haleyon Liew, director, program development; Lori Henry, special donor coordinator; Hortense T. Hall, program development; Randy M. Shulman, membership; Terry Anthony, executive assistant; and Alison Slaughter, executive assistant.

Time Inc., recipient of the Better World Society's Communication's Medal, publishes the following magazines: *Time, Fortune, People, Life, Working Woman, Money, McCall's, Asia Week, Parenting, President, Sports Illustrated (Kids), Hippocrates, Southern Accents,* and *Cooking Light.*

APPENDIX B

GUIDELINES FOR THE LOCAL CHALLENGE

In collaboration with Barrett Mosbacker, the following guidelines are offered as long-term strategy for fighting Planned Parenthood in the local community. While the strategy will need to be adapted to the local situation, success will most likely be realized by incorporating as many guidelines as possible.

Begin to gather data on the level of teenage pregnancy in your area. Be sure to separate pregnancies of married teenagers and teenagers who are 18 or older from other pregnancies. Gather information on the "effectiveness" of sex education and family planning programs in reducing teenage pregnancy rates. Such information is readily available from major Christian and conservative organizations across the country. It is important that all information gathered be factual, in context, and properly footnoted, whether presented orally or in writing.

Prepare factual and concise flyers and/or short reports for distribution to local government officials, the media, and others interested in the issue.

As feasible, set up breakfast and lunch meetings with key members of the media, local government officials, and other community leaders to discuss the problem of teenage pregnancy and Planned Parenthood in particular. Personal contact is an effective method of communicating your point of view. As you build personal relationships your credibility will grow, as will your effectiveness.

Remember that the media is not necessarily your enemy. Develop cordial, professional relationships with key media figures whenever possible and be prepared to provide them with factual information when they request it or as you deem appropriate. Let's be realistic, however. Some in the media have a political agenda they wish to advance. Consequently, you may be as professional and kind as possible and some reporters will still do whatever they can to make you look bad.

Identify and recruit as many professionals as possible (lawyers, doctors, nurses, teachers, business executives, clergy) to work with you. They can provide valuable insight, add credibility to your efforts, and are excellent spokesmen.

Form a committee. Develop a plan of action and delegate responsibilities. The plan of action should be clear and concise. Everyone should know exactly what is expected of them and, when possible, on what date it will be expected. It may be best not to identify the committee with a pro-life group as this will automatically bias the press coverage and the perceptions of elected officials.

Do not resort to unnecessary and inflammatory rhetoric. For example, do not refer to Planned Parenthood as "sex-perts" or to school-based clinics as "sex clinics." Such language only serves to detract from your credibility and does nothing to enhance your arguments. Moreover, such language is unprofessional and connotes "fanaticism" in the minds of the media and the public.

Gather factual information on the level of public spending in support of Planned Parenthood over several years and compare this with teenage pregnancy, illegitimate birth, and abortion rates over the same period. Was there an increase in both expenditures for Planned Parenthood as well as pregnancy rates? This will be the case in most areas. Use this information to demonstrate that Planned Parenthood cannot prove its programs have been effective. Such evidence does not exist because the programs do not work. Be sure to check birth rates and pregnancy rates.

Have a list of qualified individuals prepared in advance for submission to those who will be appointing members of various committees and task forces established to study teenage pregnancy and intervention strategies. Preferably, the list should be comprised of professionals. Since such committees are almost always a part of the implementation strategy employed by Planned Parenthood supporters, it is important to be prepared in advance to submit qualified nominees for committees.

Identify those who are supporting Planned Parenthood and the groups or agencies with which they are affiliated. Pay close attention to the arguments they are using to justify support of Planned Parenthood and be prepared in advance to answer their arguments with carefully reasoned responses and documented facts.

Do not use outdated information about Planned Parenthood. Gather current material and information, preferably from the local affiliate. Avoid quoting material from sources that are obviously Christian or pro-life. Unfortunately, the media and the public consider information provided from such sources as suspect because it comes from "biased" organizations. It is best to reference material from government agencies, respected journals, and from Planned Parenthood itself.

Discussions concerning Margaret Sanger should be limited or eliminated. This is because policy-makers may not see a connection between the Planned Parenthood of today and its founder. While a connection can be drawn, it is probably more profitable for you to concentrate on stronger and more contemporary issues.

Be prepared to offer alternatives to funding of Planned Parenthood. This is critical as it is difficult for elected officials to vote against a proposed "solution" to a real problem unless there is an alternative they can support. One alternative could include revising the sex education curriculum.

Compile a comprehensive list of all services available throughout the community that provide counseling, family planning, and health care to adolescents. It is not necessary that the list include only those agencies with which you are in agreement. The point is to prove that services exist and to provide the total cost of providing each service. Generally, such a list reveals that substantial sums of money are already being spent on a wide range of services available to adolescents. In such cases, funding of Planned Parenthood is an expensive and unnecessary duplication of services.

Monitor the budget process. A good time to make a concerted effort to defund Planned Parenthood is when elected officials are looking for ways to cut the budget. If Planned Parenthood becomes a controversial and time-consuming item in the budget, elected officials are more likely to cut its funding.

Set up speaking engagements with as many churches and civic groups as possible to inform them of the real nature of Planned Parenthood and its programs. Enlist their active support in opposing Planned Parenthood funding. Be sure the person speaking on behalf of your organization is well trained and knowledgeable. A poor, uneducated speaker, who relies on emotion and inflammatory rhetoric, may do you more harm than good.

Develop a comprehensive mailing list. Maintain the list on a computer with software capable of sorting data by name, address, precinct, church, and other necessary categories. This should be done from the start of your efforts.

Recruit intelligent, well-informed, and articulate people to run for elected office. Be prepared to work over several years to get these candidates elected. Remember that the effort must be persistent as victory is seldom realized during the first couple of years. This is a long-term effort. As much as possible, concentrate on off-year elections.

Be prepared to assemble a large group of individuals opposed to funding of Planned Parenthood for any public hearing on the issue. Admonish those attending to be respectful and courteous at all times—even when those supportive of Planned Parenthood are speaking. Loud outbursts from such a gathering are not helpful and only serve to reinforce stereotypes.

Identify influential political leaders, professionals, or other civic leaders to lobby elected officials privately. It is sometimes wiser for the group opposing funding of Planned Parenthood to maintain a low public profile and to work with others behind the scenes. Public officials do not like to appear to be caving in to special interest groups.

Identify elected officials opposed to the funding of Planned Parenthood. Seek and heed advice concerning how to best approach those currently supporting Planned Parenthood and those who are undecided.

Identify articulate individuals to write informative, factual columns and letters to the editors of the local newspapers.

Generate a massive letter-writing campaign and generate hundreds of telephone calls to elected officials regarding Planned Parenthood funding.

Be prepared to continue this effort until you succeed. Success will not be realized unless a commitment is made to fight public funding of Planned Parenthood every year it is considered.

Remember that Planned Parenthood never stops pushing its agenda and neither should those opposed to its funding. Regardless of the outcome of any particular battle, do not become discouraged. Be faithful. Learn from your mistakes and correct them. Even if you lose year after year, you are educating thousands of people and giving Planned Parenthood a "black eye" in the community.

APPENDIX C

ADVERTISEMENT ANALYSIS

In January 1989, the Planned Parenthood Federation of America began placing a series of copyrighted, full-page advertisements in *Time*. A description of the advertisements, including the text of each, is below. Analysis of each advertisement follows.

During the same period, Planned Parenthood placed full-page advertisements in other publications, including the *National Journal*. The placing of full-page advertisements in nationally known and widely read newspapers and magazines is a common practice of the Planned Parenthood Federation of America. Similar advertisements have also been placed in local newspapers.

❧ ❧ ❧

Date of Ad: January 23, 1989

Pictured: Joseph Scheidler, director of the Pro-Life Action League, speaking into a bullhorn.

Caption: Should a woman's private medical decisions be made by a man with a bullhorn?

Name of Advertising Series: It's time to go public for privacy.

Text of Advertisement:

Let's be absolutely clear about what leading "pro-lifers" want the government to do.

Ban abortions. No exceptions.

Not even in the case of rape. Women would just lie about it, says one activist.

Not even in the case of incest. Victims consent to incest, according to a leading theorist of the movement.

Not even to safeguard the health of the woman, no matter how young she is.

"Pro-life" organizer Joe Scheidler used a private detective to track down a 12-year-old girl scheduled for an abortion, and then, according to the Chicago Tribune, "harangued her mother" through his bullhorn, "demanding to see the child alone."

"(The mother) was almost hysterical," Scheidler is quoted as saying, "We couldn't reason with her."

But reason has nothing to do with it. Claiming to oppose abortion, "pro-lifers" attack every known way to avert abortion.

They lobby against birth control. ("I think contraception is disgusting," says Scheidler, "people using each other for pleasure.") And they oppose sex education that deals with the facts of real life.

Meanwhile, clinic bombers are celebrated as heroes of the "pro-life" cause.

Violence, intimidation, and other cruel and irrational tactics will not prevent abortion.

Responsible family planning services and information programs that respect every individual's rights, needs and convictions can do so much more.

We believe abortion is a personal and private decision. Not a chance to grandstand for political advantage.

To fight for the right to privacy, write us: PPFA, 810 Seventh Ave., New York, NY 10019. We'll make sure your voice is heard where it counts.

Analysis: Showing a man with a bullhorn creates an immediate emotional response. Add the caption and the response becomes even stronger.

The advertisement refers to "leading 'pro-lifers.'" Nothing is said about what makes a person a "leading" pro-lifer and the identity of this "leading" pro-lifer is not given.

The term "pro-lifer" is placed in quotation marks for a reason. The underlying question becomes: Are these people really "pro-life" given all of the terrible things they do? After all, some of them even support the death penalty or oppose government programs they consider to be "handouts."

The advertisement says that leading foes of abortion want to ban abortion without exception. The truth is that almost every group which opposes abortion accepts the physical life of the mother as the only case when abortion would be allowed. Planned Parenthood knows this as it is part of the proposed Human Life Amendment.

Abortion would not be allowed in the case of rape or incest because a consistent ethic would not allow it. Legal abortion activists use the rape and incest argument because it, too, evokes a strong emotional response. When asked whether they would oppose all other abortions if it were allowed for the life of the mother, rape, and incest, which account for fewer than two percent of all abortions, advocates of unrestricted abortion say "no." They are not concerned about the rape or incest victim, only about protecting unrestricted, unregulated legal abortion.

Advocates for legal abortion know that opposing abortion in such cases makes pro-lifers look uncaring. They are basically saying that those who oppose abortion for rape and incest certainly should not be listened to with regard to abortion, or anything else for that matter, period. Advocates of unrestricted abortion do not like being questioned about their support for sex selection abortion. When Molly Yard was president of the National Organization for (a few) Women, she announced her support for sex selection abortion on national television.

Notice that the statement, "Women would just lie about it," is not a quotation. It is attributed to "one activist" who is not identified, assuming someone said it at all. However, it is possible lying could take place, unless a requirement was set that the rape or incest must be reported within a short period of time. Is Planned Parenthood willing to assure that no one, who they claim will do almost anything to get a desired abortion, would lie? Those who support abortion apparently have no problem with the lie which led to the *Roe v. Wade* case in the first place.

The statement, "Victims consent to incest," is also not a quotation. The statement is ludicrous and if someone did say this the person is certainly not speaking for, nor is he or she representative of, the movement working to end legal abortion.

The advertisement says abortion is opposed even to "safeguard the health of the woman . . ." The problem is that advocates of unrestricted abortion define "health" broadly, as the Supreme Court did in *Doe v. Bolton*. Hence, the word "health" becomes meaningless.

A spokesman for Scheidler explains that only the part of the advertisement concerning the hiring of a private investigator is accurate. She said Scheidler did not "harangue" anybody with a bullhorn. In fact, Scheidler was out of town when the girl was found. Whatever the case, Planned Parenthood has taken one man and one incident and attempted to apply them to the entire movement.

The advertisement says that abortion opponents "attack every known way to avert abortion. They lobby against birth control." This is completely untrue. The mainline movement opposes abortion and only those birth control methods (abortifacients) which end the life of a human being after it has begun. Can Planned Parenthood point to any proposed legislation to outlaw true contraception? Contraception, which prevents conception, is not being opposed through legal means. Even the Roman Catholic Church does not believe true contraception should be outlawed, even though Roman Catholic leaders believe it to be wrong. By the way, abstinence, requiring parental involvement, and anti-abortion laws are known ways to "avert" abortion, too.

Scheidler's statement following this attack is his own opinion and it does not represent the movement (assuming he said it at all). The movement working to restrict abortion does not oppose any method of contraception and it certainly does not oppose abstinence. It does, however, oppose contraception for teens as studies show it does more harm (failure rate, poor use, emotional and physical trauma, etc.) than good.

It is argued that abortion foes oppose "sex education." Organizationally, anti-abortion activists only oppose so-called "value-neutral" sex education. Most do not oppose the teaching of biological facts, when done at an appropriate age. However, opponents of abortion do not want groups like Planned Parenthood doing the "teaching."

It is written that "clinic bombers are celebrated as heroes . . ." This is ridiculous. Any individual who sees a bomber as a hero is grossly irrational and inconsistent with the ethics espoused by those opposed to abortion.

The advertisement refers to "violence, intimidation, and other cruel and irrational tactics . . ." Abortion foes strongly oppose all of these. Nevertheless, Planned Parenthood seeks to take individual persons and examples and extrapolate them to the entire movement. It should be noted that even if these tactics were employed by the entire movement, that would not make the goals/cause wrong, just the methods.

The advertisement refers to, "Responsible family planning services and information programs that respect every individual's rights, needs and convictions . . ." None of these are opposed by abortion foes as a whole, as long as they do not kill anybody. They do, however, promote parental involvement for minors.

The bottom line is that Planned Parenthood is using a tactic of fear, hatred, stereotyping, and distortion in order to reach its political and social goals. The movement working to restrict abortion lacks the funds to respond to Planned Parenthood's statements by running counter-advertising. Consequently, many people believe what they read in the Planned Parenthood advertisements.

❧ ❧ ❧

Date of Ad: February 6, 1989.

Pictured: Randall Terry, director of Operation Rescue, raising his fist and speaking into a microphone.

Caption: "I don't think Christians should use birth control."

Name of Advertising Series: Don't wait until women are dying again.

Text of Advertisement:

Leading "pro-lifers" want to outlaw abortion for any woman, even in the case of rape or incest.

But they don't stop there.

They also oppose the use of birth control by millions of American couples.

Randall Terry, one of the men behind the current campaign to blockade health clinics and publicly harass and humiliate women, has stated: "I don't think Christians should use birth control. You consummate your marriage as often as you like and if you have babies, you have babies."

Another "pro-life" activist declares: "We are totally opposed to abortion under any circumstances. We are also opposed to . . . all forms of birth control with the exception of natural family planning (methods based on periodic abstinence)."

Other "pro-life" speakers denounce contraception as "disgusting," call the family planning movement "satanic," and warn that birth control will lead to the death of Western civilization.

Leading "pro-lifers" are usually careful to avoid condemning birth control in public. Yet they lobby behind the scenes, and have already succeeded in shaping federal policy and limiting family planning assistance.

The tragedy is that responsible family planning programs do much more to actually avert abortions than the "pro-life" campaign of violence and intimidation ever can.

In fact, restricting Americans' birth control options will inevitably lead to more crisis pregnancies and more abortions.

That's the exact opposite of what "pro-lifers" say they're for. And an urgent reason to ask what their leaders are really against.

Make time to save your right to choose. Before the "pro-lifers" start making your choices for you.

Take action! To join Planned Parenthood's Campaign to Keep Abortion Safe and Legal, please mail this coupon to: PPFA, 810 Seventh Ave., New York, NY 10019.

Analysis: The analysis of this advertisement is much like that of the advertisement picturing Joe Scheidler. Therefore, similar statements will not be responded to again.

Picturing Randall Terry raising his fist evokes a vision of a revolutionary anarchist. Terry's statement, "I don't think Christians should use birth control . . ." is Terry's opinion and has nothing to do with the movement to end abortion. Terry allegedly said he does not believe Christians should use birth control. This is his personal advice to Christians, not to non-Christians. Terry did not say contraception should be outlawed.

The advertisement refers to Terry as "one of the men behind the current campaign to blockade health clinics and publicly harass and humiliate women . . ." Using the term "men" implies it is only men who are supporting Terry's actions or leading the movement to stop abortion.

Calling abortion facilities "health clinics" is an attempt to make Terry look like he opposes true medical care and, of course, if Terry opposes it, all others who want to end abortion do, too. Medical care which protects human life (implied by the phrase "medical care") is not at issue. Procedures which destroy life are at issue.

Finally, harassing and humiliating women is certainly not Terry's motive. This is simply a matter of opinion and inflammatory rhetoric.

"Another 'pro-life' activist" is quoted as opposing birth control. Again, for some reason, this "activist" (whatever that means) is not identified. Nevertheless, the person speaks for him or her self, not the movement. The same is true of the "other 'pro-life' speakers." No one person speaks for the movement. It is not organized that way, which is largely untrue of the pro-legal abortion movement. The Planned Parenthood of America often distances itself from its more radical affiliates. Similarly, some affiliates attempt to distance themselves from other affiliates. When more radical affiliates are quoted, Planned Parenthood says, "Don't put us all in the same boat!" A double standard clearly exists. What's more, while distancing occurs in public, little, if anything, is done to correct the problem.

It is said that anti-abortion leaders "are usually careful to avoid condemning birth control in public. Yet they lobby behind the scenes . . ." Planned Parenthood leaders seem to see birth control opponents behind every door. As a lobbyist, I have never seen anyone lobby "behind the scenes" or otherwise against true contraception. Besides, who are "they" referred to in the ad?

Once again, all legitimate groups oppose all forms of violence and intimidation. However, no matter how many times this is made clear, Planned Parenthood relies on the attack for propaganda purposes.

Planned Parenthood argues that its programs will lead to fewer abortions. Statistics show there are more people, including teens, using contraceptives than ever before and there are also more abortions than ever before. Simply put, it is not in Planned Parenthood's best interest to prevent unwanted pregnancy.

Finally, abortion opponents do not want to make choices for anyone. They just do not want the killing of unborn human beings to be considered a legitimate "choice." Nor do they want theft, drug dealing, or rape to be considered a legitimate "choice."

❧ ❧ ❧

Date of Ad: February 20, 1989.

Pictured: A weeping Jimmy Swaggart, televangelist, pictured as seen on television while he confessed to unspecified sins.

Caption: "Sex education classes in our public schools are promoting incest."

Name of Advertising Series: Don't wait until women are dying again.

Text of Advertisement:

America has always been blessed with characters who claim to have all the answers.

The problem is, they don't always practice what they preach. And hypocrisy can be extremely harmful.

Take leading "pro-lifers," for example.

They want the government to outlaw abortion for every woman, even in the case of rape or incest.

Yet prohibition has never stopped abortion. It has only made terminating a pregnancy dangerous for the poor. And more expensive for the better-off.

"Pro-lifer" leaders claim they're ready to stop abortion by any means necessary.

Yet they violently oppose proven ways to avert abortion, like effective family planning programs and sex education that addresses young people's real-life problems and concerns.

According to Jimmy Swaggart, "Sex education classes in our public schools are promoting incest." While according to Phyllis Schlafly, "Sex education is a principle cause of teenage pregnancy."

Of course, enforcing ignorance and preventing young people from making safe, responsible decisions will only result in more unintended pregnancies and more abortions.

In fact, the "pro-lifers" couldn't do more to increase the number of abortions if they tried—while they push for measures that actually threaten women's lives.

Make time to save your right to choose. Before the "pro-lifers" start making your choices for you.

Take action! To join Planned Parenthood's Campaign to Keep Abortion Safe and Legal, please mail this coupon to: PPFA, 810 Seventh Ave., New York, NY 10019-5818.

Analysis: Now this advertisement is a low blow—linking Jimmy Swaggart to those working to end unlimited abortion.

The advertisement says that those "who claim to have all the answers [no one I know] don't always practice what they preach. And hypocrisy can be extremely harmful." True, some people do not practice what they preach. We all fall into this category to varying degrees, including Planned Parenthood leaders. It is just that most people are not shown as being hypocritical on national television. Nevertheless, being inconsistent (a hypocrite) is only harmful to the hypocrite. Moreover, being hypocritical does not mean a person is wrong about what is being preached. It only means the person is a human being—a weak human being. Even if abortion foes were the most hypocritical people on earth, that would not make the killing of preborn human beings any less wrong.

It is argued that "prohibition has never stopped abortion. It has only made terminating a pregnancy more dangerous for the poor. And more expensive for the better-off." Let me make my point on these statements by changing some words. "Prohibition has never stopped the smuggling of illicit drugs. It has only made smuggling illicit drugs more dangerous for the poor. And more expensive for the better-off." The fact that some will break a law is grossly insufficient reason not to make a law. There are no laws that go completely unbroken. Laws are made to protect people. Those who choose to break the law obviously take some risk in doing so and the wealthy will always have the ability to do things the rest of us cannot do.

It is written that anti-abortion "leaders claim they're ready to stop abortion by any means necessary." First of all, who are these "leaders?" Second, this statement implies that abortion foes would use unethical or violent means to do so. This is simply not the case, though Planned Parenthood would like people to believe otherwise.

The advertisement continues, "Yet they violently oppose proven ways to avert abortion . . ." Abortion foes "violently" oppose nothing. Jimmy Swaggart, hardly considered an anti-abortion leader, gives his opinion about sex education. If Swaggart is right in a particular locale, that should not indict all sex education programs. Neither should Swaggart's comments be considered indicative of the opinions of all abortion opponents. But is Swaggart, as hypocritical as he may be, right about this matter?

Phyllis Schlafly gives her opinion on sex education. Actually, she is right about some sex education programs contributing to teen pregnancy, but they obviously do not *cause* teen pregnancy. Schlafly obviously knows this is true. What she likely means is that some sex education programs encourage sexual experimentation.

Abortion foes are accused of "enforcing ignorance and preventing young people from making safe, responsible decisions." The truth is that they want to educate children about the "facts," but include some education as to the value of abstaining from sexual relationships outside of marriage, especially at a young age. Planned Parenthood leaders believe that a condom or a pill is equal to allowing a young person to "make a responsible decision." Abortion foes believe that abstaining from sex at age 13 is the only "responsible" decision. Planned Parenthood's own documents show it does not hold this view. It believes a teen can be sexually active and "responsible" at the same time.

It is written that abortion foes "push for measures that actually threaten women's lives." If Planned Parenthood officials believe opposing abortion threatens the lives of women, it has a low regard for the intelligence of women. If a woman cannot handle the pressures of pregnancy (billions of women have done so), how could she handle the pressures of the presidency? Women can do both. They should not be underestimated.

❧ ❧ ❧

Date of Ad: March 6, 1989.

Pictured: A teenage girl.

Caption: "Would you lie to a pregnant teenager?"

Name of Advertising Series: Don't wait until women are dying again.

Text of Advertisement:

Nationwide, "pro-lifers" have launched a campaign of violence and intimidation against women and health professionals.

But their lowest tactic is deception.

Across the country, thousands of "crisis pregnancy centers" offering "free pregnancy tests" have opened with the sole purpose of luring desperate women to a session of lies about abortion.

These outfits aren't staffed by medical professionals. The pregnancy test they offer is an over-the-counter kit available at any drugstore. The results are often withheld. And "counseling" means being left alone in a darkened room to watch a barrage of horrifying and misleading slides and films.

But the deception may not stop there. According to police, a center in California tried to lure a pregnant 14-year-old away from home, even supplying her parents with a letter saying she had been awarded an overseas scholarship. By the time her parents discovered the ruse, it was too late for an abortion.

Other women have been promised material support during their pregnancies: a referral to the local welfare office.

Meanwhile, women are being denied access to birth control that can avert an unintended pregnancy—and information about the actual medical risks of pregnancy before full maturity.

Law enforcement and public health officials have denounced these "pro-life" tactics as false and misleading. At Planned Parenthood, we discuss alternatives in a responsible way.

But "pro-lifers" who lie are endangering people in crisis. And that shows no regard for anyone's life.

Make time to save your right to choose. Before the "pro-lifers" start making your choices for you.

Take action! To join Planned Parenthood's Campaign to Keep Abortion Safe and Legal, please mail this coupon to: PPFA, 810 Seventh Ave., New York, NY 10019-5818.

Analysis: Planned Parenthood claims that abortion foes have launched a nationwide "campaign of violence and intimidation against women and health professionals." No specifics are given, though one can assume it is referring to some efforts to end legal abortion. It should be noted that anti-abortion advocates oppose both violence and intimidation. It is just that Planned Parenthood seems to label every type of action that challenges it as either "violence" or "intimidation."

"But their lowest tactic is deception," Planned Parenthood argues. Throughout the advertisement, Planned Parenthood attacks pregnancy counseling centers—all pregnancy counseling centers. Once again, all pregnancy counseling centers are placed in the same boat.

Planned Parenthood implies that if one pregnancy counseling center does something wrong, all centers must be the same. If one Planned Parenthood affiliate does something wrong, however, that does not mean all Planned Parenthood offices are the same. Of course not. It should also be noted that Planned Parenthood affiliates are under a central authority (the Planned Parenthood Federation of America) while pregnancy counseling centers are more autonomous.

Planned Parenthood argues that pregnancy counseling centers are set up "with the sole purpose of luring desperate women to a session of lies about abortion." The implication is that abortion foes have only one purpose in mind—to lie to women. That is all they are really after. This "save the baby" thing is only a vehicle used by abortion opponents so they can practice their uncontrollable urge to lie. Obviously ridiculous.

The use of the term "luring" invokes the "Ted Bundy image." Planned Parenthood uses the word "lies," but at no time are specifics given. The only reference is to a story of one person who lied to the parents of one young woman, an act opposed by reputable anti-abortion groups. The mainline movement totally opposes lying. No exceptions. But this refers to the actions taken by one individual at one center. No other information is given. Was this person a Planned Parenthood or media plant?

Planned Parenthood claims women have been promised "material support" but were only referred to a welfare office. No specifics as to who, when, or where are given. This is simply an unsubstantiated accusation.

Shortly after the *Webster* decision, I was a guest on a Washington, D.C., radio program during which a woman called to make an accusation similar to that in the Planned Parenthood ad. I asked for specifics. Which pregnancy counseling center? What was the name of the person to whom she spoke? Naturally, the woman could not remember. I told her to call me or send me this information once she remembered and I would check it out and report my findings to the host of the radio program to announce on the air. Needless to say, I never heard from the woman. My guess is that she fabricated the whole story. It is amazing how people quiet down when questioned about specifics.

It should be noted that Planned Parenthood often refers women to welfare agencies, but it is called "public assistance" or "social services" when Planned Parenthood makes the referral. It is "welfare" when pregnancy counseling centers make the referrals. Moreover, if a woman seeks an abortion, Planned Parenthood only asks for her money—up front.

Planned Parenthood argues that pregnancy counseling centers are not "staffed by medical professionals," as though only "medical professionals," many of whom have never faced an untimely pregnancy, are in a superior position to assist women than those who volunteer their time. The sole purpose of the volunteer is to help the woman so she can save the life of her offspring. Many of the "medical professionals" would, of course, be abortionists or others with a stake in the abortion industry. Pregnancy counseling center volunteers, on the other hand, have no financial interest. While Planned Parenthood has volunteers, they are trained to facilitate its multi-million dollar business.

Another important point must be made. What is so wonderful about a clinic which is staffed by medical professionals, particularly when a candidate for abortion usually does not come into contact with one of these "professionals" until she is lying on a table?

It is said the pregnancy test "is an over-the-counter kit available at any drug store. The results are often withheld." Planned Parenthood surely is not referring to Christian Action Council's 400-plus affiliated pregnancy counseling centers. The test is not available "over-the-counter" and the results are never withheld. What specific pregnancy counseling center is Planned Parenthood talking about?

Planned Parenthood asserts that pregnancy counseling center "'counseling' means being left alone in a darkened room to watch a barrage of horrifying and misleading slides and films." Once again, no specific clinics are identified. In legitimate pregnancy counseling centers, films or slides are shown only with the consent of the woman, if at all. Most films consist only of fetal development. The Planned Parenthood hierarchy believes that providing women with information on what abortion really is serves only to "horrify" women and "mislead" them. Not only are no specifics given about what is "misleading," no evidence is presented that mainline pregnancy counseling centers use such films or how such films are "misleading." It is believed that the "horrifying and misleading slides and films" are any which show what abortion does to a preborn human being.

Planned Parenthood says women are denied "information about the actual medical risks of pregnancy before full maturity." Not given in context, such "information" is patently misleading. Presented in an improper way, any teenager who chose to give birth would believe she is risking her own life. The fact is that childbirth is not more dangerous than abortion. Statistics showing otherwise are misleading as they include deaths during pregnancy and months afterwards. The deaths do not even have to be related directly to childbirth to be classified as a maternal death. On the other hand, abortion-related deaths are often reported as attributable to some other cause.

As usual, Planned Parenthood does not cite references for the, "Law enforcement and public health officials" statement. However, these officials are not the only people denouncing unethical tactics. Anti-abortion activists are doing so as well. The only problem is that Planned Parenthood is less than honest about what is really happening at pregnancy counseling centers. After all, pregnancy counseling centers are taking business away from Planned Parenthood and this means Planned Parenthood's brand of "counseling" cannot reach some people.

The most amusing part is that Planned Parenthood writes that its employees "discuss alternatives in a responsible way. But 'pro-lifers' who lie are endangering people in crisis." Any woman who chooses abortion is welcomed by Planned Parenthood. It is happy to take her money and do the procedure in its own facility. If a woman does not choose abortion, she is referred to someone else. In other words, Planned Parenthood helps women directly, but only if abortion is chosen. Moreover, Planned Parenthood's "counseling" has been found to be anything but neutral—and no wonder since Planned Parenthood is in the abortion business. One survey found that about 86 percent of Planned Parenthood clients choose abortion. Nationally, fewer than 33 percent choose abortion. What is happening in Planned Parenthood facilities that makes it have such an outrageous abortion rate?

Pregnancy counseling center workers, on the other hand, are most often volunteers. They have nothing to gain personally. Materials and services are always offered free. But remember that Planned Parenthood, which calls itself "responsible," also believes a 13-year-old can be involved in a sexual relationship and still be "responsible."

Pregnancy counseling centers offer women a real choice—one that can be made once a woman knows there are those who will stand behind her and give her the material needs and emotional support. Planned Parenthood opposes this effort and should be ashamed for doing so. Attacking the caring, selfless women and men who volunteer their time and personal resources to pregnancy counseling centers is truly the "lowest form of deception."

❧ ❧ ❧

Date of Ad: March 20, 1989.

Pictured: A woman answering her front door. Two detectives are there.

Caption: "How would you like the police to investigate your miscarriage?"

Name of Advertising Series: Don't wait until women are dying again.

Text of Advertisement:

Leading "pro-lifers" think nothing of invading women's privacy and jeopardizing their health. Their national campaign of violence and intimidation attracts plenty of media attention.

But the outrages they commit now are nothing compared to what would happen if they win.

Their Human Life Amendment to the Constitution treats the fetus as an independent human being from the very instant of fertilization. Abortion would be called murder under all circumstances. So would many effective birth control methods. And every miscarriage could be suspect.

While some "pro-lifers" declare that only health professionals who assist with an abortion should be charged with murder, countless women could be caught up in police investigations and prosecutions even if they are never arraigned.

If the right to choose abortion is limited or eliminated, women who can afford to travel could probably evade the law.

Poor women and teenagers with no resources would be forced to induce their own abortions or subject themselves to an illicit, dangerous back-alley procedure.

And thousands of them would be brutalized, maimed and killed.

How do we know what will happen if the "pro-lifers" win? Because that's the way it was before abortion was made legal and safe in 1973. The choice the "pro-lifers" present isn't whether abortion should be stopped. Prohibition never worked.

The choice is privacy . . . or punishment. Safety for women . . . or terrible danger. It's really not a choice we need to make again.

Make time to save your right to choose. Before the "pro-lifers" start making your choices for you.

Take action! To join Planned Parenthood's Campaign to Keep Abortion Safe and Legal, please mail this coupon to: PPFA, 810 Seventh Ave., New York, NY 10019-5818.

Analysis: Planned Parenthood says opponents of abortion "think nothing of invading women's privacy and jeopardizing their health." No, abortion foes just do not think destroying an unborn human being has anything more to do with privacy than does child abuse. Planned Parenthood also believes that abortion somehow preserves the "health" of women. Planned Parenthood is obviously misinformed about what abortion does—to the woman and her preborn offspring.

It is written that violence and intimidation "attracts plenty of media attention." This is true, but largely because Planned Parenthood officials call their friends in the media whenever someone allegedly does something to it.

It is alleged that under the Human Life Amendment, "Abortion would be called murder under all circumstances. So would many effective birth control methods." The truth is that laws would have to be written to determine how abortionists would be punished. No one now knows, even with the Human Life Amendment, how abortionists would be punished. Therefore, "murder" is not necessarily the term that would apply. Since Congress or state lawmakers would set the penalties, all citizens would have input as to the punishment that would be set by their elected representatives. The Human Life Amendment does not include punishment, but does call for the lawmakers to set a punishment. Furthermore, only those methods of birth control that end a life after it has begun would be outlawed. True, some of these birth control methods are effective (abortion being the most effective form of birth control), but it seems effectiveness is not reason enough to continue a practice. Torturing and dragging criminals through the streets would be an effective means of killing prisoners on death row, but there are other considerations.

Comments such as "every miscarriage could be suspect" and "countless women could be caught up in police investigations and prosecutions even if they are never arraigned" are simply scare tactics. Talk about lies and intimidation. Before 1973, women who had miscarriages were not subject to investigations. Planned Parenthood leaders should be ashamed of making such statements, especially when they know such assertions are false. Do Planned Parenthood leaders believe they need to resort to scare tactics in order to get people on their side? It seems Planned Parenthood is really the group that is frightened—frightened it is going to lose its lucrative abortion business.

It is argued that women who can afford to leave the country for abortion will do so while poor women "would be forced to induce their own abortions or subject themselves to an illicit, dangerous back-alley procedure." The wealthy have always had advantages over the poor. This is nothing new. If the wealthy want to go to a country where bigamy is allowed, or where they can use drugs, they can do so. Our laws are for people who are in our country. We are not responsible for Americans who are in another country as they are subject to the laws of the country they are visiting at the time. Is this really being presented as an argument for keeping abortion legal? Planned Parenthood cannot be serious.

The most interesting phrase is that the poor would be "forced" to self-induce an abortion or get a "back-alley" abortion. The term "back-alley" obviously induces an emotional response. Nevertheless, the fact is that no one will be forced into any back-alley and no one will be forced to self-induce an abortion. Anyone caught forcing a woman to do so should be punished. Of course, this is not what Planned Parenthood means. It means women will have no other option, which is clearly untrue. But the fact remains that women will not be forced into having abortions.

If "thousands" (who knows where they get this figure) are brutalized, maimed or killed, it will be because a person chose to participate in an illegal activity. More likely, however, the woman would just purchase an abortion pill (like RU 486) that will cause an abortion. Why would anyone self-induce abortion or go to a "back-alley" when she can just get an illegal pill? While RU 486 is not a simple abortion pill, it would likely become a primary method used by physicians performing illegal abortions. Moreover, illegal abortion would force governments to provide real, positive solutions to the problems facing women. Abortion foes should take the lead in seeking these solutions. Planned Parenthood claims it is doing more than any other group to prevent the "need" for abortion, yet it is willing to encourage women to have a "dangerous, back-alley" abortion if it becomes illegal.

When Planned Parenthood says "that's the way it was before . . . 1973," Planned Parenthood has two problems. First, how long before 1973 is it referring? Second, does it really believe that 1973 technology can be compared to 1989 (when the advertisement was published) technology? The fact is we now have new and more effective methods to kill unborn human beings—something in which Planned Parenthood is obviously interested.

"Prohibition never worked," Planned Parenthood says. Now it wants to compare the prohibition of liquor in the early part of this century to abortion today? Moreover, Planned Parenthood writes that we must choose, "Safety for women . . . or terrible danger." Abortion foes support safety for women, born and preborn. That is why they oppose abortion in the first place.

Note: All Planned Parenthood advertisements are professionally developed and are highly successful. Do not underestimate their impact. Advertising agencies are skilled at getting the desired response from the public.

APPENDIX D

SELECTED QUOTATIONS AND COMMENTARY

"The Abortion Dilemma: Rights and Lives"

The following are excerpts from "The Abortion Dilemma: Rights and Lives," aired on NBC stations following the showing of the made-for-television film, "Roe vs. Wade," on May 15, 1989.

Program Participants: Faye Wattleton, then-president, Planned Parenthood Federation of America; Anna Quindlen, author; Christopher Smith, member of Congress, R-New Jersey; Olivia Gans, director, American Victims of Abortion; and Tom Brokaw, NBC News, program moderator.

DIALOGUE

Brokaw: A lot of people in this country, however they feel about the abortion issue, believe that it's become almost too easy. Isn't that a fair judgment?

Wattleton: No, it's not a fair judgment because the ease with which abortion is available is one that permits women to consider all of the options available to them and there's no reason why obstacles should be placed as barriers to women beyond their own personal conscience and the context of their lives. For poor women, it has become increasingly difficult because funds for poor women through our national health care program have been virtually cutoff. So those people who do not have the means or the resources to have an abortion and to pay for an abortion very often must sacrifice other basic needs or forgo the abortion as a result of the cut-off of government funding.

Brokaw: But a recent *Boston Globe* poll indicated that 75 percent of the American women who were having an abortion said the baby would interfere with their work or with their school, with other responsibilities. Are you beginning to lose that argument, do you think, with the American public, because the same poll indicated that that wasn't sufficient reason for an abortion.

Wattleton: Well, I think what we've seen is that the American public believes that there are increasingly more reasons why abortion is legitimate. There's no question that there is a good deal of conflict and ambiguity among Americans for the reasons that people give in having abortions, but I think that poll also showed that while some women feel that the time may be wrong for them to, in terms of their being best suited, to have a baby, they also desire in the future to have children and feel that they can be better prepared to give a child a better life and a better family if they forgo a pregnancy at this time and I think that's the very best environment to bring a child into the world.

COMMENTARY

Brokaw did a good job following up on his first question. Wattleton still evaded it. The poll showed that Americans oppose more than 95 percent of the abortions now being done (those for personal convenience). In other words, the American public believes there are few reasons why abortion would be a legitimate decision.

Wattleton's final comment, about what the poll also shows, makes little sense. The point is that few reasons for abortion are supported by the American people and Planned Parenthood is losing this argument. Wattleton never directly responded to Brokaw's point, but Brokaw let her get away with doing so after asking the question twice.

Note Wattleton's technique of seeming to answer the question posed while making unrelated points as well. This technique shows Wattleton's skill at forcing others to discuss what she wants to discuss.

❧ ❧ ❧

DIALOGUE

Olivia Gans stated that she believes the made-for-television movie based on *Roe v. Wade* is propaganda. Brokaw challenged Gans' statement. He then asked Quindlen if she saw the program as propaganda.

Quindlen: No, I didn't see it as propaganda, but I must say, Tom, that I saw it as a very powerful case for the legalization of abortion, for women to be able to have that option, because it touched my heart to see Holly Hunter portraying this woman who so desperately needed that right.

Wattleton: Well, I disagree with that characterization [that the made-for-television movie is propaganda]. I think that the writers of this particular evening's presentation did make a very strong case for the ambiguity—the fact that these things are not clear cut, the struggles that go on, her desire to, to perhaps proceed with the pregnancy and yet her conditions that mitigated her to make a decision to have an abortion if she could've had it. And I don't think it was propaganda. I think that these are very complex issues that have no simple solution and the solution is not just simply not to have an abortion.

COMMENTARY

What else would Quindlen and Wattleton say? If the program supports their side, it was not propaganda. If it had been slanted toward the pro-life side, it would have been called propaganda. The fact that Quindlen says, "I saw it as a very powerful case for the legalization of abortion," proves that Gans was correct.

❧ ❧ ❧

DIALOGUE

Olivia Gans commented on her own abortion.

Gans: My child died because of *Roe v. Wade* and I will never be happy about that.

Brokaw: And that was a decision that you made to go [interruption] . . .

Wattleton: That was a decision you made.

Gans: That was a decision that I felt forced to make by the pressure of the abortionist involved with my case [audience laughter].

COMMENTARY

It is incredible and insensitive on the part of the audience to laugh. It is clear that the laughter came from pro-legal abortion members of the audience. It is also incredible that Brokaw challenged Gans on her comment. He should have left this to Wattleton and Quindlen. Brokaw often questioned comments made by Smith and Gans and seldom questioned those made by Quindlen and Wattleton.

Brokaw never asked Gans to elaborate on why she felt pressured by the abortionist in her case.

It is interesting to note that, as is often the case, the one priest in the audience was shown on camera. This encourages the myth that abortion is a "Catholic issue."

❧ ❧ ❧

DIALOGUE

Congressman Smith was asked about abortion in the case of rape and incest. Smith said he opposes it, but President Bush supports legal abortion in those cases.

Wattleton: But, but, but you know this is a rather remarkable conversation. That may be George Bush's view. That may be Chris Smith's view. The point is, is that if I am facing an unintended pregnancy in my life, my circumstances have nothing to do with your views, and the Constitution has continued to protect me. I must continue [audience applause], I must continue as an American citizen, who lives in a free society built on pluralism and religious liberty, to find that answer for myself and not from some politician to pass a law that dictates how I will conduct my personal life.

(Congressman Smith referred to prenatal life.)

Wattleton: Women are not stupid. Women have always known that there was a life there.

Smith: They believe, our opponents, that life begins at birth, and I think that's absurd [interruption] . . .

Wattleton: That simply is . . .

Smith: The law ought to say life [interruption] . . .

Wattleton: That simply is not true.

Smith: . . . begins at the moment of conception.

COMMENTARY

No one asked Wattleton to explain what she does actually believe if she says women "have always known that there was a life there." What kind of life? Is it human?

Wattleton denies holding the view Smith claimed she and her organization hold, but no one asked for clarification.

No one asked Wattleton about sex selection abortion.

Wattleton's "politician" comment was intended to evoke an anti-politician emotional response from the audience.

❧ ❧ ❧

DIALOGUE

Wattleton was asked whether Planned Parenthood could pay for women to go to a state where abortion was legal if some states passed laws severely restricting abortion.

Wattleton: No, there would be no possibility that we could do that. I think that we have to keep in mind that right now, 1.6 million abortions are performed in this country each year and what likely is to happen is, will happen, as was the case before *Roe v. Wade* when 17 states and the District of Columbia had already reformed their abortion laws and women were forced to travel to other states if they had the means. If they didn't have the means, they were forced to resort to unsafe circumstances. So the point is not whether abortions will go on. Abortions have been with us for 5,000 years. The question is under what circumstances will they exist. Will they be unsafe and deadly or will women be able to make that decision in the safety of their personal lives in consultation with their physician.

COMMENTARY

Wattleton is skilled at turning a question into an excuse for making a speech. If she and the supporters of her organization are so convinced that women should have access to abortion, why aren't they willing to put their money where their mouths are?

No one questioned Wattleton about her "unsafe and deadly" comment and that is unfortunate.

❧ ❧ ❧

DIALOGUE

Gans attacked Planned Parenthood for its role in advocating and providing abortion services. Wattleton gave a familiar reply.

Wattleton: Ms., Ms. Gans, I don't believe that this is a, this is a discussion, this is a program about Planned Parenthood. But since you have raised it, I think it's important to point out that Planned Parenthood is doing more than any other organization in this country to prevent the need for abortion. Why don't you join us in better sexuality education in this country, better family planning programs, and more contraceptive technology. Those are the options . . .

COMMENTARY

If I were Wattleton, I wouldn't want it to be a discussion about Planned Parenthood either. A discussion on Planned Parenthood would never take place because its leaders never agree to participate in such a forum.

The truth is that Planned Parenthood has done more to create a market for family planning and abortion than any other organization. It is appalling that Wattleton is always allowed to get away with this comment. Even experienced pro-lifers let her get away with it.

Sex education imparts knowledge. It does not reduce teen pregnancy. Family planning, a reliance on imperfect technology, is a failure. Planned Parenthood is a failure.

❧ ❧ ❧

DIALOGUE

Gans again referred to Planned Parenthood. She also referred to Dr. Mary Calderone as a past president of Planned Parenthood.

Wattleton: Well, first of, first of all, first of all I think it's, I think that once again you have engaged in a misrepresentation of the facts. Dr. Calderone was never president of Planned Parenthood, but that's beside the point. The point is [audience applause and laughter], the point is here is that women must be free to decide for themselves. Your anger and your regret should not be imposed on women as a matter of national law. We must remain free to make our own mistakes, even if we regret them.

(Gans referred to her aborted child.)

Wattleton: Not everyone perceives a fetus as a child.

COMMENTARY

Wattleton was right. The Calderone issue was beside the point, but it served to allow Wattleton to charge that the facts had been misrepresented "once again." While I have personally read at least one book which refers to Calderone as the president of Planned Parenthood, this is incorrect. Calderone was the medical director of the Planned Parenthood Federation of America, which makes her a high-ranking Planned Parenthood official. She founded and served as executive director for the Sex Information and Education Council of the United States (SIECUS) until her retirement. But since Calderone was never president of Planned Parenthood, Wattleton thought she would use the misstatement to attack Gans' credibility instead of Gans' argument—a typical Wattleton trick. It is clear that Calderone was, at the very least, a high-ranking Planned Parenthood official, one with great authority, yet Wattleton did not volunteer this minor correction. By ignoring Gans' specific attacks against Planned Parenthood, Wattleton changed the issue around to make Gans look uninformed.

Just because a fetus is not yet an infant, not yet a teenager, not yet an adult, that does not mean we have a license to kill him or her. A "fetus" is no less homo sapien. Those who claim otherwise are espousing a political philosophy, not a biological fact.

❧ ❧ ❧

DIALOGUE

Congressman Smith explained his opposition to RU 486. Quindlen's response was quite remarkable.

Quindlen: Isn't part of your opposition to the [RU 486] pill, Congressman, that it wouldn't punish the woman [interruption] . . . The so-called pro-life movement seems to be very interested in seeing that women are punished [interruption] . . . At the end of their pregnancy, if they go through with it, they should have to give their children away . . . They should have abortions where they will be the least accessible to them. It seems that punishment is the name of the game and so is paternalism.

COMMENTARY

Absolutely incredible. Just once I would like to see pro-legal abortion activists defend abortion without resorting to these tactics. They seldom actually talk about abortion, however. Supporters of unrestricted abortion talk around the actual subject.

Women who carry to term are not forced to "give their children away," but it's better than killing them to avoid this hardship. "Punishment" has nothing to do with it. These people are simply anti-adoption and, in some cases, anti-birth.

❧ ❧ ❧

DIALOGUE

Wattleton: Well, unfortunately, unfortunately what you're trying to do is take away the rights of women and you know that if this drug [RU 486] comes to the U.S. market, that the decision to terminate a pregnancy will truly be between a woman and her physician.

(Congressman Smith attempted to respond, but he was interrupted.)

Wattleton: Congressman Smith, if I may, if I may finish. If I may finish. Women are indeed moral entities. We were not excluded from the moral process that makes up the fabric of our society. If we are sufficiently moral to bear children and to raise them and to bring up the future of America, we certainly ought to be entrusted with our morality to decide whether we want to continue a pregnancy and to preserve our health and our future [interruption]. If I may finish. If I may finish, Congressman . . . Always, always, women's concerns must be considered paramount. Women are more than fetuses and that must be a matter of individual self-determination. Even you say that in cases of a woman on her death bed an abortion is okay. Mr. Bush says in cases of rape and incest an abortion is okay. Well, there are other reasons that are totally, ethically appropriate for the individual to decide and we've got to continue a society that permits this.

COMMENTARY

As for Wattleton's first comment, abortion foes are trying to save the lives of preborn children *and* their mothers, not take away so-called rights.

Wattleton often interrupts pro-life speakers and they most often let her get away with doing so. When Wattleton appeared to be finished, Smith started to respond (twice). Wattleton then uses the condescending, "If I may finish." The problem is, as one can tell by the length of her comments, that it seems Wattleton will never finish. Wattleton uses every question as a license to make a speech. The speech sometimes addresses the question, but almost always adds material outside of the question.

Comments like, "Women are indeed moral entities," are also condescending, as though Smith is anti-women. No one questions that women are moral entities. Every human being has that capacity. That fact does not mean that we allow everyone to make decisions as to what is and what is not moral based on their own personal lives and belief systems. Wattleton said, "Women are more than fetuses." This is not true. Women are at a different stage of development but they are not "more." Are men "more" than boys? Are women "more" than girls?

As for allowing abortion for the life of the mother, pro-lifers cannot placate anyone with this argument. If they do not allow abortion for the life of the mother, we are accused of being anti-woman and insensitive. If they do allow it, doing so is used against pro-lifers as some kind of acknowledgement that women are more important than their children.

❧ ❧ ❧

DIALOGUE

Context: Congressman Smith began to explain how some abortions are performed. He described salt poisoning.

Wattleton: As a matter of fact, very few abortions are performed in that way, as a matter of fact.

COMMENTARY

What's the difference? Scraping, poisoning, suctioning, all produce the same end—a dead baby. Faye, how many are "very few?"

APPENDIX E

SELECTED QUOTATIONS AND COMMENTARY

Abortion: For Survival *and "Abortion: An Issue Forum"*

The following are excerpts from *Abortion: For Survival*, produced by the Fund for the Feminist Majority, as well as the subsequent panel discussion. The program was broadcast on the Turner Broadcasting System on July 20, 1989, and rebroadcast on July 22 and 23, 1989. The special was a presentation of the Better World Society.

While it is tempting to respond to every quotation, only a few have commentary provided due to space and time constraints. In addition, it is difficult to get a real feel for the program unless you have seen it. You are encouraged to do so. If nothing else, the program will motivate you to action.

SECTION 1
ABORTION: FOR SURVIVAL

Identifiable Program Participants

Byllye Y. Avery, founder and president, National Black Women's Health Project; Maria Elena Blackwell, regional project administrator, Pathfinder Fund; Sharon Camp, Ph.D., vice-president, Population Crisis Committee; Francine Coeytaux, associate, Population Council; Joan B. Dunlop, president, International Women's Health Coalition; Kenneth C. Edelin, M.D., professor, Obstetrics and Gynecology, Boston University (then-chairman of the board of the Planned Parenthood Federation of America—not identified as such in the program); Praema Rachavan-Gilbert, M.D., director of medical services, Pathfinder Fund; David Grimes, M.D., professor, Obstetrics and Gynecology, University of Southern California (also on the board of the Planned Parenthood Federation of America—not identified as such in program); Katie E. McLaurin, president, International Projects Assistance Services (IPAS); Christina Pickles, actress, program host; Ruth Roemer, J.D., adjunct professor of health law, School of Public Health, University of California at Los Angeles; Allan Rosenfield, M.D., dean, School of Public Health, Columbia University (also on the board of the Planned Parenthood Federation of America—

not identified as such in program); and Keith Russell, M.D., professor, Obstetrics and Gynecology, University of Southern California.

Christina Pickles (Program Host)

> "In 1973, the historic Supreme Court decision *Roe v. Wade* made abortion legal in the United States. From that time until now, a strong majority of Americans have supported that decision, despite massive propaganda efforts by the anti-abortion minority . . . We've all heard the hysteria of those who would see these rights taken away and emotional voices can often distort issues. The voices you are about to hear are rational ones. Voices of professionals and experts who have seen firsthand life with legal abortion and life without it. They are the voices of people who understand that for women, their children, and even for our planet, the right to legal, safe abortion is a matter of survival."

Commentary: If pro-life advocates are an "anti-abortion minority," why are abortion apologists so afraid of letting the elected representatives of the people decide these issues?

At least one of these "experts" has performed abortions. Others have played a major role in working to keep abortion legal. These "professionals" are hardly neutral and their voices are hardly "rational." A number of them make money off legal abortion. How neutral is that?

Saying that a "strong majority of Americans" have supported *Roe v. Wade* is ludicrous. Most Americans could not tell you what was decided in the case or how the *Doe v. Bolton* companion decision plays a part in the issue. Polls show that most Americans oppose more than 95 percent of all abortions performed.

❧ ❧ ❧

> "Abortion has existed in every society, regardless of restrictions, since 2500 B.C. It is one part of a solution to a universal human need—the need for people to control their family size. Worldwide there are between 55 and 60 million abortions each year."

Commentary: Let me see if I understand this one. Since abortion has been around so long, we should keep it legal. Right. Was being an abortionist really the oldest profession?

Controlling family size is a "universal human need?" Since when?

❧ ❧ ❧

> "Research shows that the more contraceptive options available to a society, along with the education necessary to use them, the less that society needs to depend on abortion as a backup."

Commentary: Whose research? Besides, if abortion is so good, what's wrong with using it as a primary means of birth control?

❧ ❧ ❧

> "But even when birth control is available and affordable, it still can fail."

Commentary: True, so why is birth control pushed as the answer to our problems? Since no method is 100 percent effective, people will still get pregnant and still get AIDS or other sexually transmitted diseases. Are we going to tell these people, mostly young people, that at least the statistics showed that these problems were unlikely? That's fine, so long as you or your children are not the victim of one of these "failures."

❧ ❧ ❧

"Making abortion illegal does not reduce its incidence. In fact, it may increase it. Compare the abortion rates for the United States where abortion is legal to that of Brazil where it is illegal. Brazil, with 58 percent of the population of the United States, has twice as many abortions."

Commentary: The source of this information appears to be the Population Crisis Committee, hardly a neutral organization. Brazil (a lesser developed country) is compared to the United States (a First World country) to prove this point? Sorry, but the entire argument is quite ridiculous on its face. How do supporters of legal abortion know how many illegal abortions are done in Brazil?

❧ ❧ ❧

"At the peak of the Depression with two children, no home, and an unemployed husband, she became one of the millions of American women to resort to an illegal abortion, and to die from it."

Commentary: Now it's "millions" (plural) who resorted to illegal abortion, and died from it." And to think pro-lifers are often criticized for using emotional stories and exaggerating alleged statistics.

❧ ❧ ❧

"Today, doctors and public health officials . . . are again working to dispel the barrage of misinformation that the anti-abortion movement continues to spread about the [abortion] procedure. . . ."

"A persistent myth is that abortions usually take place quite late in pregnancy. Actually, 91 percent of all abortions in this country take place before the 12th week, 8 percent in the second trimester, and less than 1 percent in the third, and those exclusively for medical reasons . . . This is the contents of an emptied uterus after an eight week abortion, before which 50 percent of all abortions occur. It is clearly not a baby, despite what anti-abortionists say in their propaganda."

Commentary: It is true that 91 percent of abortions are done in the first trimester, as though that makes much difference since regardless of when the abortion is performed the result is the same. However, it is absolutely untrue that the late-term abortions (second and third trimester) are done "exclusively for medical reasons." In addition, the remaining 9 percent—of 1.6 million—is not a small number.

The abortion victim they showed looked like strawberry jam. Put me through a blender or giant vacuum cleaner and I probably won't look too good either. True, it's not a baby (yet), and a baby is not a teenager (yet), and an embryo is not a fetus (yet). These terms only refer to different stages of human development. It is, however, human—a human that has been destroyed. Supporters of abortion want to make a judgment of human worth based on the stage of development. For abortions done in the eighth through 12th week (still first trimester), they count body parts.

❧ ❧ ❧

"Overseas, as we speak, as many as 200,000 women die each year from botched illegal abortions. This is not only a grim prediction of what could happen here . . . "

Commentary: There is no way anyone could show that there would be 200,000 deaths from illegal abortion in the United States if abortion became illegal again. There were not before 1973 and there will never be, unless groups such as Planned Parenthood and the National Organization for Women urge women to seek illegal abortions. Most deaths would come from Third World countries where general medical conditions would make death more likely from every disease, operation and the like. In addition, we must question the 200,000 figure in the first place. It is simply fabricated.

❧ ❧ ❧

"The United States has been providing 40 percent of the family planning funds for developing nations."

Commentary: What makes leaders of pro-legal abortion groups think the United States owes these monies to anyone or that past foreign appropriations policy locks the government into supporting these groups?

❧ ❧ ❧

"IPAS [International Projects Assistance Services] is doing something about abortion deaths in the developing world. IPAS produces and distributes the aspiration syringe that can correct botched abortions or perform early abortions under the most primitive of medical conditions."

Commentary: IPAS is not doing anything about abortion deaths. Not for the preborn, that is. Are we expected to believe no complications leading to death can arise from the IPAS method?

❧ ❧ ❧

"An aspiration abortion with a syringe takes only a minute or two, requires no anesthesia, and can be performed without a physician by trained nurses, midwives or birth attendants. Again, what you're seeing is the contents of a uterus after an early IPAS abortion. . . ."

"But pressure from anti-abortion forces threatens the research and use of RU 486 in this country and internationally. The Moral Majority, in a March 1989 press release, claims that the anti-abortion forces had succeeded in blocking the distribution of RU 486, even for its live-saving medical applications."

Commentary: I knew they would eventually bring up the now-defunct Moral Majority. RU 486 was not invented and is not being marketed to "save lives," but to end them. At this time, there are no proven life-saving applications of the deadly drug.

❧ ❧ ❧

"Is the fight to outlaw abortion also a crusade against birth control? It seems such a contradiction since reliable contraception decreases the need for abortion. But one look at the literature of anti-abortion groups tells the story. They do want to take away your right to effective contraception . . . And they've made inroads overseas where the United States has poured millions of dollars into natural family planning programs that teach only the Catholic Church sanctioned method of periodic abstinence."

Commentary: Congressman Dornan answers this accusation below. The mainline pro-life movement is not opposed to true contraception. It is, however, opposed to abortifacients. Mentioning the Catholic Church is an attempt to make people believe that if pro-lifers have their way, they will make everyone behave the "Catholic way." It is nothing but an appeal to anti-Catholic bigotry.

❧ ❧ ❧

"In what could be termed a rash of domestic terrorism, factions of the anti-abortion minority have turned to tactics of increasing violence and harassment."

Commentary: The way they talk about the pro-life movement being so small, I am shocked that they have enough people to have "factions."

Using the term "terrorism" is an attempt to evoke an emotional response similar to one generated when people think of overseas hijackings and bombings. All legitimate pro-life groups have condemned such "terrorism." Pro-legal abortion groups don't want to be held responsible for everything done in the name of "abortion rights," but pro-lifers are all held responsible for the acts of individuals when done in the name of the pro-life movement.

❧ ❧ ❧

"The realities of adoption are heartbreaking. In the United States, 34,000 children wait to be adopted. Eighty-two percent of them are older, handicapped, or have special needs. Fifty-one percent are minority. Those seeking to adopt overwhelmingly request healthy white babies. An additional 450,000 children wait in state facilities and foster homes after being removed from their parents for abuse or neglect—part of the 2.2 million children who are abused every year."

Commentary: Aborting babies is not a solution to the problem stated. This statement actually encourages abortion over adoption (nothing new) which makes these people pro-abortion, not pro-choice. There is currently about a five year waiting list for adopting babies. Shockingly, child abuse (another adult problem) is given as a reason for killing the child before he or she is born. First, we cannot say, before a child is born, whether he or she will be abused. Second, the problem is with the abusive adult, not the child. Third, killing is not a solution. Fourth, no parent gets pregnant for the purpose of having someone around whom the parent can abuse. Why are children still abused even though we've had many years of legal abortion? The Lenowski study showed that 90 percent of abused children were planned pregnancies—wanted by their parents.

❧ ❧ ❧

"We are living on a planet where the words 'quality of life' have no meaning to billions of people. The World Health Organization estimates that 430 million people do not have enough to eat and suffer from malnutrition. Ten million children under the age of five suffer from the most severe form which is usually fatal if not treated. Can we continue to keep from women in these desperate straits modern fertility control, including safe abortion? Can we tell them they have no right to limit their family size and no right to survival?"

Commentary: If tax dollars pay for a program or any part of a program, the government has the right to put restrictions on its use. People in Third World countries can do anything they want with their own money, but we don't owe them the money that will be used to kill their children. Population growth decreases with industrialization. Population growth can be curbed by bringing Third World countries up to First World standards, not by killing Third World children.

❧ ❧ ❧

"Abortion is a necessity for millions of women worldwide—for their health, for their well-being, for their dreams of a better tomorrow. The reality is that a woman will seek an abortion, legal or illegal, almost instinctively, and in self-defense. A woman will do this when an unwanted pregnancy presents an excessive strain on her or her family's physical, emotional, or economic resources. Throughout the ages, courageous women have made it their right and indeed their responsibility. In a civilized society, we owe women the legal right to make this decision safely. It is a matter of survival."

Commentary: Abortion is not a "necessity." The most incredible statement in the whole program is that a woman will seek an abortion "almost instinctively." What an attack on women. These so-called feminists are doing nothing but selling women short. This is not a case of self-defense with the preborn human being as the enemy.

Margot Kidder, BWS Host, Actress

"The program is presented by the Better World Society, a non-profit organization which produces and televises programs to help people understand the critical global problems we face and how to solve them. Reducing population growth is one of the most important goals facing our planet today."...

"The [Better World] Society believes that all women must have access to all available methods for controlling their own fertility, including abortion."

Commentary: In a telephone call made by me to the Society following its first program (when I first heard of the group), I was told that the Society did not take a position on abortion. I see we now know the truth.

Sharon Camp, Ph.D.

"Maybe 46 percent of all American women will have an abortion sometime in their lifetime."

Commentary: Where did this statistic come from? If it has any basis, it is certainly not accounting for repeat abortions or population growth. Could it be that Camp starts the statement with "maybe" for a reason? Maybe Saddam Hussein will win the Nobel Peace Prize.

❧ ❧ ❧

"Last year we did a study of access to birth control in 115 countries. Abortion is more frequently used as a method of birth control than all but a few methods of contraception."

Commentary: At least those supporting legal abortion now admit it's simply another form of birth control, but saying it's the most common form of birth control used today is nothing to brag about. Of course, the implication is that "everybody's doing it," so we certainly could not outlaw abortion.

❧ ❧ ❧

"We estimate that worldwide perhaps 30 million unwanted pregnancies result just from contraceptive failure. These are not people who are promiscuous. These are people who are trying to limit their family size and their contraceptives fail them."

Commentary: No source was cited for the estimated 30 million unwanted pregnancies, unless one considers "we" to be an acceptable citation. Many "estimates" turn out to be wild guesses. How does Camp know whether these people are promiscuous? Maybe we have different definitions of the term. Eighty percent of all abortions are performed on single women.

❧ ❧ ❧

"Population growth is the common denominator under virtually all of the world's problems . . ."

Commentary: No, adult irresponsibility is the common denominator for virtually all of the world's problems. Babies, born or preborn, are not an inherent problem, and no problems are solved by killing them.

Ruth Roemer, J.D.

"We want abortion for the sake of our children."

Commentary: Doublespeak. It sounds like, "We want gas chambers for the sake of the Jews," or, "We want lynching for the sake of blacks."

❧ ❧ ❧

"Before abortion was legalized there were estimates that there were 200,000 to a million illegal abortions performed per year in the United States."

Commentary: Sure there were estimates—all from unreliable, pro-legal abortion sources. These statistics are totally fabricated. First, an "estimate" between 200,000 and one million provides a whopping margin. This alone should make us suspicious. Second, illegal activity is not reported so such "estimates" (read, guesses) are unreliable. The source is most likely the Alan Guttmacher Institute.

❧ ❧ ❧

"They have no right, really, to impose their views on the rest of society, and certainly no right in a country that has a constitutional ban against merger of religion and state, to impose the views of one religion on other people."

Commentary: At the time this statement was being made on the program, two Catholics were shown holding a rosary and one person was shown holding a crucifix.

Was Roemer's comment also said to abolitionists during slavery? Was this said to the Rev. Martin Luther King, Jr.? Religion is not the issue. Killing human beings is the issue. The value of a democracy is that individuals can air and work to see their views become law. Moreover, just because an opinion on a particular subject concurs with that of a religion, that does not mean the opinion is automatically a religious one. Otherwise, supporting legal abortion is a religious opinion because some denominations have taken an active stand for legal abortion.

Joan B. Dunlop

"To think that this is something for which we must apologize. We have forgotten that this is a moral right. . . ."

"Abortion is a positive good."

Commentary: The big lie. "War is peace."

Maria Elena Blackwell

"The harsh reality is that a woman will seek an abortion anyway, whether legal or not."

Commentary: Tragically, this is true. Some will seek abortion. Most will not as the vast majority of people obey the law. Most will seek positive solutions. Do we legalize rape because some will do it whether it's illegal or not? How about drug abuse? How about theft? How about murder? How about spousal abuse?

David Grimes, M.D.

"Where will abortions take place? In safe, legally compassionate surroundings, or in the back alley?"

Commentary: Planned Parenthood executives have admitted that most illegal abortions were done by qualified physicians. The "back-alley" argument is designed to get an emotional response from the listener. Besides, thanks to groups like Planned Parenthood telling women of the dangers of back-alley abortion, who would go there? I hope Planned Parenthood will continue to spread the word on this, even after abortion is outlawed.

❧ ❧ ❧

"One cannot have effective fertility control without abortion as a backup. It's never been accomplished in any society to my knowledge. . . ."

"The lesson is very simple. When you legalize abortion, the nation's health improves. If you restrict abortion, the nation's health suffers. . . ."

"It's important to understand that by legalizing abortion in the United States, we almost eliminated deaths from illegal abortion so that by 1979, the federal government could not identify a single woman anywhere in this country who died from illegal abortion."

Commentary: Let me see if I've got this straight. After abortion was made legal, there were no deaths from illegal abortion. No kidding. It doesn't take a doctor to figure this one out. What Grimes does not say is that there were 18 deaths attributed to legal abortion in 1979. Since deaths caused by abortion are often listed as some other cause (heart failure, hemorrhaging, etc.), and sometimes even listed as a maternal death, this number is surely higher. After all, an abortionist has nothing to gain from listing a death as abortion related. It only gives abortion foes more ammunition. Few women return to their abortionist when complications occur. Why return to the person who caused the problem in the first place?

❧ ❧ ❧

"I'm hesitant to label any drug a miracle drug, but there are a number of potential uses of RU 486."

Commentary: RU 486 a miracle drug? This is an attempt to get approval. Grimes refers to "potential uses" for the drug. No use, other than its definite killing ability, has been demonstrated. Moreover, RU 486 is currently being marketed (and was invented) for one reason and one reason only—its effectiveness in killing preborn human beings.

❧ ❧ ❧

"It really is an example of medical McCarthyism in which we see an entire doctrine or school of thought pushing itself on the practice of medicine and science."

Commentary: The latest fad seems to be to mention either McCarthyism or terrorism against those who disagree with you. These are rational voices? Some in the medical and scientific communities want to work without government "interference" so controversial, immoral experiments can be done.

❧ ❧ ❧

". . . these persons are also opposed to sexuality in general, and sex education in particular, so there's a broader under-current that underlies the abortion debate."

Commentary: "These persons" are opposed to neither. They just don't want certain people teaching their children without permission and they want sexual activity to take place under certain circumstances. Free sex has proven to be a failure—a source of countless problems.

❧ ❧ ❧

"I predict that when medical historians of the future look back on the 20th century, the legalization of abortion will stand as one of the real triumphs of our times."

Commentary: I believe that as God looks on the twentieth century, the legalization of abortion stands as one of the real tragedies of our times.

Kenneth C. Edelin, M.D.

"We can try to make it illegal. We can try and turn back the clock. And women will die. Women will die. . . ."

"And that woman who died didn't care whether it was legal or illegal, and she did not ask a judge, or a jury, or her minister, or her state legislature. She knew that she was pregnant and did not want to be, and was willing to take the risk, and she is just representative of thousands and millions of women who were desperate enough to put their lives on the line to do that."

Commentary: Now is it thousands or millions? Women need real help, not dead children.

❧ ❧ ❧

"What really frightens me is that the men who will make that decision don't care. Don't care. They will sit in that marble structure in Washington and hand down this decision and won't see the consequences . . . The most vulnerable, the weakest in our society, poor women, will be the first affected and the most severely affected."

Commentary: This is interesting coming from a man who was convicted by a jury of manslaughter after he botched a late-term abortion (see *The Press and Abortion, 1838–1988*, by Marvin N. Olasky, pages 124–130). Edelin cares? Besides, I always thought the preborn were the "most vulnerable, the weakest in our society."

We must care for the preborn and their mothers. Abortion solves no problem. It is a problem.

While Edelin negatively refers to "the men who will make that decision," he certainly did not think so when seven men on the Supreme Court issued *Roe v. Wade*. Moreover, Sandra Day O'Connor may not like being ignored when Edelin refers to "men" making these important decisions.

❧ ❧ ❧

"Black women in Georgia died four times more frequently from illegal abortion than white women, and black teenagers died eleven times more frequently than their white counterparts."

Commentary: This is interesting since, today, government reports say about one-third of all abortions are done on African-Americans. Is it any wonder that one African-American writer called abortion "black genocide?"

Allan Rosenfield, M.D.

"The organizations that are supporting the current position on *Roe v. Wade*, and are against changing that status, include the American Medical Association, the American College of Obstetricians and Gynecologists, the American Academy of Pediatrics, the American Psychiatric Association, the American Public Health Association. Our President [George Bush], during the debates in the campaign, said he won't put women in jail, but he'll put doctors in jail. I was offended by that statement. We should have all risen up against that statement. We have a duty to provide this service to women and I defy them to put us in jail in providing this medical service."

Commentary: The groups listed are reflecting a political, good-old-boy agenda, not a moral or scientific opinion. It's interesting to note that the American Medical Association was one of the first groups to lobby for abortion restrictions early in the twentieth century.

Rosenfield defies the government to jail him if he breaks the law? Well, I'll visit you in jail, Allan. What would Rosenfield say to a doctor who does not want to do abortions? Would he say the doctor is not doing his duty? Would Rosenfield offer the same support to doctors jailed for other reasons if the doctors really believe they are right?

❧ ❧ ❧

"This drug, RU 486, and that class of drugs, may have an impact on breast cancer, may have an impact on prostate cancer. They [abortion foes] don't care. They want it off the market because it can be an abortifacient. It's an immoral, almost obscene stance."

Commentary: RU 486 can be an abortifacient? It is an abortifacient. There is no reason to believe the drug will be useful for any other purpose, but raising the hopes of millions of people who suffer from deadly diseases and who are desperately seeking a cure, will, in an obscene way, gain more support for the legalization of RU 486.

❧ ❧ ❧

"Another example of the fact that children are not wanted in many instances because women simply can't take care of them are the figures we're seeing from Latin America of the so-called street children. There are estimates that in Brazil there are as many as 11 million abandoned children living in the streets. What better testimony is there to the need for family planning, for abortion services, and for a variety of other services, for these women who are so desperate as to abandon their children."

Commentary: More "estimates." The women in Latin America are acting out of economic hardship, not because they do not want their children. "Solution" to street children: kill them before they're born. How about after they're born?

Katie E. McLaurin

"Access to safe abortion services is frequently a matter of a woman's survival."

Francine Coeytaux

"We all talk as if we can get along without abortion, that we have perfect contraception."

Praema Rachavan-Gilbert, M.D.

"You know, we have to think very seriously about this. What are the consequences of forcing a woman to have a child that she just doesn't want? Is she gonna hate this child?"

Commentary: Not wanting to be pregnant does not translate into not wanting a child. Not wanting a child does not translate into hate. Has Rachavan-Gilbert ever heard of adoption?

Other Statements Made During The Program

"[Abortion is] A simple, safe procedure that no one needs to be ashamed of or embarrassed about. . . ."

"Is it the one inch tissue that we are concerned about, or is it the dead woman on the motel floor, and this is the dead woman . . . "

Commentary: A photograph is shown of a naked woman, dead on the floor.

Pro-lifers are usually verbally attacked when they show photographs that are designed to get an emotional response. We grieve for the dead woman who tried to abort herself. But must we only be concerned for the woman or her unborn baby?

How many one inch pieces of tissue have a beating heart and brain waves?

Byllye Y. Avery

"Why does the government want hungry children in the world?"

Commentary: No one wants children to be hungry. Hunger is the result of distribution problems which are most often caused by politics. Hunger is a problem created by adults, yet we punish innocent preborn human beings for our failures. Abortion does not solve (and has not solved) the problem of hunger in the world. Of course, if we kill all hungry people, that would be one "solution," wouldn't it? Of course not. We don't kill an entire class of human beings as a "solution" to social problems. Should we kill all of the homeless until we find homes for everyone? Obviously ridiculous. Abortion allows lawmakers to escape finding real, long-term solutions to the problems created by adults.

❧ ❧ ❧

"The anti-choice are the no choice people. They really don't care about people and they really don't care about children."

Commentary: That's easy for anyone to say. Pro-life people are the only truly disinterested parties in the abortion debate. They are standing up for others and will never receive thanks or praise from those they seek to protect. This is not true of pro-legal abortion activists who want their personal rights, their freedom of choice, control over their bodies, and their income from performing abortions.

SECTION 2
"ABORTION: AN ISSUE FORUM"

Following the showing of "Abortion: For Survival," a panel discussion was held. The discussion included occasional taped reports done in a news format. The quotations below have been edited to eliminate repetition. For example, one person said Nellie Gray's name four times when asking her a question. Her name is used only once below.

Identifiable Program Participants:

Martin Agronsky, moderator; Robert K. Dornan, member of Congress, R-California; Nellie Gray, president, March for Life; Eleanor Smeal, Fund for the Feminist Majority; and Faye Wattleton, then-president, Planned Parenthood Federation of America.

General Comments:

It is important to notice how each participant reacted while being introduced as it shows training for a television presence. Wattleton looked right into the television camera and smiled. She smiled throughout most of the program as well. Smeal gave a brief, slight smile and nodded her head. Gray gave a slight nod and did not smile at all. Dornan gave a nod but no smile.

Faye Wattleton:

> "The point, Nellie, that I'm trying to make is that your view is, and I don't know if you've ever been pregnant. I don't know if you're married [interruption], I don't know if you've ever been a mother. I don't know if you've ever had these experiences. But the point is that, that's your view. We respectfully acknowledge your right to hold that view. There are a range of views on these issues and your dogma cannot be imposed. The fact that you have declared that women will not is really the essence here, is that people must be left to decide for themselves. You among them must decide for yourself and that I want you to grant me the dignity of my ability to decide for myself. And by the way, even though you declare it not to be existing, it will happen anyway. The only question is whether women will die, and that's really the essence. . . ."
>
> "The Supreme Court [in *Webster*] did not make abortion illegal. It's important to remember that, but what it did [interruption] was to say that states can now regulate the availability of abortions and the people who will suffer the most are those people who have the least resources or the fewest resources to get around the regulations. . . ."
>
> "I think it's rather remarkable now about, and the fallaciousness of your position, is that you somehow think that the sperm and the egg are dead before they meet. If we took this out to the logical extension [interruption] . . . "
>
> "Nellie, not every fertilized egg becomes a baby, Mr. Dornan. As a matter of fact [interruption] there are a great numbers of fertilized eggs that are aborted spontaneously. The great maker in the sky makes certain that they don't continue."

Commentary: Dornan and Gray did an excellent job responding to these points.

An egg or sperm alone do not become a baby. They are not unique, individual human beings.

Comparing a spontaneous abortion to an induced abortion is ludicrous.

❧ ❧ ❧

> "As a matter of fact, Mr. Dornan, no one, no one backs away from the reality that if a woman selects a method of birth control that is not highly effective, she must consider the option of abortion [interruption] . . . Mr. Dornan, I believe that a woman must consider that, must consider that, as a method of backup, if she considers a method that is not as effective. Now, if you want that to stop, why don't you join us in working for better birth control technology, so that people do not have to face that problem."

Commentary: This last sentence is Wattleton's common strategy. Pro-lifers can't join Planned Parenthood because pro-lifers disagree over abortifacients and more basic issues. Wattleton almost always gets applause when she uses the "why don't you join us" line. Unfortunately, her opponents often let her get away with it. They seem to be left without a response. This shows poor preparation since Wattleton almost always uses the line.

A relative of this argument is that pro-lifers should be more concerned about homeless, abused, and starving children (as well as countless other issues)—people already born. The same argument was used by an opponent of animal rights who wrote a letter to the editor of *People*. "The activists should get their facts straight," wrote Karry Ward of Snohomish, Washington, whose letter was printed in the October 21, 1991, edition. "They should put their efforts toward helping abused, abandoned, starving animals . . . "

❧ ❧ ❧

"You have no reason to come here and say to us if you're going to give us assistance but you're going to put strings on it."

Commentary: If it's American taxpayer money, the giver has every right to place strings on it. Wattleton doesn't complain when corporations place restrictions on the donations made to Planned Parenthood.

Dornan's comment was great: "Oh, just give us the money to kill our babies. Don't put strings on it."

❧ ❧ ❧

"Shall we regulate your sperm production? Shall we start regulating your sperm production?"

Commentary: Are we expected to believe that Wattleton thinks that laws protecting prenatal life (from outside forces) are comparable to regulating sperm production (a bodily function)? If she really does believe they are comparable, Wattleton had better take a good sex education course.

❧ ❧ ❧

"The part that is so unfortunate is that you seem to only see the world through the prism of your life experience. There are many situations—I am a nurse midwife by profession and training—there are many situations in which those circumstances, those particular elements, do not exist and we must let people alone and leave them to their own situation."

Commentary: Everyone sees everything based on their life experiences. How can we punish a child molester or drug kingpin if we haven't had his or her life experience and been there?

❧ ❧ ❧

". . . I believe that our position is the compromise position, which is to say that we hold very different points of view, and we must leave it to the individual to decide."

Commentary: This is the latest strategy—claim they are the compromise. Wrong.

Robert K. Dornan

"Here's a line in there that I personally resent. That anybody who's pro-life really doesn't care about children. I wouldn't say that about you folks. And I know it's not true about Nellie and I hope it's not true about this grandfather of seven. It's just not true. . . ."

"One of those doctors said that birth control was our hidden agenda . . . not one [federal lawmaker], across the whole political spectrum, do I know, has a bill or even an idea, to thwart birth control in any way at all, let alone what Dr. Grimes says."

Commentary: You tell 'em, Congressman.

❧ ❧ ❧

[Quoting film] "'Only those should be born who have a fair chance at life.' Let's come back to who decides that."

Commentary: A good issue, Congressman, since that's essentially the line that closed the film. What was Smeal's response? She attacked Dornan for "quoting a woman who died." Smeal continued, "You don't have any compassion."

Another common technique is for those who support legal abortion to use emotion when a pro-life advocate addresses something they said. Dornan wanted to comment on the statement made by the woman who later died from an illegal abortion. Is this sacrilegious? Of course not, but at least Smeal never did have to respond to Dornan's initial question—or most others, for that matter.

❧ ❧ ❧

"You don't kill babies before or after they're born to solve a world food problem. . . ."

"I say it's not birth control, it's abortion."

Commentary: Dornan made this latter comment about abortifacient birth control. What was Smeal's response? "Well, now you're getting into semantics, but most people say that this is a birth control method."

Semantics, Eleanor? Semantics? Actually, both Dornan and Smeal are right in one respect. Dornan is right when he argues that certain forms of birth control are abortifacients, which effectively makes the result an abortion. Smeal is right when she says they are simply birth control, but then again, according to Smeal's film, so is abortion.

Eleanor Smeal

"You just saw some of the most articulate national spokespeople for the medical profession [interruptions]. They're esteemed doctors [interruptions] . . . "

Commentary: These people were not "spokespeople for the medical profession" as many in the profession oppose abortion. Gray responded to the "esteemed doctors" comment by saying something along the lines that some of those in the film are "butchers." Smeal's response: "Don't say that about a Kenneth Edelin. Don't say that about a Keith Russell. Do you know who he is?" Well, we certainly do (see above).

APPENDIX F

SUBMITTERS OF WEBSTER CASE AMICUS BRIEFS

The following is a partial list of individuals and organizations submitting an *amicus* ("friend of the court") brief to the United States Supreme Court in the case of *Webster v. Reproductive Health Services*.

Submitting brief in support of Reproductive Health Services (supporting unrestricted legal abortion):

140 members of Congress
Attorneys general of California, Colorado, Massachusetts, New York, Texas, and Vermont
167 scientists and physicians
608 state legislators from 32 states
896 American law professors
281 American historians
57 bioethicists
6 deans of medical schools
37 chairmen of medical school departments of obstetrics and gynecology
64 health care professionals
women who have had abortions
Abortion Rights Mobilization
AFL-CIO, Public Employees Division
American Federation of State and County Municipal Employees
Alan Guttmacher Institute
All-People's Congress
American Academy of Pediatrics
American Association of Reproductive Health Professionals
American Association of University Women
American Civil Liberties Union
American College of Obstetricians and Gynecologists
American College of Preventive Medicine
American Fertility Society
American Friends Service Committee
American Indian Health Care Association
American Jewish Committee
American Jewish Congress

American Medical Association
American Medical Women's Association
American Nurses Association
American Psychiatric Association
American Psychological Association
American Public Health Association
American Society for Adolescent Medicine
American Veterans Committee
Americans for Democratic Action
Americans for Religious Liberty
Americans United for Separation of Church and State
Asian American Legal Defense and Education Fund
Association of Latino Attorneys
Association of Sex Educators and Therapists
B'nai B'rith Women
Black Women's Agenda
Catholics for a Free Choice
Center for Constitutional Rights
Center for Law and Social Justice
Center for Population Options
Center for Women Policy Studies
Coalition of College Campus Ministers
Committee for Hispanic Children and Families
Committee to Defend Reproductive Rights
Coalition of Labor Union Women
Federally Employed Women
Federation of Feminist Women's Health Centers
Hispanic Health Council
Human Rights Campaign Fund
Institute for Women's Policy Research
International Center for Research on Women
International Fund for Health and Family Planning
International Women's Health Coalition
Lawyers for Reproductive Rights
League of Women Voters, USA
Mexican-American Legal Defense and Education Fund
Mexican-American Women's National Association
Ms. Foundation for Women
National Abortion Federation
National Abortion Rights Action League
National Assembly of Religious Women
National Association of Nurse Practitioners in Reproductive Health
National Association of Public Hospitals
National Association of Social Workers
National Association of Women Lawyers
National Black Women's Health Project
National Center for Lesbian Rights

National Coalition Against Domestic Violence
National Coalition of American Nuns
National Conference of Black Lawyers
National Conference of Women's Bar Association
National Council of Jewish Women
National Council of Negro Women
National Education Association
National Family Planning and Reproductive Health Association
National Federation of Business and Professional Women's Clubs
National Gay and Lesbian Task Force
National Institute for Women of Color
National Latin Health Organization
National Lawyers Guild
National Minority AIDS Council
National Organization for Women
National Society of Genetic Counselors
National Urban League
National Women's Health Network
National Women's Law Center
National Women's Political Caucus
National Writers' Union
Native American Community Board
New Jewish Agenda
Newspaper Guild
Organization of Asian Women
Organization of Pan-Asian Women
People for the American Way
Planned Parenthood Federation of America
Population Council
Population Crisis Committee
Population Services International
Presbyterian Church of the USA
Presbyterian Church of the USA, Committee of Women of Color
Program for Introduction and Adaptation of Contraceptive Technology
Puerto Rican Legal Defense and Education Fund
Religious Coalition for Abortion Rights
Religious Coalition for Abortion Rights, Women of Color Partnership Program
Republicans for Choice
Sex Information and Education Council
Sierra Club
Transnational Family Research Institute
Union of American Hebrew Congregations
Unitarian Universalist Association
Unitarian Universalist Association, Women's Federation
United Church of Christ, Coordinating Center for Women
United Church of Christ, Office of Church in Society
United Methodist Church, General Board of Church and Society

Voters for Choice/Friends of Family Planning
Women for Racial and Economic Equality
Women's AIDS Prevention Project
Women's Equity Action League
Women's Law Project

Submitting brief in support of *Webster*, the attorney general for the State of Missouri (against unrestricted legal abortion):

108 members of Congress
State legislators from Pennsylvania and Missouri
The State of Louisiana, joined by the attorneys general of Arizona, Idaho, Pennsylvania, and Wisconsin
Agudeth Israel of America
Alabama Lawyers for Unborn Children
American Academy of Medical Ethics
American Association of Pro-life Obstetricians and Gynecologists
American Family Association
American Life League
Birthright International
Catholic Health Association
Catholic League for Religious and Civil Rights
Center for Judicial Studies
Christian Action Council
Christian Advocates Serving Evangelism
Christian Life Commission of the Southern Baptist Convention
Doctors for Life
Elliott Institute for Social Sciences Research
Family Research Council
Feminists for Life of America
International Right to Life Federation
Knights of Columbus
Legal Defense Fund for Unborn Children
Lutheran Church, Missouri Synod
Missouri Catholic Conference
National Association of Evangelicals
National Association of Pro-Life Nurses
National Legal Foundation
National Right to Life Committee
Orthodox Christians for Life
Rutherford Institute
Southern Center for Law and Ethics
United States Catholic Conference
Women Exploited by Abortion

(From *Washington Memo*, Alan Guttmacher Institute, April 19, 1989.)

APPENDIX G

NATIONAL ORGANIZATIONS SUPPORTING TITLE X REAUTHORIZATION

National organizations endorsing the reauthorization of the Title X program include:

Alan Guttmacher Institute
American Academy of Child and Adolescent Psychiatry
American Academy of Pediatrics
American Association of University Women
American Baptist Churches
American Civil Liberties Union
American College of Nurse-Midwives
American College of Obstetricians and Gynecologists
American Federation of State, County and Municipal Employees
American Fertility Society
American Jewish Committee
American Medical Association
American Medical Student Association
American Nurses Association
American Psychiatric Association
American Psychological Association
American Public Health Association
American Public Welfare Association
American Youth Work Center
Americans for Democratic Action
Association of American Medical Colleges
Association of Maternal and Child Health Programs
Association of State and Territorial Health Officers
Catholics for a Free Choice
Center for Population Options
Center for Women Policy Studies
Child Welfare League of America
National Abortion Federation
National Abortion Rights Action League

National Association of Nurse-Practitioners in Family Planning
National Association of Social Workers
National Audubon Society
National Council of Jewish Women
National Education Association
National Family Planning and Reproductive Health Association
National Urban League
National Women's Health Network
National Women's Political Caucus
Nurses Association of the American College of Obstetricians and Gynecologists
Planned Parenthood Federation of America
Sierra Club California Population and Growth Issues Committee
Union of American Hebrew Congregations
Unitarian Universalist Association of Congregations in North America
United States Conference of Mayors
United States Local Health Officers
Women's Equity Action League
Young Women's Christian Association of USA, national board

(From Washington Memo, Alan Guttmacher Institute, February 10, 1989.)

APPENDIX H

CELEBRITY SUPPORTERS

Many celebrities have expressed support for legal abortion, Planned Parenthood and/or the Better World Society. Some are members of the National Leadership Committee, part of Planned Parenthood's Campaign to Keep Abortion Safe and Legal. Some have merely lent their names to the pro-legal abortion effort. Others are actively involved, donating money as well as time.

This list is presented to underscore Planned Parenthood's influence in the entertainment industry and with other well-known individuals. These people do not need our condemnation, for we, too, could have been listed herein were circumstances different:

Singers, singing groups, and musicians supporting legal abortion, Planned Parenthood and/or the Better World Society include: Anita Baker, Harry Belafonte, Tony Bennett, Betty, Mary Chapan Carpenter, Cher, Judy Collins, Sheena Easton, Ronnie Gilbert, Kim Gordon (Corina and Sonic Youth), Arlo Guthrie, Deborah Harry, Lady Miss Kier, Cyndi Lauper, Lisa Lisa and Cult Jam, Yo-Yo Ma, MC Lyte, MC Peaches, Madonna (Louise Ciccone), Maureen McGovern, Melissa Manchester, Wynton Marsalis, Holly Near, Sinead O'Connor, Kate Pierson (B-52s), Lou Rawls, Helen Reddy, Della Reese, REM, Linda Ronstadt, Peter Seeger, Bobby Short, Phoebe Snow, Paul Stookey (Peter, Paul and Mary), Barbara Streisand, James Taylor, Mary Travers (Peter, Paul and Mary), Wendy and Lisa (formerly with Prince and the Revolution), Tina Weymouth (Tom Tom Club), Peter Yarrow (Peter, Paul and Mary), and Frank Zappa.

Actors and actresses include: Alan Alda, Anthony Alda, Anne Archer, Roseanne Arnold (formerly Roseanne Barr, also a comedian)), Edward Asner, Kim Basinger, Justine Bateman, Polly Bergen, Meredith Baxter, Corbin Bernsen, Valerie Bertenelli, Beau Bridges, Matthew Broderick, Ellen Burstyn, LaVar Burton, John Callahan, Keith Carradine (has spoken in support of making condoms available in schools), Rae Dawn Chong, Glenn Close, Nicholas Coster, Hume Cronyn, Jane Curtain (also a comedian), Blythe Danner, Ossie Davis, Richard Dreyfuss, Griffin Dunne, Jill Eikenberry, Douglas Fairbanks, Jr., Morgan Fairchild, Mike Farrell, Louise Fletcher, Jane Fonda, Jodie Foster, Arlene Francis, Bonnie Franklin, Estelle Getty, Robert Gintry, Sharon Gless, Whoopi Goldberg (also a comedian), Nancy Lee Grahan (founder of Daytimers for Choice), Linda Gray, Michele Greene, Jasmine Guy (also a singer), Veronica Hamel, Valerie Harper, Cathryn Hartt, Goldie Hawn, Eileen Heckart, Katharine Hepburn, Holly Hunter, Celeste Holm, Amy Irving, Erica Jong, Joanna Kerns, Margot Kidder, Richard Kiley, Jack Lemmon, Cleavon Little, Susan Lucci, Ali MacGraw, Robin Mattson, Kelly McGillis,

Elizabeth McGovern, Marcia McKenna, Kristy McNichol, Dudley Moore, Mary Tyler Moore, Laraine Newman, Paul Newman, Denise Nicholas, Leonard Nimoy, Sarah Jessica Parker, Estelle Parsons, Gregory Peck, Christina Pickles, Martha Plimpton (daughter of Keith Carradine), Margaret Reed, Christopher Reeve, Tim Robbins, Ester Rolle, Charlotte Ross, Susan Sarandon, Ally Sheedy, Cybill Shepherd, Ron Silver, Jimmy Smits, Roderick Spencer, Mary Steenburgen, Rod Steiger, Dee Wallace Stone, Peter Strauss, Meryl Streep, Marlo Thomas, Robert Townsend (also a comedian), Michael Tucker, Kathleen Turner, Cicely Tyson, Blair Underwood, Sam Wanamaker, Malcolm Jamal Warner, Lesley Ann Warren, Sam Waterston, Raquel Welch, Robin Williams (also a comedian), Shelley Winters, D.B. Wong, and Joanne Woodward.

Writers include: Maya Angelou, Judy Blume, Berke Breathed (comic strip), Miriam Claire, Paul R. Ehrlich, Ph.D., Albert Ellis, Ph.D. (psychologist), Diane English, Susan Fales (television), Susan Faludi, Susan Faludi, Betty Friedan (also involved with the American Humanist Association), Arthur Frommer (travel), Ursula K. LeGuin, Eda LeShan, Rod McKuen, Robert K. Merton (sociologist), Edward P. Morgan (journalist), Robert Nisbet, Ph.D. (psychology), George Plimpton, Harold Prince, Thomas Tyron, Anna Quindlen, Abigail Van Buren ("Dear Abby" columnist who is also active in the pro-euthanasia movement), and Alice Walker.

Other supporters include: Steve Allen (comedian, singer), Susan Anton (model), Richard Belzer (comedian, actor), Linda Bloodworth-Thomason (producer), Julian Bond (political activist), Josh Brand (producer), Hodding Carter (columnist/commentator), Wilt Chamberlain (former basketball player), Julia Child (cook, television program host), Ramsey Clark (former U.S. attorney general), Juliet Cuming (producer, director), Phyllis Diller (comedian), Phil Donohue (talk show host), Hugh Downs (co-host of "20/20," ABC News), Kenneth C. Edelin, M.D. (professor, Obstetrics and Gynecology, Boston University), Linda Ellerbee (news reporter and program host), Betty Ford (former First Lady), Kenneth Galbraith (economist), David Geffen (Geffen Entertainment), Paul Harvey (newscaster, commentator), Christie Hefner and Hugh Hefner (Playboy Enterprises), Buck Henry (comedian, actor), Larry Holmes (boxer), Virginia Huldekoper (competitive skier), Joel Hyatt (Legal Services), Lee Iacocca (business executive), Robert Iger (ABC entertainment chief), Jesse Jackson (political activist), Ben Jones (former actor, member of Congress), Callie Khouri (screenwriter), John Landis (director), Norman Lear (producer, director, screenwriter, founder of People for the American Way), Spike Lee (producer, director, screenwriter), Sidney Lumet (director), Carol Mann (professional golfer), Penny Marshall (director, actress), Jayne Meadows (comedian, singer), Mike Medavoy (executive president, Orion Pictures), Lorne Michaels (producer), Michael Milken (financier), Earl Monroe (president, Pretty Pearl Records), Martina Navratilova (tennis player), Joseph Papp (producer), Gordon Parks (photographer, writer,director), Rosa Parks (political activist), Ron Reagan (son of the former president), Carl Reiner (screenwriter, producer, director), Joan Rivers (talk show host, comedian), Jeff Sagansky (CBS entertainment chief), Arthur Schlesinger, Jr. (former U.S. secretary of defense), William Schulz (president, Unitarian Universalist Association), Aaron Spelling (producer), Cheryl Tiegs (model), R. E.

"Ted" Turner (Turner Broadcasting), Robin Tyler (comedian, producer), and Ruth Westheimer, Ph.D. (sexuality counselor).

Somewhat ***less prominent public figures*** have also expressed support including: Josephine Abercrombie, James G. Abourezk, Mrs. Vincent Astor, Letitia Baldrige, Red Barber, Joe Louis Barrow, Jr., T. Berry Brazelton, M.D., Rabbi Balfour Brickner, Yvonne B. Burke, Betty Lou Carter, M. C. Chang, Ph.D., Kenneth B. Clark, Ph.D. (also involved with the American Humanist Association), William L. Clay, William Sloane Coffin, Johnnetta B. Cole, Mary Dent Crisp, Constance Curry, Suzanne de Passe, Patricia Derian, Peter Duchin, Richard W. Edelman, James Farmer, Frances D. Fergusson, Ph.D., Henry W. Foster, Jr., M.D., Judith Frey, Willard Gaylin, M.D., Stephen Gillers, Esq., Allen Ginsberg, Lynn F. Glaze, Hazel Gluck, Stephen Jay Gould, Patricia Albjerg Graham, Ph.D., Rosalind Redfern Grover, Lena Guerrero, Robert Guillaume, Ph.D., Roger Guillemin, David Halberstam, Bob Hall, LaDonna Harris, Susan Harris, Richard Gordon Hatcher, Eugenie C. Havemeyer, Alexander Heard, Jean K. Heard, Aileen C. Hernandez, Elsie H. Hillman, Elizabeth Holtzman, Mr. and Mrs. James R. Houghton, Alice Stone Ilchman, Ph.D., John E. Jacob, Cornelia D. Jahncke, Vernon E. Jordan, Jr., Esq., Lawrence Kasdan, Wendy Wallace Kelsey, Nan Kempner, Donald Kennedy, Ph.D., Nannerl O. Keohane, Mary E. King, Robert C. Kolodny, M.D., Deborah Landis, Edward Lewis, Robert Longo, Kenneth R. R. Gros Louis, Ph.D., John E. Mack, M.D., Jean Bronson Mahoney, Peter N. McCloskey, Jr., Donald F. McHenry, Dina Merrill, Joyce D. Miller, Diane Nash, Arthur C. Nielsen, Jr., Federico Pea, Brock Peters, Muriel M. Petioni, M.D., George H. Pfau, Jr., Carolyn F. Piel, M.D., Rabbi Sally J. Priesand, Joseph L. Rauh, Jr., Bernice Johnson Reagon, Mrs. John F. Riddell, Jr., Lee Salk, Ph.D., Rev. William F. Schulz, Albert Shanker, William L. Shirer, Ann Johnston Singh, Constance Iona Slaughter-Harvey, John E. Smith, Candy Spelling, Paula Steiger, Alan R. Sweezy, Ph.D., Edward F. Swenson, Jr., Howard J. Tatum, M.D., Ph.D., Susan L. Taylor, William L. Taylor, Lionel Tiger, Ph.D., David B. Truman, Joseph D. Tydings, Julia A. Walker, Roger Wilkins, William Julius Wilson, Ph.D., and Leah Wise.

Those generally confirmed as abortion foes include the following ***actors and actresses:*** Woody Allen, Scott Bacula, Kirk Cameron, Mia Farrow, Mel Gibson, Helen Hayes, Charlton Heston, Ricardo Montalban, Kate Mulgrew, Jack Nicholson, Frank Runyon (one of the few soap opera stars who did not join Daytimers for Choice), Martin Sheen, Brooke Shields, and Lisa Whelchel.

Singers, singing groups, and musicians generally confirmed as against abortion include: Bob Ayala, Ray Boltz, Pat Boone, Scott Wesley Brown, Anita J. Bryant, Glen Campbell, Carman, Rick Cua, Dion, In Effect, Lola Falana, Amy Grant, Steve Green, Kathi Hart, Jacob's Trouble, Gordon Jensen, Phil Keaggy, Newsboys, Marie Osmond, Sandi Patti, Michael Peace, Cliff Richard, Sandy Rios, Ricky Skaggs, Michael W. Smith, Randy Stonehill, Donna Summers, Russ Taff, Steve Taylor, Whitecross, and Deneice Williams.

Several ***sports figures*** (some of whom have retired) are confirmed opponents of abortion. Football: Mark Bavaro, Mike Ditka, Joe Gibbs, J. D. Hill, Jeff Kemp, Joe

Kulbacki, Tom Landry, Steve Largent, Pete Metzelaars, Frank Reich, Phil Simms, Steve Young, and Jim Zorn.

Baseball: Bill Almon, Jesus Alou, Jose L. Alvarez, Sparky Anderson, Rob Andrews, Rick Auerbach, Chuck Baker, Reginald Baldwin, Jim Barr, Juan Berenguer, Dwight Bernard, Larry Bittner, Doug Blair, Barry Bonnell, Mike Bruhert, Mike Brumley, Ray Burris, Rick Camp, John Candelaria, Doug Capilla, Phil Caravetta, Gene Clines, Dave Concepcion, Marty Conejo, Joe Deer, Adrian Devine, Duffy Dyer, Nino Espinosa, Jim Ewell, Sergio Ferrer, Rollie Fingers, Mike Fischlin, Tim Foli, Pepe Frias, Jerry Fry, Tony Garofalo, Steve Garvey, Casar Geronimo, Fernando Gonzalez, Tom Grieve, Ken Griffey, Dave Hamilton, Preston Hanna, Larry Herndon, Ed Herrmann, Ron Hodges, Tom Hume, Roy Lee Jackson, Randy Jones, Tommy John, Junior Kennedy, Bruce Kison, Bob Knepper, Ray Knight, Darrold Knowles, Jerry Koosman, Mike Krukow, Tony Kubek, Dennis Lamp, Tom Lasorda, Gary Lavelle, John Lemaster, Skip Lockwood, Gary Maddox, Rudy May, Lee Mazilli, Andrew J. McGaffigan, Lynn McGlothen, Tom McKenna, Roger Metzger, George Mitterwald, Omar Moreno, Dale Murray, Fred Norman, Ed Ott, Bob Owchinko, Jose Pagan, Rick Parker, Frank Pastore, Broderick Perkins, Tony Perez, Gerry Pirtle, Terry Puhl, Rick Reuschel, Jerry Reuse, Don Reynolds, J.R. Richard, Dave Roberts, Bill Robinson, Phil Roof, Chico Ruiz, Joe Sambito, Manny Sanguillen, Manny Sarmiento, George Scherger, Jim Sexton, Larry Sheets, Larry Shepard, Eric Show, Chris Speier, Willie Stargell, Rennie Stennett, Jim Sundberg, Bruce Sutter, Craig Swan, Rick Sweet, Kent Tekulve, Gene Tenace, Darrell Thomas, Jerry Turner, Mike Vail, Bob Valentine, Dick Williams, Rick Williams, and Joel Youngblood.

Other sports figures include Isiah Thomas, Don Heinkel (basketball), Burt Adams (hockey) and Julie A. Cole (golf).

Others generally confirmed as anti-abortion include: Patrick Buchanan (columnist, television commentator), Caesar Chavez (labor leader), General Charles Duke (astronaut), Dick Gregory (comedian, social activist), Bob Hope, Tunch Ilken, Michael O'Martian (music producer), Eunice Kennedy Shriver (Special Olympics, sister of Senator Kennedy and the late President Kennedy, mother of Maria Shriver and, most importantly, mother-in-law of Arnold Schwarzenegger), LaGard Smith (author), Cal Thomas (columnist, commentator), and Lech Walesa (Polish leader).

Several individuals are ***"rumored"*** to be opposed to abortion. This means that some evidence exists, but no clear statements have been made. This list includes: Robert Blake (actor), Nel Carter (actress, singer), Michael Chang (professional tennis player), Harry Connick, Jr. (singer, actor), Kevin Costner (actor, producer, director, screen writer), Fred Grandy (former actor, "The Love Boat," member of Congress, R-Iowa), Richard Harris (actor, producer), Mary Hart (television program co-host), Peter Himmelman, Ann Jilian (actress, singer), Ken Kesey (author), Gavin McCloud (actor, author), Patricia Neal (actress), Merlin Olson (actor, sportscaster), Tom Selleck (actor), John Stamos (actor), and Robert Urich (actor).

Note: The sources for the information included in Appendix G are numerous including media reports and programs, Feminists for Life, Planned Parenthood documents, Athletes for Life, and the American Life League. Some groups report that Jordan Knight of New Kids on the Block is against abortion, but significant doubt left him off the list. Even Madonna is listed as being against abortion by one group. This is completely false.

NOTES

Chapter 1: Foundation for Social Change

1. Madeline Gray, *Margaret Sanger: A Biography of the Champion of Birth Control* (New York: Richard Marek Publishers, 1979), p. 10.
2. Virginia Coigney, *Margaret Sanger: Rebel With a Cause* (Garden City, NY: Doubleday and Company, 1969), p. 66.
3. Gray, *Margaret Sanger: A Biography of the Champion of Birth Control*, p. 14.
4. Joan Dash, *A Life of One's Own: Three Gifted Women and the Men They Married* (New York: Harper and Row, 1973), p. 4.
5. Donald K. Pickens, *Eugenics and the Progressives* (Nashville, TN: Vanderbilt University Press, 1968), p. 72.
6. Elyse Topalian, *Margaret Sanger* (New York: Franklin Watts, 1984), pp. 4–5.
7. Margaret Sanger, *My Fight for Birth Control* (New York: Farrar and Rinehart, 1931), p. 7.
8. Coigney, *Margaret Sanger: Rebel With a Cause*, p. 21.
9. Dash, *A Life of One's Own: Three Gifted Women and the Men They Married*, p. 4.
10. Sanger, *My Fight for Birth Control*, p. 4.
11. Margaret Sanger, *Margaret Sanger: An Autobiography* (New York: W.W. Norton and Company, 1938), pp. 14 and 29.
12. Gray, *Margaret Sanger: A Biography of the Champion of Birth Control*, p. 17.
13. Coigney, *Margaret Sanger: Rebel With a Cause*, p. 36.
14. Gray, *Margaret Sanger: A Biography of the Champion of Birth Control*, p. 25.
15. Sanger, *Margaret Sanger: An Autobiography*, p. 182.
16. Ibid., p. 55.
17. Coigney, *Margaret Sanger: Rebel With a Cause*, p. 61.
18. David M. Kennedy, *Birth Control in America: The Career of Margaret Sanger* (New Haven: Yale University Press, 1970), p. 17.
19. Coigney, *Margaret Sanger: Rebel With a Cause*, p. 66.
20. Ibid., p. 80.
21. James Reed, *The Birth Control Movement in American Society: From Private Vice to Public Virtue*, (Princeton, NJ: Princeton University Press, 1983), p. 131.
22. Coigney, *Margaret Sanger: Rebel With a Cause*, p. 67.
23. Sanger, *Margaret Sanger: An Autobiography*, p. 109.
24. Coigney, *Margaret Sanger: Rebel With a Cause*, p. 68.
25. Gray, *Margaret Sanger: A Biography of the Champion of Birth Control*, p. 44.
26. Coigney, *Margaret Sanger: Rebel With a Cause*, p. 98.
27. Gray, *Margaret Sanger: A Biography of the Champion of Birth Control*, p. 142.
28. Margaret H. Sanger, "The Case for Birth Control: A Supplementary Brief and Statement of Facts," May 1917, p. 8.
29. Sanger, *My Fight for Birth Control*, p. 80.
30. Ibid., p. 84.
31. Ibid., pp. 86–87.
32. Sanger, *Margaret Sanger: An Autobiography*, p. 121.
33. Sanger, *My Fight for Birth Control*, p. 125.
34. Margaret Sanger, *Woman and the New Race* (New York: Brentano's, 1920), p. 222.
35. Peter Fryer, *The Birth Controllers* (New York: Stein and Day, 1965), p. 213.
36. Coigney, *Margaret Sanger: Rebel With a Cause*, p. 93.
37. Topalian, *Margaret Sanger*, p. 68.

38. Sanger, *Margaret Sanger: An Autobiography*, p. 366.
39. Ibid., p. 367.
40. Ibid., p. 110.
41. Sanger, *My Fight for Birth Control*, p. 200.
42. Coigney, *Margaret Sanger: Rebel With a Cause*, p. 91.
43. Lawrence Lader and Milton Meltzer, *Margaret Sanger: Pioneer of Birth Control* (New York: Thomas Y. Crowell, 1969), p. 100.
44. Ibid., p. 104.
45. Sanger, *My Fight for Birth Control*, p. 331.
46. Coigney, *Margaret Sanger: Rebel With a Cause*, p. 132.
47. Ibid., p. 133.
48. Ibid., p. 132.
49. Ibid., p. 128.
50. Ibid., p. 129.
51. Ibid., p. 146.
52. Ibid., p. 175.
53. Ibid., pp. 175–176.
54. Gray, *Margaret Sanger: A Biography of the Champion of Birth Control*, p. 336.
55. Coigney, *Margaret Sanger: Rebel With a Cause*, p. 138.
56. Reed, *The Birth Control Movement in American Society: From Private Vice to Public Virtue*, p. 85.
57. Sanger, *Margaret Sanger: An Autobiography*, p. 141.
58. Coigney, *Margaret Sanger: Rebel With a Cause*, p. 156.
59. Gray, *Margaret Sanger: A Biography of the Champion of Birth Control*, p. 166.
60. Coigney, *Margaret Sanger: Rebel With a Cause*, p. 159.
61. Dash, *A Life of One's Own: Three Gifted Women and the Men They Married*, p. 69.
62. Alice Groff, "The Marriage Bed," *Woman Rebel*, July 1914, p. 39.
63. Kennedy, *Birth Control in America: The Career of Margaret Sanger*, p. 23.
64. Sanger, *Woman and the New Race*, p. 170.
65. Coigney, *Margaret Sanger: Rebel With a Cause*, p. 40.
66. Ibid., p. 143.
67. Kennedy, *Birth Control in America: The Career of Margaret Sanger*, p. 76.
68. Reed, *The Birth Control Movement in American Society: From Private Vice to Public Virtue*, p. 98.
69. Sanger, *My Fight for Birth Control*, p. 199.
70. Sanger, *The Pivot of Civilization*, p. 281.
71. Reed, *The Birth Control Movement in American Society: From Private Vice to Public Virtue*, p. 115.
72. Kennedy, *Birth Control in America: The Career of Margaret Sanger*, p. 104.
73. Ibid., p. 224.
74. Reed, *The Birth Control Movement in American Society: From Private Vice to Public Virtue*, p. 265.
75. Dash, *A Life of One's Own: Three Gifted Women and the Men They Married*, p. 106.
76. Reed, *The Birth Control Movement in American Society: From Private Vice to Public Virtue*, p. 265.
77. Kennedy, *Birth Control in America: The Career of Margaret Sanger*, p. 257.
78. Ibid., pp. 106–107.
79. Dash, *A Life of One's Own: Three Gifted Women and the Men They Married*, p. 110.
80. Ibid., p. 31.
81. Gray, *Margaret Sanger: A Biography of the Champion of Birth Control*, p. 326.
82. Kennedy, *Birth Control in America: The Career of Margaret Sanger*, pp. 19–20.
83. Ibid., p. 127.
84. Emily Taft Douglas, *Margaret Sanger: Pioneer of the Future* (Garrett Park, MD, Garrett Park Press, 1975), p. 146.

85. "Margaret Sanger and the Battle for Birth Control," *Washington Star*, interview with Madeline Gray, author of *Margaret Sanger: Biography of the Champion of Birth Control*, April 21, 1979.
86. Dash, *A Life of One's Own: Three Gifted Women and the Men They Married*, p. 79.
87. Ibid., p. 80.
88. Gray, *Margaret Sanger: A Biography of the Champion of Birth Control*, p. 250.
89. Coigney, *Margaret Sanger: Rebel With a Cause*, p. 83.
90. Gray, *Margaret Sanger: A Biography of the Champion of Birth Control*, p. 266.
91. Ibid., p. 306.
92. Aegyptus, "The Pauline Ideals vs. Woman," *Woman Rebel*, May 1914, vol. 1, no. 3, p. 20.
93. Ibid.
94. Ibid.
95. Theodore Schroeder, "Witchcraft and Obscenity," *Woman Rebel*, May 1914, vol. 1, no. 3, p. 21.
96. *Woman Rebel*, May 1914, vol. 1, no. 3.
97. "Intelligent or Unintelligent Birth Control?: An Editorial from American Medicine," *Birth Control Review*, May 1919, p. 12.
98. "Unity!," *Birth Control Review*, November 1921, vol. 5, no. 11, p. 3.
99. Sanger, *Woman and the New Race*, pp. 62–63.
100. Sanger, *Margaret Sanger: An Autobiography*, pp. 374–375.
101. Sanger, *Woman and the New Race*, p. 229.
102. Margaret Sanger, *The Pivot of Civilization* (New York: Brentano's, 1922), p. 189.
103. Mark H. Haller, *Eugenics: Hereditarian Attitudes in American Thought* (New York, Rutgers University Press, 1968), p. 92.
104. Sanger, *The Pivot of Civilization*, p. 187.
105. Ibid., p. 176.
106. Ibid., p. 108.
107. Ibid., pp. 116–117.
108. Margaret Sanger, speech before the Institute of Euthenics [sic] at Vassar College, August 5, 1926, as printed in "The Function of Sterilization," *Birth Control Review*, October 1926, p. 299.
109. Ibid.
110. Ibid.
111. Sanger, *The Pivot of Civilization*, p. 91.
112. Ibid., p. 263.
113. Ibid., pp. 263–264.
114. Ibid., p. 264.
115. Ibid., pp. 264–265.
116. Ibid., pp. 101–102
117. Havelock Ellis, *The Problem of Race Regeneration* (New York: Moffet, Yard & Co., 1925), p. 65, as cited in Elasah Drogin, T.O.P., *Margaret Sanger: Father of Modern Society* (New Hope, KY: CUL Publications, 1986), p. 18.
118. Arthur Calder-Marshall, *The Sage of Sex: A Life of Havelock Ellis* (New York: G.P. Putnam's Sons, 1959), p. 272.
119. Leon F. Whitney, "Religion and the Birth Rate," *Birth Control Review*, April 1932, p. 103.
120. Ibid., p. 104.
121. Margaret Sanger, "Birth Control and Racial Betterment," *Birth Control Review*, February 1919, p. 11.
122. Ibid.
123. Ibid.
124. Margaret Sanger, "The Eugenic Value of Birth Control Propaganda," *Birth Control Review*, October 1921, p. 5.
125. Ibid.
126. Ibid.

127. Ibid.
128. Ibid.
129. Havelock Ellis, "Birth Control in Relation to Morality and Eugenics," *Birth Control Review*, February 1919, p. 7.
130. Marc Hillel and Clarissa Henry, *Of Pure Blood* (New York: McGraw-Hill, 1951), p. 148.
131. Ibid.
132. Comment made by John Lofton at the 1987 Arizona Right to Life Conference, October 1987.
133. Robert C. Cook, "Birth Rates in Fascist Countries," *Birth Control Review*, November 1939, p. 8.
134. Sanger, "The Case for Birth Control: A Supplementary Brief and Statement of Facts," May 1917, p. 8.
135. "Abortion in the United States," *Woman Rebel*, May 1914, vol. 1, no. 2, p. 24.
136. Sanger, *Margaret Sanger: An Autobiography*, p. 217.
137. Angus McLaren, *A History of Contraception: From Antiquity to the Present Day* (Cambridge, MA: Basil Blackwell Ltd., 1990), p. 230.
138. Sanger, "The Case for Birth Control: A Supplementary Brief and Statement of Facts," May 1917, p. 8.
139. Margaret Sanger, "A License for Mothers to Have Babies: A 'Code to Stop the Overproduction of Children'—Based on Common Sense Instead of Sentiment," American Weekly, 1934, as quoted in Drogin, *Margaret Sanger: Father of Modern Society*, pp. 70–71.
140. Linda Gordon, *Woman's Body, Woman's Right: A Social History of Birth Control in America* (New York: Grossman, 1976), p. 332.
141. Letter from Margaret Sanger to Dr. Clarence J. Gamble, December 10, 1939, as cited in "'Negro Project' Letters and Memorandums," African-Americans Agaisnt Black Genocide, undated.
142. Gordon, *Woman's Body, Woman's Right: A Social History of Birth Control in America*, p. 333.
143. Letter from Margaret Sanger to Florence Rose, March 8, 1941, as cited in "'Negro Project' Letters and Memorandums," African-Americans Against Black Genocide, undated.
144. Gordon, *Woman's Body, Woman's Right: A Social History of Birth Control in America*, p. 353.
145. Sanger, *Woman and the New Race*, p. 44
146. Ibid., pp. 44–45.
147. Coigney, *Margaret Sanger: Rebel With a Cause*, p. 173.
148. Ibid., pp. 171 and 173.
149. Ibid., p. 172.
150. Ibid., p. 174.
151. Ibid.
152. Ibid., p. 177.
153. Gordon, *Woman's Body, Woman's Right: A Social History of Birth Control in America*, p. 290.
154. Drogin, *Margaret Sanger: Father of Modern Society*, p. 28.
155. Margaret Sanger, "Address of Welcome to the Sixth International Neo-Malthusian & Birth Control Conference," *Birth Control Review*, April 1925, vol. 9, no. 4, p. 100.
156. Drogin, *Margaret Sanger: Father of Modern Society*, p. 28.
157. Kennedy, *Birth Control in America: The Career of Margaret Sanger*, p. 12.
158. Margaret Sanger, "Intelligence Tests for Legislators," *Birth Control Review*, May 1923, vol. 7, no. 5, p. 107.
159. Ibid.
160. *Washington Star*.
161. Ibid.
162. Nadine Brozan, "Another Sanger Leads Planned Parenthood," *New York Times*, January 1991.

163. "Mrs. Sanger Named 'Humanist of the Year,'" *Planned Parenthood News*, Planned Parenthood Federation of America, Winter 1958, no. 20, p. 6.
164. Gray, *Margaret Sanger: A Biography of the Champion of Birth Control*, p. 443.
165. "Around the Nation: Arizona," *USA Today*, September 13, 1991.
166. Brozan, *New York Times*.
167. Ibid.
168. Ibid.
169. Kennedy, *Birth Control in America: The Career of Margaret Sanger*, p. 277.
170. William Vogt, "A New Journal," *Planned Parenthood News*, Planned Parenthood Federation of America, Spring 1954, no. 7, p. 4.
171. "Special Offer: An Autographed Copy of The Margaret Sanger Story . . . ," *Planned Parenthood News*, Planned Parenthood Federation of America, Winter 1955, no. 10, p. 2.
172. "Planned Parenthood in the 60s: The Pill and the Population Crisis," *Planned Parenthood Press*, Planned Parenthood of Central and Northern Arizona, Summer 1987.
173. "Planned Parenthood in the 80s: Fulfilling the Dream," *Planned Parenthood Press*, Planned Parenthood of Central and Northern Arizona, Winter 1987.
174. Coigney, *Margaret Sanger: Rebel With a Cause*, p. 11.
175. Ibid., p. 12.
176. Ibid., pp. 12–13.
177. Enny Cramer Seabrook and Jack Hillary Smith, "Sexual Counseling With Adult Retarded: An Integral Part of a Planned Parenthood Clinic Services," *Papers 1975*, Planned Parenthood Federation of America, p. 93.
178. Ibid., p. 85.
179. Katharine Hepburn, fund-raising letter, Planned Parenthood, undated, pp. 1 and 4.
180. Faye Wattleton, fund-raising letter, Planned Parenthood-World Population, undated (circa January 1979), p. 2.
181. Ibid., p. 5.
182. Faye Wattleton, annual luncheon of Planned Parenthood Federation of America affiliate, St. Louis Missouri, February 5, 1979.
183. "Home Show," October 16, 1991.
184. "Robertson Attacks Planned Parenthood," *Washington Times*, February 3, 1988, p. A6.
185. Ibid.
186. Comment made by Pat Robertson, "The 700 Club," 1991.
187. *Washington Times*.
188. Ibid.
189. "Robertson vs. PPF [Planned Parenthood Federation]," *Washington Times*, February 8, 1988.
190. "A Close Look at Planned Parenthood," "Focus on the Family" radio program, October 26–27, 1989.

Chapter 2: A New Direction

1. Marianne Szegedy-Maszak, "Calm, Cool and Beleaguered," *New York Times Magazine*, August 6, 1989, p. 62.
2. Dana Micucci, "Faye Wattleton Calls Career Move a Plan for Action," *Chicago Tribune*, February 2, 1992, section 6, p. 9.
3. "A Family Story," "PrimeTime Live," Fall 1991.
4. Patricia Adams, "Faye Wattleton Resigns as President of PPFA," *INsider*, January 15, 1992, p. 1.
5. Patricia McCormack, "Her Weeping Anger Thrust Faye Wattleton To Action," *San Jose Mercury News*, February 15, 1978.
6. Christopher John Farley, "Wattleton: Time for TV: Moving on from Planned Parenthood," *USA Today*, February 24, 1992, p. 2D.
7. Elizabeth Kolbert, "Faye Unfazed," *Vogue*, January 1992, p. 142.

8. Ibid, p. 143.
9. Patricia McCormack, "New Planned Parenthood Head Opens Drive for Teen Abortions," *Kent-Ravenna Record-Courier*, February 3, 1978, p. 3.
10. Kolbert, *Vogue*, p. 143.
11. Felicity Barringer, "Planned Parenthood: Quiet Cause to Focus of Fury," *New York Times*, October 30, 1990, p. A16.
12. "A Little Publicity Can't Hurt," *Business Week*, March 26, 1990.
13. Barringer, *New York Times*.
14. Szegedy-Maszak, *New York Times Magazine*, p. 18.
15. Kolbert, *Vogue*, p. 143.
16. Szegedy-Maszak, *New York Times Magazine*, p. 62.
17. Kolbert, *Vogue*, p. 143.
18. Szegedy-Maszak, *New York Times Magazine*, p. 62.
19. Ibid.
20. *Business Week*, p. 69.
21. 1990 Annual Report, Planned Parenthood Federation of America, 1991, p. 36.
22. Ibid., pp. 2 and 35.
23. Kolbert, *Vogue*, pp. 142 and 143.
24. Ibid, p. 143.
25. Ibid.
26. Ibid.
27. Ibid., p. 196.
28. Speech by Faye Wattleton, *The Humanist*, July/August 1986, p. 5.
29. Ibid.
30. Barringer, *New York Times*.
31. "Compensation for Top Executives at Selected Non-Profits," *Chronicle of Philanthropy*, May 24, 1992, vol. 4, no. 11, p. 30.
32. McCormack, *Kent-Ravenna Record-Courier*.
33. Szegedy-Maszak, *New York Times Magazine*, p. 65.
34. Farley, *USA Today*, p. 2D.
35. Adams, *INsider*.
36. Farley, *USA Today*, p. 2D.
37. Ibid.
38. Ibid.
39. Lois Romano, "Faye: The Leader Women Are Waiting For?," *Glamour*, February 1990, p. 195.
40. Edgar Williams, "She Speaks for Planned Parenthood," *Philadelphia Inquirer*, May 17, 1984, p. 10-B.
41. Sylvia Chase, "PrimeTime Live," specific air date unknown (August or September 1991).
42. Richard Stengel, "Tough Choice," *Detroit News*, January 2, 1990.
43. Kolbert, *Vogue*, p. 142.
44. Szegedy-Maszak, *New York Times Magazine*, p. 62.
45. Romano, *Glamour*, p. 226.
46. Ibid., p. 225.
47. Laurie Belin, "The Real Issue: Choice," *Washington Post*, November 25, 1989.
48. Bud Norman and Judy Lundstrom Thomas, "Abortion Debaters Clash Over Racial Issue: Operation Rescue Chief Says Planned Parenthood Head 'Betrays' Blacks," *Buffalo News*, September 8, 1991.
49. Kolbert, *Vogue*, p. 142
50. "The Abortion Dilemma: Rights and Lives," NBC News Special Report, May 15, 1989.
51. Ibid.
52. Ibid.
53. Norman and Thomas, *Buffalo News*.

54. Linda Layton, "Beware Using Death as a Social Cure," *Rockford Register Star*, June 6, 1991.
55. Faye Wattleton, "Planned Parenthood's Leader Blasts Untruths," guest columnist, *Rockford Register Star*, August 10, 1991.
56. Ibid.
57. "U.S. Population Growth and Family Planning: A Review of the Literature," *Family Planning Perspectives*, October 1970, p. ix.
58. Layton, *Rockford Register Star*.
59. Wattleton, *Rockford Register Star*.
60. "Strategic Plan 1989–1993: Baseline Data," Planned Parenthood Federation of America.
61. "A Five Year Plan: 1976–1980," Planned Parenthood Federation of America, 1975, p. 8.
62. Layton, *Rockford Register Star*.
63. Wattleton, *Rockford Register Star*.
64. Layton, *Rockford Register Star*.
65. Wattleton, *Rockford Register Star*.
66. Ibid.
67. "The Joan Rivers Show," broadcast in 1991.
68. Norman and Thomas, *Buffalo News*.
69. Spokesman for the National Right to Life Committee, in a telephone interview, August 1989.
70. Gary J. Gillespie, Assistant Professor, Department of Speech Communication, Northwest College, in a telephone interview, August 1989.
71. Ibid.
72. Ibid.
73. Judd Rose, correspondent, "Behind the Scenes," "PrimeTime Live," 1989.
74. Marcia Ann Gillespie, "Repro Woman," interview with Faye Wattleton, *Ms.*, October 1989, p. 51.
75. Ibid.
76. Marcia Ann Gillespie, *Ms.*, p. 50.
77. David Kupelian and Jo Ann Gasper, "Abortion, Inc.," *New Dimensions: The Psychology Behind the News*, September/October 1991, p. 13.

Chapter 3: Targeting Youth

1. "A Five Year Plan: 1976–1980," Planned Parenthood Federation of America, 1975, p. 8.
2. Jo Ann Gasper, "Planned Parenthood and Sex Education, Part I: Raping Our Children's Minds," *Concerned Women*, May 1989.
3. "WAITT Celebrates 10th Anniversary," *PPMW* [Planned Parenthood of Metropolitan Washington, D.C.] *News*, Fall 1988.
4. "The 700 Club," CBN, recorded April 9, 1991.
5. "President Awards National Honor to Nashville's PG 13 Teen Troupe," *Tennessean*, April 11, 1989.
6. Letter from Richard C. Mock, deputy executive director for communications, National Volunteer Center, to a man opposed to the programs of the PG 13 Players, September 18, 1991.
7. Proclamation adopted by the House of Representatives of the State of Tennessee, December 16, 1988.
8. Ibid.
9. "Organizing a Campus-for-Choice Group: First Steps," Campus-for-Choice organizing materials, Planned Parenthood, undated (1990).
10. Ibid.
11. "Campus-for-Choice: Contents," Campus-for-Choice organizing materials, Planned Parenthood, undated (1990).
12. Conor Gallagher, telephone interview, March 24, 1992.
13. Ibid.

14. Ibid.
15. *Teen Sex? It's Okay to Say: No Way!*, Planned Parenthood Federation of America, September 1987, p. 2.
16. Ibid.
17. "American Teens Speak: Sex, Myths, TV, and Birth Control—The Planned Parenthood Poll," (Louis Harris and Associates), 1985/1986. Analysis by Michael Schwartz, "Planned Parenthood Sells Lifestyle, Not Enlightenment," *Our Sunday Visitor*, March 1, 1987.
18. "Love and Sex in the '90s: Our National Survey," nationally representative survey, *Seventeen*, November 1991, p. 64.
19. Robert Bahr, "How to Make Love to a Virgin," MGF [Men's Guide to Fashion], March 1986, p. 68.
20. Sadja Goldsmith, M.D., M.P.H., "San Francisco's Teen Clinic: Meeting the Sex Education and Birth Control Needs of the Sexually Active Schoolgirl," *Family Planning Perspectives*, October 1969, vol. 1, no. 2.
21. Joyce Price, "Safe Sex for Teens Hinges on Peers' Lead," *Washington Times*, April 16, 1990.
22. *Teen Sex? It's Okay to Say: No Way!*, p. 2.
23. *What Teens Want to Know but Don't Know How to Ask*, Planned Parenthood Federation of America, 1987, p. 5.
24. *Seventeen*, p. 64.
25. *Teen Sex? It's Okay to Say: No Way!*, p. 4.
26. Ibid., p. 5.
27. *Making Responsible Decisions About SEX*, Planned Parenthood of Lincoln (Nebraska), undated.
28. Ibid.
29. Freya L. Sonenstein, Joseph H. Pleck and Leighton C. Ku, "Levels of Sexual Activity Among Adolescent Males in the United States," *Family Planning Perspectives*, July/August 1991, vol. 23, no. 4, p. 166.
30. Gail Ireland, "Change in Sexual Attitudes Seen as Key to Fewer Teen Pregnancies," *Cedar Rapids Gazette*, May 18, 1991, p. 2B.
31. *Seventeen*, p. 14.
32. *Choices . . .* , Rocky Mountain Planned Parenthood, 1977.
33. *Ten Heavy Facts About Sex . . .* , The Institute for Family Research and Education, September 1975. (Not published by Planned Parenthood but used by Planned Parenthood.)
34. Ibid.
35. *The Great Orgasm Robbery*, Rocky Mountain Planned Parenthood, 1981.
36. *You've Changed the Combination!!!*, Rocky Mountain Planned Parenthood, 1977.
37. *Planned Parenthood: A Strong Voice for the Most Personal of Human Rights*, Planned Parenthood, undated.
38. *Sex Facts*, Planned Parenthood Center of Syracuse (New York), 1977, p. 4.
39. Ibid., p. 22.
40. Ibid., p. 24.
41. Ibid., pp. 24–25.
42. Ibid., p. 30.
43. Ibid., pp. 30–31.
44. "Abortion, Inc.," *New Dimensions: The Psychology Behind the News*, September/October 1991, p. 18.
45. Ibid.
46. *Sex Facts*, p. 41.
47. Ibid., p. 42.
48. "Books to Aid Parents in Their Task as Sex Educators," Planned Parenthood Association of San Diego County, undated.
49. Ruth Bell, *Changing Bodies, Changing Lives: A New Book for Teens on Sex Relationships*, revised and updated (New York: Vintage Books [division of Random House], 1988), p. 86.

50. Ibid.
51. Ibid., p. 81.
52. Ibid., p. 79.
53. Ibid.
54. Ibid., p. 80.
55. Ibid., pp. 81–82.
56. Ibid., p. 83.
57. Ibid.
58. Ibid., p. 109.
59. Ibid., p. 133.
60. The Boston Women's Health Book Collective, *Our Bodies, Ourselves: A Book By and For Women* (New York: Simon and Schuster, 1976), p. 42.
61. Ibid.
62. Ibid., p. 53.
63. Ibid., p. 165.
64. Ibid., p. 167.
65. The Boston Women's Health Book Collective, *The New Our Bodies, Ourselves: A Book By and For Women* (New York: Simon and Schuster, 1984), p. 121.
66. Ibid., p. 122.
67. Ibid.
68. Ibid., p. 141.
69. *Resource Guide: Audio-Visual, Print and Educational Information*, Planned Parenthood of Buffalo and Erie County (New York), undated (circa 1991), p. 7.
70. Ibid., pp. 14–15.
71. *Resource Catalog*, Planned Parenthood of Central and Northern Arizona, 1985.
72. List of recommended films, Planned Parenthood of Seattle-King County (Washington), 1977.
73. "Start Smart," audiotape transcript, Berlex Canada Inc. and Planned Parenthood of Manitoba, undated, p. 1.
74. Ibid., p. 2.
75. Ibid.
76. Ibid.
77. Ibid., p. 3.
78. Ibid., p. 4.
79. Ibid., p. 5.
80. Ibid., p. 8.
81. Ibid., p. 9.
82. Patrick Tivy, "False Ideas About Sex Common Among Young," *Calgary Herald*, January 24, 1991.
83. Ibid.
84. Ibid.
85. *A Man's Guide to Sexuality*, Planned Parenthood Federation of America, 1980, rev. February 1989, p. 2.
86. Ibid., p. 6.
87. Ibid., pp. 3–4.
88. Ibid., pp. 10 and 12.
89. Ibid., pp. 10 and 13.
90. "Then I Got That Awful Phone Call," full-page copyrighted advertisement, Planned Parenthood Federation of America, undated (circa 1986).
91. Darryl Hale and Mary-Jane R. Snyder, "Male Motivation/Education: A Pilot Program Designed to Disseminate Family Planning Information Exclusively to Males," *Papers 1975*, 1975, p. 82.
92. Alice Yarish, "Condom Contest Causes Embarrassing Ruckus," *San Francisco Examiner*, February 5, 1978.

93. Ibid.
94. Barbara Hoover, "Study: For Poor Teens, Pregnancy Isn't a Disaster," *Lansing State Journal*, June 25, 1990.
95. Ibid.
96. Ibid.
97. Ibid.
98. Barbara Kantrowitz, "Breaking the Poverty Cycle," *Newsweek*, May 28, 1990, p. 78.

Chapter 4: Conflicting Philosophies

1. "Abortion: An Issue Forum," discussion following the airing of *Abortion: For Survival*, WTBS (Atlanta), July 20, 1989, and rebroadcast on July 22 and July 23, 1989.
2. Susan Newcomer, director of education, Planned Parenthood Federation of America, "Is It O.K. for PPFA to Say 'No Way'?," Planned Parenthood Federation of America, undated (1986 or 1987), p. 2.
3. Ibid., pp. 2–3.
4. Ibid., p. 3.
5. Ibid., pp. 3–4.
6. Ibid., p. 4.
7. Ibid.
8. Radio debate between Susan Newcomer, director of education, Planned Parenthood Federation of America, and Doug Scott, executive director, Arizona Right to Life, Champaign, Illinois (University of Illinois), February 5, 1988.
9. Ibid.
10. Newcomer, "Is It O.K. for PPFA to Say 'No Way'?," p. 2.
11. *Sex Facts*, Planned Parenthood Center of Syracuse (New York), 1977.
12. Susan N. Wilson and Catherine A. Sanderson, "The Sex Respect Curriculum: Is 'Just Say No' Effective?," *SIECUS Report*, September/October 1988, p. 10.
13. Ibid.
14. Ibid.
15. Ibid.
16. "Abortion, Inc.," *New Dimensions: The Psychology Behind the News*, September/October 1991, p. 18.
17. Wilson and Sanderson, *SIECUS Report*, p. 11.
18. Ibid.
19. Thomas L. Jipping, J. D., personal interview, April 22, 1992.
20. "Beware!!! 'Sex Respect' May Be Coming to Your Child's School," *Springfield Memo*, Illinois Planned Parenthood Council, 1988.
21. Memo from Susan Newcomer, director of education, Planned Parenthood Federation of America, to "Interested Individuals," August 20, 1987, p. 1.
22. Ibid., p. 2.
23. Beverly Beyette, "Teen Sex Education Campaign Launched: Planned Parenthood Targets Youth, Parents and Three Networks' Contraceptive-Ad Ban," *Los Angeles Times*, October 17, 1986.
24. Ibid.
25. "The New Cold War," *New Dimensions: The Psychology Behind the News*, June 1990, p. 34.
26. Faye Wattleton, "From the President," 1985 Annual Report, Planned Parenthood Federation of America, 1986, p. 5.
27. Gloria Feldt, "A Positive Force to Prevent Teen Pregnancy," *Planned Parenthood Press*, Planned Parenthood of Central and Northern Arizona, Summer 1987, p. 2.
28. Julie Housewright, clinic manager, Planned Parenthood of Southeast Iowa, "Care, Not Judgments Offered at Clinics," letters to the editor, *The Hawk Eye*, December 18, 1991.
29. Ibid.
30. Joyce Price, "Safe Sex for Teens Hinges on Peers' Lead," *Washington Times*, April 16, 1990.

31. Mercedes Arzu Wilson, "The Risky Business of Adolescence: How to Help Teens Stay Safe," Family of the Americas Foundation, testimony before the Select Committee on Children, Youth and Families, July 18, 1991, p. 3.
32. Ibid., p. 4.
33. Ibid., pp. 4–5.
34. Faye Wattleton, fund-raising letter, Planned Parenthood-World Population, undated (circa January 1979).
35. Warren M. Hern, M.D., "Is Pregnancy Really Normal?," *Family Planning Perspectives*, Alan Guttmacher Institute, January 1971, vol. 3, no. 1.
36. Willard Cates, Jr., M.D., M.P.H., David A. Grimes, M.D., and Jack C. Smith, M.S., "Abortion as a Treatment for Unwanted Pregnancy: The Number Two Sexually Transmitted 'Disease,'" U.S. Department of Health, Education, and Welfare, Public Health Service, Centers for Disease Control, Bureau of Epidemiology, Family Planning Evaluation Division, presented at the 14th annual scientific meeting of the Association of Planned Parenthood Physicians, Miami Beach, Florida, November 11, 1976, pp. 1–2.
37. Ibid., p. 4.
38. Ibid., pp. 6–7.
39. Ibid., pp. 7–8.
40. Ibid., p. 8.
41. Mary S. Calderone, M.D., *Medical Morals*, February-March 1968, as cited in "The Two Faces of Planned Parenthood," by Robert G. Marshall, 1984.
42. Rebecca Schmidt, "Sex Education Urged to Combat Pregnancies," *Colorado Springs Gazette Telegraph*, July 20, 1978.
43. *Facts About Birth Control*, Planned Parenthood Federation of America, July 1990, p. 1.
44. Ibid, p. 2.
45. Ibid, pp. 6, 11 and 17.
46. Ibid., pp. 17, 24, 20, 30 and 14.
47. Ibid, p. 22.
48. "The Cosmo Guide to Healthy Sex and Family Planning," p. 2.
49. Stephen Whitty, "AIDS: Facts and Fallacies," MGF *(Men's Guide to Fashion)*, date unknown (circa 1990), p. 32.
50. Louise B. Tyrer, M.D., then-vice president, medical division, Planned Parenthood Federation of America, letter to the editor, *Wall Street Journal*, April 26, 1991.
51. Barbara Kantrowitz, "The Dangers of Doing It," *Newsweek*, special edition, Summer/Fall 1990, p. 56.
52. "It Happened to Me: I Had an Abortion," *Sassy*, January 1992, p. 74.
53. Linda Gase, "Pregnant Teens," *'Teen*, December 1991, p. 22.
54. *Newsweek*, special edition, p. 57.
55. "Planned Parenthood Presents 'The Cosmo Guide to Healthy Sex and Family Planning,' (Special Advertising Section)," Association of Reproductive Health Professionals advertisement, 1988, p. 11.
56. "On the Cover," *Self*, April 1992, p. 10.
57. Phillips Cutright, Ph.D., "Illegitimacy: Myths, Causes and Cures," *Family Planning Perspectives*, January 1991, vol. 3, no. 1, p. 39.
58. *The American Heritage Dictionary of the English Language*, New College Edition, 1976.
59. Ibid.
60. Michael Schwartz, *Arizona Right to Life News*, October/November/December 1987.
61. Ibid.
62. Ibid.
63. Ibid.
64. Michael Schwartz, in a speech at the Christian Action Council Activist Summit, August 1991.
65. Ibid.
66. Ibid.

67. Ibid.
68. Ibid.
69. Ibid.
70. Announcement for the "Family Life Education: Are We Prepared?," conference, May 12, 1989, sponsored by Planned Parenthood of Northern New England and the Vermont Department of Education (includes accompanying material by the PPFA), 1989.
71. Ibid.
72. Ibid.
73. Ibid.
74. Ibid.
75. Ibid.
76. "Countering Homophobia," program literature, undated (event held on March 8, 1991).
77. Ibid.
78. Ibid.
79. Ibid.
80. Betsy Crane, "Let's Get Heterosexism Out of Sexuality Education," *Resources, Research and Reviews*, Planned Parenthood of Thompkins County, September 1988, vol. 5, no. 4, p. 1.
81. *Resources, Research and Reviews*, Planned Parenthood of Thompkins County, September 1988, vol. 5, no. 4, p. 1.
82. "Out of the Closet and Into the Classroom," *Resources, Research and Reviews*, Planned Parenthood of Thompkins County, September 1988, vol. 5, no. 4, p. 2.
83. Notes of two participants (identity withheld) in "Countering Homophobia" program, March 8, 1991.
84. Ibid.
85. Ibid.
86. Ibid.
87. Ibid.
88. Ibid.
89. Ibid.
90. Ibid.
91. Ibid.
92. Ibid.
93. Ibid.
94. Diane Ravitch, "They're Not Learning How to Teach," "Bookshelf," *Wall Street Journal*, a book review of *Ed School Follies: The Miseducation of America's Teachers*, by Rita Kramer (The Free Press, 1991), October 28, 1991.
95. Ibid.
96. Jo Ann Gasper, "Planned Parenthood and Sex Education, Part I: Raping Our Children's Minds," *Concerned Women*, May 1989, p. 5.
97. Ibid.
98. Ibid.
99. Ibid, p. 21.
100. Debra W. Haffner, "Safe Sex and Teens," *SIECUS Report*, September/October 1988, p. 9.
101. Ibid.
102. Kate Fillion, "Sex in the Schools," *Canadian Living*, September 1991, p. 149.
103. Ibid., pp. 149–150.
104. Ibid., p. 150.
105. Ibid.
106. Ibid.
107. Ibid., p. 151.
108. Ibid.
109. Ibid.
110. *Human Sexuality: What Children Should Know and When They Should Know It*, Planned Parenthood Federation of America, 1987.

111. Ibid.
112. Ibid.
113. Ibid.
114. Ibid.
115. Ibid.
116. Ibid.
117. Ibid.
118. Ibid.
119. Letter addressed to "School Board Chairperson," from Jeff Gill, president, and Ray Tomalty, vice president, Planned Parenthood Ontario, October 21, 1991.
120. Ibid.
121. "The Effectiveness of Current Sexuality Education in the Ontario School System," Planned Parenthood Ontario, February 1991, p. 1.
122. Ibid., pp. 1–2.
123. Ibid., pp. 3–5.
124. Kathleen Parker, "Cure For What Ails Us: A Little Prudery and a Lot of Prudence," *Buffalo News*, December 31, 1991, p. C1.
125. Ibid.
126. Ibid.
127. Ibid.
128. Earvin "Magic" Johnson, "PrimeTime Live," March 26, 1992, from a program first aired on Nickelodeon.
129. "Review and Outlook: The Joy of What?," editorial, *Wall Street Journal*, December 12, 1991.
130. Ibid.
131. Ibid.
132. Ibid.
133. Ibid.
134. Janice Castro, "Watching a Generation Waste Away," interview with Sylvia Ann Hewlett, *Time*, August 26, 1991, p. 10.
135. Ibid.
136. Ibid., pp. 10 and 12
137. Ibid., p. 12

Chapter 5: "Stupid" Parents

1. "Meet: Faye Wattleton: Cool Woman, Hot Topic," *NEA Today*, March 1991, p. 9.
2. *The Perils of Puberty*, Rocky Mountain Planned Parenthood, 1974, pp. 8–9.
3. Ibid., p. 9.
4. Ruth Bell, *Changing Bodies, Changing Lives: A New Book for Teens on Sex Relationships*, revised and updated (New York: Vintage Books, 1988), p. 90.
5. *Ten Heavy Facts About Sex . . .* , The Institute for Family Research and Education, 1975. (Not published by Planned Parenthood but used by Planned Parenthood.)
6. "Since Your Parents Are Afraid to Talk to You and Your School's Hands Are Probably Tied, Here's Some Hard Facts," advertisement, Planned Parenthood, *Dallas Observer*, January 30, 1986.
7. Ibid.
8. *Be an Askable Parent: The Family Survival Kit*, Planned Parenthood for Central and Northern Arizona (PPCNA), undated (circa 1987), p. 1.
9. Ibid.
10. Ibid.
11. Ibid, p. 3.
12. *How to Talk to Your Teenagers About the Facts of Life*, Planned Parenthood Federation of America, July 1986, p. 4.

13. *Be An Askable Parent: The Family Survival Kit*, p. 3.
14. Ibid., p. 7.
15. Ibid., p. 12.
16. Ibid., p. 14.
17. *How to Talk With Your Teenager About the Facts of Life*, Planned Parenthood Federation of America, November 1988 (revised edition), p. 4.
18. *How to Talk to Your Teenagers About the Facts of* Life.
19. *What Teens Want to Know But Don't Know How to Ask*, p. 16.
20. *How to Talk With Your Teenager About the Facts of Life*, pp. 5 and 14.
21. *How to Talk to Your Teenagers About the Facts of Life.*
22. *How to Talk With Your Teenager About the Facts of Life*, p. 16.
23. *What Teens Want to Know But Don't Know How to Ask*, Planned Parenthood Federation of America, March 1987, p. 15.
24. Ibid, p. 16.
25. *How to Talk to Your Teenagers About the Facts of Life.*
26. *How to Talk With Your Teenager About the Facts of Life*, p. 20.
27. Ibid., p. 31.
28. Ibid., p. 28.
29. *What Teens Want to Know But Don't Know How to Ask*, p. 23.
30. *How to Talk to Your Teenagers About the Facts of Life.*
31. "Books to Aid Parents in Their Task as Sex Educators," Planned Parenthood Association of San Diego County, undated.
32. Wardell B. Pomeroy, Ph.D., *Boys and Sex: A Long-Needed Modern Sexual Guide for Boys* (Delacorte Press New York: Delacorte Press, 1968), p. 107.
33. Ibid., pp. 107–108.
34. Ibid., back cover.
35. Wardell B. Pomeroy, *Girls and Sex* (New York: Delacorte Press, 1981), pp. 95–96.
36. Ibid., p. 96.
37. Ibid., p. 88.
38. "Books to Aid Parents in Their Task as Sex Educators."
39. Rebecca Schmidt, "Sex Education Urged to Combat Pregnancies," *Colorado Springs Gazette Telegraph*, July 20, 1978.
40. Ibid.
41. Faye Wattleton, *How to Talk With Your Child About Sexuality: A Parent's Guide* (Garden City, NY: Doubleday and Company, 1986), pp. 120–121.
42. Cindy Brown, education director, Planned Parenthood of Southeast Iowa, "Sex Educators Must Think Long Term," letter to the editor, *The Hawk Eye*, January 8, 1992.
43. Ibid.
44. *How to Talk With Your Teenager About the Facts of Life*, p. 2.
45. *NEA Today*, p. 9.
46. *What Teens Want to Know But Don't Know How to Ask.*
47. 1989 Service Report, Planned Parenthood Federation of America, 1989, p. 17.
48. Ibid.
49. Jacqueline Kasun, "Sex Education: A New Philosophy for America?," *The Family in America*, July 1989, p. 3.
50. *Resource Guide: Audio-Visual, Print and Educational Information*, Planned Parenthood of Buffalo and Erie County (New York), undated (circa 1991).
51. Barbara Kantrowitz, "The Push for Sex Education," *Newsweek*, special edition, Summer/Fall 1990, p. 52.
52. Kasun, *The Family in America.*
53. "A Close Look at Planned Parenthood," "Focus on the Family" radio program, October 26–27, 1989.
54. Ibid.
55. Ibid.

56. Ibid.
57. Ibid.
58. Ibid.
59. Ibid.
60. Ibid.
61. Ibid.

Chapter 6: Public Relations and the Media

1. Elyse Topalian, *Margaret Sanger* (New York: Franklin Watts, 1984), p. 65.
2. "A Five Year Plan: 1976–1980," Planned Parenthood Federation of America, 1975, p. 10
3. "Arden Conference Pinpoints Social Research Needs," *Planned Parenthood News*, Spring 1954, no. 7, p. 3.
4. *Family Planning Perspectives*, October 1971, vol. 3, no. 4, pp. 65–67.
5. "An Unexpected Child Can Really Rock the Cradle," advertisement, Planned Parenthood Federation of America, *Family Planning Perspectives*, October 1971, vol. 3, no. 4, p. 65.
6. "How Many Children Should a Couple Have?," advertisement, Planned Parenthood Federation of America, *Family Planning Perspectives*, October 1971, vol. 3, no. 4, p. 66.
7. "Get to Know the Two of You Before You Become the Three of You," advertisement, Planned Parenthood Federation of America, *Family Planning Perspectives*, October 1971, vol. 3, no. 4, p. 67.
8. Mary Beth Murphy, "$1 Million Drive Backs Abortion," *Milwaukee Sentinel*, June 6, 1979.
9. "Planned Parenthood Shifting to a Patriotic Theme," *New York Times*, October 5, 1980, p. 25.
10. Ibid.
11. "The Strength of America is its People and Their Right to Choose," full-page copyrighted advertisement, Planned Parenthood Federation of America, *Washington Post*, January 20, 1981.
12. Frederick C. Smith, board member, Planned Parenthood Federation of America, in a letter addressed to members of Congress and state legislators, Planned Parenthood Federation of America, January 26, 1981.
13. "We Believe in Planned Parenthood Because We Love Children," full-page signature advertisement, Planned Parenthood of Central and Northern Arizona, *Phoenix Gazette*, November 13, 1987.
14. Ibid.
15. Katharine Hepburn, fund-raising letter, Planned Parenthood, undated.
16. "Teen Pregnancy Television Campaign: Father," Planned Parenthood Federation of America, produced by the Public Media Center, undated (circa 1990).
17. "Teen Pregnancy Television Campaign: Mother," Planned Parenthood Federation of America, produced by the Public Media Center, undated (circa 1990).
18. "Teen Pregnancy Television Campaign: Brother," Planned Parenthood Federation of America, produced by the Public Media Center, undated (circa 1990).
19. "Teen Pregnancy Television Campaign: Should Have Said #1," Planned Parenthood Federation of America, produced by the Public Media Center, undated (circa 1990).
20. "Teen Pregnancy Television Campaign: Son," Planned Parenthood Federation of America, produced by the Public Media Center, undated (circa 1990).
21. "What Every Teenager's Parents Need to Know. A Candid Talk With a Planned Parenthood Counselor," full-page copyrighted advertisement, Planned Parenthood Federation of America, *New York Times*, March 19, 1991, p. A20.
22. "When JR Took Mandy for a Little Roll in the Hay, Which One Had the Condom?," print copyrighted advertisement, Planned Parenthood Federation of America, *USA Today*, December 3, 1986.
23. "They Did It 20,000 Times on Television Last Year," print copyrighted advertisement, Planned Parenthood Federation of America, *USA Today*, December 8, 1986.

24. "Sex, TV and Your Kids—PPMW [Planned Parenthood of Metropolitan Washington, D.C.] Symposium," *Action*, Planned Parenthood of Metropolitan Washington, D.C., September 1986, vol. 1, no. 79, p. 3.
25. Faye Wattleton, fund-raising letter, Planned Parenthood Federation of America, undated (circa 1986), p. 1.
26. Ibid., p. 2.
27. Ibid.
28. Ibid., pp. 4–5.
29. "They Did It 20,000 Times on Television Last Year. How Come Nobody Got Pregnant?," print advertising copy sent with fund-raising materials, Planned Parenthood Federation of America, 1986.
30. Ibid.
31. "Donahue," specific air date unknown (1991).
32. "Doogie Hauser, M.D.," broadcast on CBS, September 25, 1991.
33. Martha T. Moore, "Ads from the Round File," *USA Today*, October 31, 1991.
34. Victoria Graham, "Condoms Becoming More Accessible, Widely Advertised," *Arizona Republic*, July 3, 1978, p. C2.
35. Mary Beth Murphy, *Milwaukee Sentinel*.
36. Graham, *Arizona Republic*.
37. Ibid.
38. Ibid.
39. "Increase and Multiply?," program of the Better World Society, aired on WTBS, November 1987.
40. "Increase and Multiply?," "Action Guide," Better World Society, undated (circa 1987).
41. Robert Marshall and Charles Donovan, *Blessed Are the Barren: The Social Policy of Planned Parenthood* (San Francisco: Ignatius, 1991), p. 280.
42. "Choice, Challenge, Continuity," 1981 Annual Report, Planned Parenthood Federation of America, 1982, p. 34.
43. Ibid.
44. "Action Guide."
45. "Harnessing the Power of Television to Make a Better World," Better World Society, undated (circa 1987).
46. Ibid.
47. Ibid.
48. Ibid.
49. Better World Society awards program, aired on WTBS, December 10, 1988.
50. R. E. "Ted" Turner, chairman, Better World Society, 1988 Better World Society Awards program, aired on WTBS, December 10, 1988.
51. *National and International Religion Report*, November 6, 1989.
52. 1988 Better World Society Awards program, aired on WTBS, December 1988.
53. Ibid.
54. Ibid.
55. Ibid.
56. Ibid.
57. Ibid.
58. "Abortion Led to Ballad: O'Connor Sings of the Child Who Would Have Been," Associated Press report, undated (1990 or 1991).
59. Ibid.
60. *Spin*, November 1991, as cited in "Quote of the Month," *Christian American*, January/February 1992, p. 9.
61. Ibid.
62. "The New Cold War," *New Dimensions: The Psychology Behind the News*, June 1990, vol. 4, no. 6, p. 23.

63. Adrian Deevoy, "If You're Going to Reveal Yourself, Reveal Yourself!: Madonna Talks Tough About Life and Truth or Dare," *US*, interview, June 13, 1991, p. 23.
64. Nancy Griffin, "Cher," *US*, interview, October 1991, p. 46.
65. Norman Mailer, in an interview with David Frost, as cited in "Pro-Choice Hostages Speak Out," *Citizen*, March 16, 1992, p. 8.
66. "Family Feud," broadcast June 1991.
67. Ibid.
68. Karen Thomas, "Brooke Shields on Virginity's Virtues," *USA Today*, July 23, 1991.
69. Mel Gibson, as told to the Spanish magazine *El Pais*, as cited in "Pro-Choice Hostages Speak Out," *Citizen*, March 16, 1992, p. 8.
70. Liz Smith, as cited in "Pro-Choice Hostages Speak Out," *Citizen*, March 16, 1992, p. 8.
71. *US*, April 16, 1990, p. 49.
72. "Sex in the '90s" and "More Sex in the '90s," Music Television News Special Reports, Music Television, broadcast on April 20, 1991.
73. "Sex in the '90s," Music Television News Special Report, Music Television, broadcast on April 20, 1991.
74. "More Sex in the '90s," Music Television News Special Report, Music Television, broadcast on April 20, 1991.
75. "Sex in the '90s."
76. Ibid.
77. Ibid.
78. Ibid.
79. Ibid.
80. Ibid.
81. Ibid.
82. Ibid.
83. Ibid.
84. Ibid.
85. Ibid.
86. Ibid.
87. Ibid.
88. Ibid.
89. Ibid.
90. Ibid.
91. Ibid.
92. "More Sex in the '90s."
93. Ibid.
94. Ibid.
95. Ibid.
96. Ibid.
97. Ibid.
98. Ibid.
99. Ibid.
100. Mötley Crüe album, as cited by Thomas L. Jipping, "A Generation at Risk: What Can Be Done?," *The World and I*, April 1992, vol. 7, no. 4., p. 106.
101. "Rock 'n' Roll Banned," "A Current Affair," aired on December 31, 1991.
102. Music Television "Video Awards," Music Television, rebroadcast on specific broadcast date unknown (rebroadcast in December 1991).
103. "Awarding God?," *You!*, May 1991, Vol. 91, no. 5, p. 4.
104. "Raising a Voice for Choice," *Newsweek*, July 1, 1991.
105. "Federal Funds Used for Pro-Abortion Commercial," *New York Guardian*, January 1992.
106. Ibid.
107. Thomas L. Jipping, J.D., personal interview, April 24, 1992.

108. Marvin N. Olasky, *The Press and Abortion, 1838–1988* (Hillsdale, NJ: Lawrence Erlbaum Associates, 1988), p. xii.
109. Ibid.
110. Lawrence Lader, *Abortion II: Making the Revolution* (Boston: Beacon Press, 1973), p. ix, as cited by Olasky in *The Press and Abortion, 1838–1988*.
111. Bernard N. Nathanson, *Abortion America* (Toronto: Life Cycle Books: 1979), p. 51.
112. Olasky, *The Press and Abortion, 1838–1988*, p. 99.
113. Ibid., p. 190.
114. Laurence Zuckerman, "To March or Not to March," *Time*, August 14, 1989, p. 45.
115. David Shaw, "Bias Seeps Into News on Abortion," *Los Angeles Times*, July 1, 1990, p. A48.
116. Zuckerman, *Time*.
117. "Abortion Inc.," *New Dimensions: The Psychology Behind the News*, September/October 1991, p. 88.
118. Ibid.
119. Barbara Reynolds, "Inquiry" editor, *USA Today*, August 16, 1991, as cited in *Notable Quotables*, *MediaWatch*, Media Research Center, December 23, 1991, vol. 4, no. 26, p. 8.
120. "This Week," May 26, 1991, as cited in *Notable Quotables*, p. 6.
121. "CBS Evening News," July 1, 1991, as cited in *Notable Quotables*, p. 2.
122. John Daniszewski, "Doctors Adopt Pro-Life Stance," *Washington Times*, December 17, 1991.
123. "20/20," ABC News, broadcast on April 7, 1989.
124. Joseph Sobran, "Abortion as Genocide? Now Skeptics are 'Not So Sure,'" *Palm Beach Post*, October 30, 1989, p. 3F.
125. Ibid.
126. "Pro-Choice 1990: Skeletons in the Closet," *New Dimensions: The Psychology Behind the News*, pp. 22–23.
127. *INsider*, Planned Parenthood Federation of America, November 1, 1991, p. 6.
128. Zuckerman, *Time*.
129. Olasky, *The Press and Abortion, 1838–1988*, p. 147.
130. Zuckerman, *Time*.
131. S. Robert Lichter, Stanley Rothman and Linda S. Lichter, *The Media Elite: America's New Powerbrokers* (Bethesda, MD: Adler and Adler, 1986), p. 29.
132. Cal Thomas, "Conspiring Magazine Editors," *Washington Times*, August 21, 1989.
133. Ibid.
134. Ibid.
135. Ibid.
136. Ibid.
137. Cal Thomas, "Abortion and the Press," *Washington Times*, April 2, 1990.
138. 1985 Annual Report, Planned Parenthood Federation of America, 1986, p. 20.
139. 1989 Annual Report, Planned Parenthood Federation of America, 1990, p. 18.
140. "PPFA Annual Conference Events Open to the Press," Planned Parenthood Federation of America, October 1990, p. 3.
141. *INsider*, p. 7.
142. "3 'Republic' Staffers Get Awards from Planned Parenthood for Writing," *Arizona Republic*, December 20, 1987.
143. Shaw, "Bias Seeps Into News on Abortion," *Los Angeles Times*, p. A48.
144. Ibid.
145. John Elvin, "Inside the Beltway: Got Your #," *Washington Times*, March 13, 1991.
146. "'Rights' It Is," "Style and Substance," *Wall Street Journal* bulletin, December 18, 1989, vol. 2, no. 14.
147. *Chicago Sun-Times*, November 20, 1978, as cited by Olasky in *The Press and Abortion, 1839–1988*.

148. *Kansas City Star*, March 11, 1976, as cited by Olasky in *The Press and Abortion, 1838–1988*, p. 122.
149. *Kansas City Times*, February 4, 1978, as cited by Olasky in *The Press and Abortion, 1838–1988*, p. 122.
150. Richard LaCayo, "Abortion: The Future is Already Here," *Time*, May 4, 1992, p. 27.
151. Ibid.
152. Ibid., p. 28.
153. Ibid.
154. Ibid.
155. Ibid., p. 29.
156. Ibid., p. 30.
157. Ibid., p. 32.
158. Ibid., p. 30.
159. Ibid., pp. 30–32.
160. Ibid., p. 32.

Chapter 7: The Abortion Connection

1. "A Close Look at Planned Parenthood," "Focus on the Family" radio program, October 26–27, 1989.
2. Richard Stengel, "Tough Choice," *Detroit News*, January 2, 1990.
3. Alan F. Guttmacher, M.D., president, Planned Parenthood Federation of America, *Family Planning Perspectives*, January 1971, p. 55.
4. "A Five Year Plan: 1976–1980," Planned Parenthood Federation of America, 1975, pp. i and 4.
5. "Planned Parenthood in the 70's: Expanding the Vision," *Planned Parenthood Press*, Planned Parenthood of Central and Northern Arizona, Fall 1987.
6. *Doe v. Bolton (410 US 179)*, decision of the United States Supreme Court, January 22, 1973.
7. *Facts and Figures on Legal Abortion of Importance to All Americans*, Planned Parenthood Federation of America, 1973.
8. Ibid.
9. Ibid.
10. Ibid.
11. Barbara Calfee, "CAPS Project, Beginning Third Year, Achieves '75 in 75,'" *INsider*, Planned Parenthood Federation of America, September 1, 1991, p. 12.
12. "Nine Reasons Why Abortions Are Legal," full-page copyrighted advertisement, Planned Parenthood Federation of America, *New York Times*, October 17, 1988, p. A37.
13. Ibid.
14. Mary S. Calderone, M.D., "Illegal Abortions as a Public Health Problem," *American Journal of Health*, July 1960.
15. Marvin Olasky, *The Press and Abortion, 1838-1988*, p. 90.
16. "Five Ways to Prevent Abortion (And One That Won't)," full-page copyrighted advertisement, Planned Parenthood Federation of America, *New York Times*, October 18, 1988.
17. Ibid.
18. "What Every Man Should Know About Abortion," full-page copyrighted advertisement, Planned Parenthood Federation of America, *Time*, December 16, 1985.
19. Ibid.
20. Ibid.
21. "The Right to Choose Abortion Makes All My Other Rights Possible," full-page copyrighted advertisement, Planned Parenthood Federation of America, *Time*, 1985.
22. Ibid.
23. "A Five Year Plan: 1976–1980," p. 3.

24. "'Til Victory is Won . . . An Action Agenda for 1982–84," Planned Parenthood Federation of America, 1982.
25. Faye Wattleton, annual luncheon of Planned Parenthood Federation of America affiliate, St. Louis, Missouri, February 5, 1979.
26. *Ten Heavy Facts About Sex . . .* , The Institute for Family Research and Education, 1975. (Not published by Planned Parenthood but used by Planned Parenthood.)
27. *They Learn History at Yale . . . Economics at Harvard . . . Sex Education at State Street and Main*, Planned Parenthood-World Population, undated (circa 1977).
28. "'Til Victory is Won . . . An Action Agenda for 1982–84."
29. Ibid.
30. George Langmyhr, M.D., "The Role of Planned Parenthood-World Population in Abortion," *Implementation of Legal Abortion: A National Problem*, December 1971, p. 1190.
31. *Planned Parenthood: A Strong Voice for the Most Personal of Human Rights*, Planned Parenthood, undated.
32. *Pro-Child, Pro-Family, Pro-Choice*, Planned Parenthood/Orange and San Bernadino Counties, California, undated (1988 or 1989).
33. Ibid.
34. *So You Don't Want to Be a Sex Object*, Rocky Mountain Planned Parenthood, 1984.
35. Virginia Coigney, *Margaret Sanger: Rebel With a Cause* (Garden City, NY: Doubleday and Company, 1969), p. 178.
36. "Impact on . . . Abortion," policy statement of Planned Parenthood of Central and Northern Arizona, September 1988.
37. Louise B. Tyrer, M.D., FACOG, and Julie E. Salas, M.A., "Contraceptive Problems Unique to the United States," *Clinical Obstetrics and Gynecology*, June 1989, vol. 32, no. 2, p. 313.
38. Katharine Hepburn, fund-raising letter, Planned Parenthood, undated.
39. Ibid.
40. Faye Wattleton, fund-raising letter, Planned Parenthood-World Population, undated (circa January 1979), p. 2.
41. Faye Wattleton, fund-raising letter, Planned Parenthood-World Population, undated, p. 2.
42. "The Facts Speak Louder: Planned Parenthood's Critique of 'The Silent Scream,'" Planned Parenthood, undated.
43. Ibid.
44. Ibid.
45. Ibid., pp. 8 and 9.
46. Ibid.
47. Dena Kleiman, "Debate on Abortion Focuses on Graphic Film," *New York Times*, January 23, 1985.
48. James W. Prescott, *The Abortion of* The Silent Scream: *A False and Wrongful Cry for Human Pain, Suffering, and Violence*, American Humanist Association, 1986, p. 3.
49. Ibid., p. 4.
50. Ibid., p. 10.
51. Sue Woodman, "The Decision No Woman Wants to Make: Clearing Up the Mounting Distortions About 'Late' Abortions," *Self*, September 1987, p. 147.
52. Ibid.
53. Ibid., p. 148.
54. Ibid.
55. Ibid.
56. Calfee, *INsider*.
57. Barbara Calfee, "CAPS [Consortium of Abortion Providers] Project Update," *News From CAPS*, October 1990, p. 3.
58. Calfee, *INsider*.
59. Ibid.
60. Ibid.

61. Ibid.
62. Calfee, *News From* CAPS.
63. Calfee, *INsider*.
64. "'Hats Off' to the Newest Members of CAPS [Consortium of Abortion Providers]," *News From* CAPS, October 1990, p. 1.
65. "A Tradition of Choice for 75 Years," 1991 Service Report, Planned Parenthood Federation of America, 1991, p. 10.
66. 1990 Service Report, Planned Parenthood Federation of America, 1990, p. 14.
67. Carol Everett, letter sent to the editor of the *Belleville News Democrat*, September 20, 1990.
68. Ibid.
69. "Abortion and Women's Health," Alan Guttmacher Institute, 1990.
70. Richard LaCayo, "Abortion: The Future is Already Here," *Time*, May 4, 1992, p. 29.
71. Memorandum from Eve W. Paul, Planned Parenthood Federation of America, to Joan McCracken, executive director of a Planned Parenthood affiliate, December 12, 1980.
72. Marianne Szegedy-Maszak, "Calm, Cool and Beleaguered," *New York Times Magazine*, August 6, 1989, p. 62.
73. 1991 Service Report.
74. Ibid.
75. Ibid.
76. "CAPS [Consortium of Abortion Providers] Survey '90," Consortium of Abortion Providers, confidential report, undated (1991).
77. Ibid.
78. Ibid.
79. Ibid.
80. Ibid.
81. Ibid.
82. Ibid.
83. Ibid.
84. Ibid.
85. "Family News in Focus" radio program, October 22, 1990.
86. "PPL [Planned Parenthood League] Offers Loan Fund, Abortion Service," *Options*, Planned Parenthood League (Detroit, MI), Fall 1990, p. 2.
87. "Planned Birth, the Future of the Family and the Quality of American Life," June 1977, p. 31.
88. Ibid., p. 32.
89. Elizabeth Hrenda-Roberts, "Oversexed," letter to the editor, *New Republic*, April 6, 1992.
90. Abraham Stone, M.D. and Norman E. Himes, Ph.D., revised by Joseph J. Rovinsky, M.D., *Planned Parenthood: A Practical Handbook of Birth-Control Methods*, 1965.
91. *Plan Your Children for Health and Happiness*, Planned Parenthood, August 1963.

Chapter 8: "What Women Don't Know . . ."

1. "Pregnancy Counseling Standards for Parenthood Federation of America," Planned Parenthood of Seattle-King County, November 1983.
2. Ibid.
3. "Abortion, Inc.," *New Dimensions: The Psychology Behind the News*, September/October 1991.
4. Based on an article by Carol C. Gilbert and Clare Brightman, "A Marketing Perspective for Planned Parenthood," *Papers 1975*, Planned Parenthood Federation of America, 1975, p. 64.
5. Carol C. Gilbert and Clare Brightman, "A Marketing Perspective for Planned Parenthood," *Papers 1975*, Planned Parenthood Federation of America, 1975, p. 64.

6. Memorandum and attachments from David J. Andrews, executive vice president, Planned Parenthood Federation of America, to affiliate executive directors and board presidents, September 21, 1990.
7. *Planned Parenthood . . . The Career of Choice! . . . "It's More Than a Living . . . It's Living Your Ideals,"* recruitment brochure of the Planned Parenthood Federation of America, undated (1990).
8. Lee Minto, "Executive Director's Report [1981]," Planned Parenthood of Seattle-King County [Washington] newsletter, Spring 1982, p. 2.
9. Lee Minto, "Executive Director's Report [1983]," Planned Parenthood of Seattle-King County [Washington] newsletter, Spring 1984.
10. Audit of the United States General Accounting Office, as reported by Jo Ann Gasper, "Planned Parenthood: The Professional Killers," *Concerned Women*, August 1989.
11. "Abortion Factbook," National Committee for Adoption, 1989, as cited in "Abortion Inc.," *New Dimensions: The Psychology Behind the News*, September/October 1991, p. 44.
12. Faye Wattleton, *How to Talk With Your Child About Sexuality: A Parent's Guide* (Garden City, NY: Doubleday and Company, 1986), p. 120.
13. Linda Gase, "Pregnant Teens," *'Teen*, December 1991, p. 98.
14. "Providing Prenatal Care Services at Family Planning Clinics: Problems and Opportunities," *Family Planning Perspectives*, Special Report, May/June 1989, vol. 21, no. 3, p. 127.
15. Ibid.
16. Richard Stengel, "Tough Choice," *Detroit News*, January 2, 1990.
17. Felicity Barringer, "Planned Parenthood: Quiet Cause to Focus of Fury," *New York Times*, October 30, 1990, p. A16.
18. 1990 Service Report, Planned Parenthood Federation of America, 1990, pp. 6, 10–12.
19. "A Tradition of Choice for 75 Years," 1991 Service Report, Planned Parenthood Federation of America, 1991, p. 12.
20. 1990 Service Report, p. 12.
21. "Promiscuous Teen Paying Price," *Mogollan Advisor*, March 25, 1987.
22. Ibid.
23. "Lies Don't Bother Planned Parenthood . . . ," *ALL About Issues*, March 1986, p. 26.
24. Ibid, pp. 26–27.
25. Tina (last name withheld), telephone interview, March 1987.
26. Ibid.
27. Personal letter to the Christian Action Council, undated (1991).
28. "Facts About Planned Parenthood," *The Precious Feet People*, October 1986.
29. Gloria Feldt, executive director, Planned Parenthood of Central and Northern Arizona, at a public meeting held to take comment on a proposed family planning clinic for Payson, Arizona, March 27, 1987.
30. *The Precious Feet People*.
31. Ibid.
32. "It Happened to Me: I Had An Abortion," *Sassy*, December 1992, p. 74.
33. "A Close Look at Planned Parenthood," "Focus on the Family" radio program, October 26–27, 1989.
34. Peter T. Knoepfler, M.D. and Lee S. Minto, "A Psychiatrist Volunteers at a Planned Parenthood Clinic," *Papers 1975*, Planned Parenthood Federation of America, 1975, p. 140.
35. Report of a woman (name withheld) who investigated a number of abortion facilities for an article she was writing. All were investigated in 1989. The woman posed as a 16-year-old client. Quotations taken from written report.
36. Ibid.
37. Ibid.
38. Ibid.
39. Ibid.
40. Ibid.

41. Ibid.
42. Ibid.
43. Ibid.
44. "The 700 Club," CBN News, 1991.
45. Ibid.
46. "Focus on the Family" radio program.
47. Ibid.
48. "Early Pregnancy Termination (Abortion)," Planned Parenthood of Seattle-King County (Washington), November 1984.
49. Ibid.
50. Robert H. Ruff, *Aborting Planned Parenthood*, 1988, pp. 97–138.
51. Ibid.
52. David C. Reardon, *Aborted Women: Silent No More*, 1987.
53. "Department of Education 3-Year Plan and Long Range Goals," 1990–1993, Planned Parenthood Federation of America (authenticity unconfirmed), undated, p. 29.
54. Michele Breslauer, "Opposition Update: Origins of Phony PPFA Document Sought," *INsider*, February 1, 1992, p. 2.
55. Cristine Russell, special health correspondent for the *Washington Post*, "NOVA: Controversial Dr. Koop," Public Broadcasting System, broadcast in June 1990.
56. C. Everett Koop, M.D., former United States surgeon general, "NOVA: Controversial Dr. Koop," Public Broadcasting System, broadcast in June 1990.
57. Gasper, *Concerned Women*.
58. "Focus on the Family" radio program.
59. Ibid.
60. Ibid.
61. Ibid.
62. Ibid.
63. Karen Goldwater, "Exception to the Rule: How Some Women Opposed to Abortion Face a Crisis Pregnancy," *INsider*, December 1, 1991, p. 4.
64. Ibid.
65. Graphics included with Goldwater article, *INsider*, December 1, 1991, p. 4.

Chapter 9: Millions of Dollars

1. "Choice, Challenge, Continuity," 1981 Annual Report, Planned Parenthood Federation of America, 1982, p. 16.
2. A *Five Year Plan: 1976–1980*, Planned Parenthood Federation of America, 1975, p. 6.
3. Based on an average of $251 for a first trimester abortion.
4. 1990 Annual Report, Planned Parenthood Federation of America, 1991, p. 36.
5. "The 1991 NP [*NonProfit Times*] 100: America's Biggest Charities," supplement to the *NonProfit Times*, November 1991.
6. "A Tradition of Choice for 75 Years," 1991 Annual Report, Planned Parenthood Federation of America, 1992.
7. Annual Reports, 1988–1991, Planned Parenthood Federation of America, 1989, 1990, 1991, and 1992, respectively.
8. Kathleen Teltsch, "Foundations Expand Family Planning Aid Abroad," *New York Times*, September 5, 1988.
9. Ibid.
10. Faye Wattleton, fund-raising letter, Family Planning International Assistance, Planned Parenthood, undated.
11. Ibid.
12. Katharine Hepburn, fund-raising letter, Planned Parenthood Federation of America, undated.

13. Faye Wattleton, fund-raising letter, Planned Parenthood-World Population, undated (circa January 1979).
14. "That's a Lot of Points of Light, George," Ms., June 1989.
15. Al Neuharth, founder, *USA Today*, "Why Women Need a New NOW Now," *USA Today*, January 10, 1992, as cited in "NOW Lives on Hype Alone," *Citizen*, March 16, 1992, p. 8.
16. "Our Country Has a Program . . . ," full page copyrighted advertisement, Planned Parenthood Federation of America, *Washington Post*, May 17, 1981.
17. "Fact Sheet: Title X: The Nation's Family Planning Program," Planned Parenthood Federation of America, September 1990, pp. 2–3.
18. Faye Wattleton, statement, press release, Planned Parenthood Federation of America, October 18, 1990.
19. Faye Wattleton, "Should the Government Fund Abortion Advocacy," *New Dimensions: The Psychology Behind the News*, September/October 1991, p. 26.
20. Ibid.
21. Ibid.
22. "Abortion, Inc.," *New Dimensions: The Psychology Behind the News*, September/October 1991, p. 12.
23. Curtis Pesmen, "The Abortion Decision," *Seventeen*, September 1991, p. 62.
24. "Changing the Rules on Family Planning," *USA Today*, May 29, 1991, p. 8A.
25. "They Want to Take Your Tax Dollars . . . ," print advertisement, The Abortion is Not Family Planning Coalition, *USA Today*, July 25, 1991, p. 7A.
26. "Do You Think Abortion is Just Another Method of Birth Control," print advertisement, The Abortion is Not Family Planning Coalition, advertising copy, undated (1991).
27. "When Planned Parenthood Says 'FREE' Speech You Pay . . . $37,000,000," print advertisement, The Abortion is Not Family Planning Coalition, advertising copy, undated (1991).
28. "As a Woman and As a Doctor . . . ," print advertisement, The Abortion is Not Family Planning Coalition, advertising copy, undated (1991).
29. "VETO . . . ," full-page copyrighted advertisement, Planned Parenthood Federation of America, *USA Today*, November 18, 1991, p. 7A.
30. Ibid.
31. Ibid.
32. "Planned Parenthood Adds New Fees to Make Up Lost Funds," *Intelligencer Journal*, November 27, 1991, p. B-1.
33. Ibid.
34. Mimi Hall, "Some Clinics Plan to Reject 'Gag' Money," *USA Today*, November 20, 1991, p. 3A.
35. Mimi Hall, "Clinics Sidestep Counseling Ban: Title X Rule Wording May Leave Loophole," *USA Today*, May 29, 1991, p. 8A.
36. Ibid.
37. "Maryland Planned Parenthood Will Not Obey Gag Rule, Director Says," Associated Press wire story, March 25, 1992.
38. "Planned Parenthood President Criticizes Bush's Gag Rule," Associated Press wire story, March 25, 1992.
39. John Walker, Family Research Council, telephone interview, March 26, 1992.
40. Ibid.
41. Robert J. Conrad, Jr., "Planned Parenthood A Radical, Pro Abortion Fringe Group," *Charlotte Observer*, June 14, 1988.
42. Bruce Millar, "'Donor Choice' Gains Ground in United Ways," *Chronicle of Philanthropy*, March 12, 1991, p. 25.
43. Ibid.
44. "A Victory for Good Sense: Settling the Abortion Clinic Dispute is Good News for the Community," *Democrat and Chronicle*, February 3, 1992.

45. Ibid.
46. Ibid.
47. Gloria Feldt, fund-raising letter, Planned Parenthood of Central and Northern Arizona, September 6, 1988.
48. "Planned Parenthood to Sell Own Brand of Prophylactics," *Arizona Republic*, July 31, 1983.
49. Robert H. Ruff, *Aborting Planned Parenthood*, 1988, p. 13.
50. Ruff, *Aborting Planned Parenthood*, p. 17.
51. Ibid., pp. 27–28.
52. Reported by Timothy Glazewski, an aide to Congressman Jon Kyl, R-Arizona, July 1989.
53. Letter to Richard P. Kusserow, inspector general, Department of Health and Human Services, to the Honorable Jon Kyl, R-Arizona, undated (January 1990).
54. "Review of Family Planning Services in the State of New Jersey," undated (later 1989 or early 1990), which accompanies letter to Richard P. Kusserow, inspector general, Department of Health and Human Services, to the Honorable Jon Kyl, R-Arizona, undated (January 1990).

Chapter 10: Public Policy Advocacy

1. "A Five Year Plan: 1976–1980," Planned Parenthood Federation of America, 1975, pp. 4 and 5.
2. Susan Manuel, "Abortion Battle is Launched," *USA Today*, April 15, 1987.
3. Donald Kauber, Jean Stabell, and Clare Brightman, "Zen and the Art of Planned Parenthood Maintenance (An Inquiry Into Values)," *Papers 1975*, Planned Parenthood Federation of America, 1975, p. 34.
4. Andrea Wemette, Planned Parenthood, speech at the Information and Education Conference, California Office of Family Planning, June 1986.
5. Frederick C. Smith, letter, Planned Parenthood, January 26, 1981.
6. "Preaching Hasn't Stopped Teenage Pregnancy. Teaching Might," full-page copyrighted advertisement, Planned Parenthood Federation of America, *New York Times*, October 7, 1984.
7. "A Happy Baby is the Best Argument for Birth Control," full-page copyrighted advertisement, Planned Parenthood of New York City, *New York Times*, November 4, 1984.
8. Katharine Hepburn, fund-raising letter, Planned Parenthood, undated.
9. Ibid.
10. Katharine Hepburn, fund-raising letter, Planned Parenthood, undated.
11. Faye Wattleton, fund-raising letter, Planned Parenthood-World Population, undated (circa January 1979).
12. "Outlook," Planned Parenthood-World Population, *Washington Memo*, Alan Guttmacher Institute, January 18, 1980.
13. "Patient Advocacy," *PPFA* [Planned Parenthood Federation of America] *Public Affairs Manual*, 1981.
14. Faye Wattleton, fund-raising letter, Planned Parenthood Federation of America, undated (circa 1988).
15. Faye Wattleton, fund-raising letter, Planned Parenthood Federation of America, undated (circa 1989).
16. "Some Women Are Silent on the Horrors of Illegal Abortion," full-page copyrighted advertisement, Planned Parenthood Federation of America, *New York Times*, April 27, 1989.
17. Ibid.
18. Ibid.
19. Ibid.
20. "For Millions of Women, the 20th Century Began on a Quiet Brooklyn Street in 1916," full-page copyrighted advertisement, Planned Parenthood Federation of America, *New York Times*, March 26, 1991, p. A15.
21. Ibid.

22. "Robert Bork's Position on Reproductive Rights: You Don't Have Any," full-page copyrighted advertisement, Planned Parenthood Federation of America, *Washington Post*, September 14, 1987, p. A9.
23. Ibid.
24. "A Close Look at Planned Parenthood," "Focus on the Family" radio program, October 26–27, 1989.
25. Ibid.
26. 1989 Annual Report, Planned Parenthood Federation of America, 1990, p. 17.
27. "His Choice or Hers?," print advertisement, Canadians for Choice, *Vancouver Province*, September 25, 1989.
28. Ibid.
29. Anglican Journal/Journal Episcopal, March 1989, as cited in "Around and About: Civil Disobedience No Answer," *About Us*, Planned Parenthood Association of British Columbia, June 1989, p. 3.
30. Ibid.
31. Ibid.
32. "Grab Bag: Long Range Plan, *About Us*, Planned Parenthood Association of British Columbia, June 1989, p. 4.
33. "Grab Bag: Services to New Canadians," *About Us*, Planned Parenthood Association of British Columbia, June 1989, p. 4.
34. "About Us," *About Us*, Planned Parenthood Association of British Columbia, June 1989, p. 5.
35. "'Til Victory is Won . . . An Action Agenda for 1982–84," Planned Parenthood Federation of America, 1982.
36. Ibid.
37. Ibid.
38. Ibid.
39. Ibid.
40. Ibid.
41. Ibid.
42. "3 White House Conferences Take Positive Stand on Family Planning," *Planned Parenthood News*, Winter 1966, no. 42, p. 3.
43. "Literature and Comment: U.S. Population Growth Reprojected," *Family Planning Perspectives*, Planned Parenthood-World Population, October 1970, vol. 2, no. 4, p. 43.
44. Larry Dumpass, Ph.D., and Charles F. Westoff, Ph.D., "Unwanted Births and U.S. Population Growth," *Family Planning Perspectives*, October 1970, vol. 2, no. 4, p. 11.
45. Ibid.
46. *Your Right to Reproductive Health Care Services Should Not Be Left to Chance: You Can Protect Your Rights. We Can Help*, Planned Parenthood of Buffalo (New York), undated (circa 1991).
47. "Public Affairs," 1989 Annual Report, Planned Parenthood Federation of America, 1990, p. 28.
48. 8 *Arguments for Keeping Government Out of Your Family's Life*, Planned Parenthood Federation of America, 1989.
49. Ibid.
50. Ibid.
51. Faye Wattleton, "Politics of Reproductive Choice," speech delivered at Behrend College (Pennsylvania State, Erie Campus), March 4, 1992.
52. Ibid.
53. Faye Wattleton, *How to Talk With Your Child About Sexuality: A Parent's Guide*, Planned Parenthood (Garden City, NY: Doubleday and Company, 1986), p. 34.
54. "Women and Smoking," "Good Morning America," ABC television, October 25, 1991.
55. Ibid.

56. Nancy Myers, "Parents, Teens Lobby for *Real* Parents' Rights," *National Right to Life News*, September 24, 1991, vol. 18, no. 16., pp. 1 and 10.
57. "A Ten-Year Strategic Plan for Securing Abortion Rights," confidential report, conducted for the Planned Parenthood Federation America by Hamilton and Staff, October 1990.
58. Ibid., pp. 1–2.
59. Ibid., p. 2.
60. Ibid., pp. 2–3.
61. Ibid., p. 3.
62. Ibid., p. 1.
63. Ibid., pp. 4–7.
64. Ibid., p. 1.
65. Ibid., pp. 8–10.
66. Ibid., p. 1.
67. Ibid., pp. 12–16.
68. Ibid., p. 1.
69. Ibid., pp. 17–23.
70. Ibid., p. 25.
71. Ibid., p. 24.
72. Letter to Ronald Brown, chairman, Democratic National Committee, signed by 50 Democrats in the House of Representatives, undated (circa April 1989).
73. Governor Robert P. Casey, D-Pennsylvania, as cited in "Pro-Choice Hostages Speak Out," *Citizen*, March 16, 1992, p. 8.
74. William W. Hamilton, Jr., director, Washington, D.C., office, Planned Parenthood Federation of America, "A Kinder, Gentler Party," Ms., Letters, June 1989.
75. Ibid.
76. "Abortion Stance Threatens to Divide Republicans," *USA Today*, September 27, 1991, p. 9A.
77. Patricia Adams, "New Organization Urges African-American Men to Support Choice," *INsider*, Planned Parenthood Federation of America, November 15, 1991, p. 3.
78. *INsider*, November 15, 1991.
79. Ibid.
80. Ibid.
81. Ibid.
82. Ibid.
83. Rev. Jesse Jackson, as quoted in *National Right to Life News*, January 1977.
84. Joseph Sobran, "Abortion as Genocide? Now Skeptics Are 'Not So Sure,'" *Palm Beach Post*, October 30, 1989, p. 3F.
85. Ibid.
86. Ibid.
87. 1991 Service Report, Planned Parenthood Federation of America, 1991, p. 10.
88. "Dear Colleague" letter, Physicians for Choice, Planned Parenthood (Buffalo, New York) January 1990.
89. David A. Grimes, M.D., "Medical Aspects of RU 486," part of the "New Birth Control in the Next Century" seminar at the 1990 annual conference, Planned Parenthood Federation of America, October 19, 1990.
90. "New Birth Control in the Next Century," seminar presented at the 1990 annual conference, Planned Parenthood Federation of America, October 19, 1990.
91. Marcia Ann Gillespie, "Repro Woman," interview with Faye Wattleton, then-president of the Planned Parenthood Federation of America, Ms., October 1989, p. 52.
92. "20/20," ABC, April 7, 1989.
93. Ibid.
94. Ibid.
95. Ibid.
96. Ibid.

97. Ibid.
98. Ibid.
99. "The French Pill (RU 486)," Fact Sheet, Planned Parenthood Federation of America, July 1990, p. 2.
100. Ibid.
101. "France Bans Abortion Pill for Women Over 35, Smokers," *Buffalo News*, April 21, 1991.
102. Ibid.
103. "Around the Nation: New Hampshire," *USA Today*, May 9, 1991.
104. *Cedar Rapids Gazette*.
105. 1989 Annual Report, Planned Parenthood Federation of America, 1990, p. 18.
106. *INsider*, November 1, 1991, p. 6.
107. "PRO-CHOICE 1991: Skeletons in the Closet," *New Dimensions: The Psychology Behind the News*, September/October 1991, p. 46.
108. Ibid.
109. "Abortion: Help for RU-486," *Newsweek*, October 7, 1991, p. 8.
110. Diane Culbertson, "My View: Down the Abortion Rat Whole," *USA Today*, October 7, 1991.
111. Ibid.
112. Ibid.
113. George Grant, *The Quick and the Dead: RU-486 and the New Chemical Warfare Against Your Family* (Wheaton, IL: Crossway Books, 1991), p. xiv.
114. Philip F. Lawler, "Counterpoint: An Issue This Paper Can't Sidestep," *Wall Street Journal*, August 29, 1991, p. A13.
115. Ibid.
116. Gloria Feldt, "From the Executive Director . . . 'Over Half a Million Served,'" *Planned Parenthood Press*, Planned Parenthood of Central and Northern Arizona, Spring 1987.

Chapter 11: Beyond North America

1. Frederick S. Jaffee, "Activities Relevant to the Study of Population Policy for the U.S.," Memorandum to Bernard Berelson, *Family Planning Perspectives*, October 1970, vol. 2, no. 4, p. ix.
2. "Standards of Affiliation," Article XI, Section 4, p. 23 (B-25).
3. Ibid., Section 2, p. 22 (B-24).
4. "PPFA's Involvement in International Family Planning," Planned Parenthood Federation of America, policy statement adopted by membership, October 2, 1980.
5. Memorandum outlining amendments to the Planned Parenthood Federation of America By-Laws, membership meeting, October 2, 1980, Article XII—Standards of Affiliation, December 10, 1980.
6. "FPA-Regional-Central Links in Policy-Making," section of a document of the International Planned Parenthood Federation, unknown date.
7. "Special Report on the United Nations Population Conference-Tribune," U.S. Coalition for Life, 1974.
8. Ibid.
9. *Human Right to Family Planning*, Planned Parenthood Federation, London, England, 1984.
10. Ibid.
11. "Direct Demand Creation," Three Year Plan, Planned Parenthood, undated.
12. Three Year Plan, Planned Parenthood, undated.
13. "Report of the Working Group on the Promotion of Family Planning as a Basic Human Right," International Planned Parenthood Federation, November 1983, p. 28–29.
14. Ibid., p. 28.
15. Ibid., p. 29.
16. "Public Education: National Office Activities," 1985 Annual Report, Planned Parenthood Federation of America, 1986, p. 20.

17. "PPFA Annual Conference Events Open to the Press," Planned Parenthood Federation of America, October 1990, p. 3.
18. "The Great Romanian Condom Airlift of '89," *World Watch*, May-June 1990.
19. "Despite Ban, Contraceptives Are Advertised at Italian Soccer Arenas," *Planned Parenthood News*, Winter 1959, no. 23, p. 7.
20. "Family Planning International Assistance," 1989 Annual Report, Planned Parenthood Federation of America, 1990, p. 12.
21. Jacqueline Kasun, *The War Against Population: The Economics and Ideology of Population Control*, 1988, p. 169.
22. James L. Buckley, "All Alone at the U.N.," *National Review*, December 14, 1984, p. 25.
23. "Court Allows Suit Over U.S. Bar to Abortion Aid," *New York Times*, January 31, 1988.
24. "The Reagan Administration is Promising the World to the Anti-Abortionists," full-page copyrighted advertisement, Planned Parenthood Federation of America, *New York Times*, August 2, 1984, p. A21.
25. Ibid.
26. "How Can You Explain That Her Mother Died of Politics?," full-page copyrighted advertisement, Planned Parenthood Federation of America, *National Journal*, February 11, 1989.
27. Susan Manuel, "Abortion Battle is Launched," *USA Today*, April 15, 1987.
28. "Abortion Fund Fight Promised," *Phoenix Gazette*, April 15, 1987.
29. Manuel, *USA Today*.
30. "The Right-Wing Coup in Family Planning," full-page copyrighted advertisement, Planned Parenthood Federation of America, *Washington Post*, February 18, 1987.
31. Ibid.
32. "White House Extremists and the Clause That Kills," full-page copyrighted advertisement, Planned Parenthood Federation of America, *Washington Post*, February 26, 1987.
33. Ibid.
34. Manuel, *USA Today*.
35. Planned Parenthood source quoted by Rita Marker, the Human Life Center, April 1986.
36. Letter to Ping Hong Li from her mother, Li-Ran, People's Republic of China, August 18, 1987.
37. Letter to Ping Hong Li from Li Gao of the Walfantia Bearings Company, People's Republic of China, August 17, 1987.
38. Letter to Ping Hong Li from an official of the Walfantia Bearings Company, People's Republic of China, September 18, 1987.
39. Letter to Ping Hong Li from an official of the Walfantia Bearings Company, People's Republic of China, September 25, 1987.
40. Letter to Dr. and Mrs. Li from Yong Hua, sister to Dr. Li, People's Republic of China, September 16, 1987.
41. Message from a cadre in charge of the birth control program, as related by Mrs. Li, September 27, 1987.
42. Letter from Congressman Jon Kyl (R-AZ) to Ruth Anne Myers, district director, Immigration and Naturalization Service, December 4, 1987.
43. Letter from Congressman Christopher H. Smith (R-NJ) to all members of the House of Representatives, April 15, 1988.
44. Ibid.
45. Letter signed by Congressmen Christopher H. Smith (R-NJ), Jon D. Kyl (R-AZ), Henry J. Hyde (R-IL) and John J. Rhodes III (R-AZ), to Attorney General Edwin Meese III, April 21, 1988.
46. Dr. Julia J. Henderson, board of directors, Better World Society, 1988 Better World Society Awards program, aired on WTBS, December 10, 1988.
47. The 1988 Better World Society Awards program, aired on WTBS, December 10, 1988.
48. "China's Birth Control Policy Drives Some to Kill Baby Girls," *Washington Post*, January 8, 1985.

49. "Female Infanticide," *Pro-Life News*, November/December 1988.
50. "The New Cold War," *New Dimensions: The Psychology Behind the News*, June 1990.
51. *Human Numbers, Human Needs*, International Planned Parenthood Federation, undated.
52. "China Moves Toward Compulsory Abortions for Retarded," *Washington Times*, December 1, 1988.
53. Ibid.
54. Ibid.
55. Ibid.
56. Faye Wattleton, "Planned Parenthood Blasts Untruths," *Rockford Register Star*, August 10, 1991.
57. *SIECUS Circle*, 1977.
58. Amendment prepared by Senator Paul Simon, D-Illinois, to a bill which would send American dollars to the United Nations Population Fund.
59. Statement made by the chairman of a congressional subcommittee, as reported by another member of Congress. All names are withheld.

Chapter 12: Attacking the Critics

1. *Defend Your Freedom to Choose*, Rocky Mountain Planned Parenthood, undated.
2. Ibid.
3. Ibid.
4. "Planned Parenthood Shifting to a Patriotic Theme," *New York Times*, October 5, 1980, p. 25.
5. "The 1986 Humanist of the Year on the Continuing Challenges for Reproductive Freedom," *The Humanist*, American Humanist Association, July/August 1986, p. 6.
6. Ibid.
7. Gail Ireland, "Head of Planned Parenthood Says Issue Is Freedom," *Cedar Rapids Gazette*, May 18, 1991, p. 1B.
8. Faye Wattleton, "Planned Parenthood's Leader Blasts Untruths," *Rockford Register Star*, August 10, 1991.
9. "The Facts Speak Louder: Planned Parenthood's Critique of *The Silent Scream*," Planned Parenthood, undated.
10. Frederick C. Smith, letter, Planned Parenthood, January 1981.
11. "When I Was Fifteen, Planned Parenthood Saved My Life," full-page copyrighted advertisement, Planned Parenthood Federation of America, *Time*, November 4, 1985.
12. "Do I Look Like a Mother to You?," full-page copyrighted advertisement, Planned Parenthood Federation of America, *Time*, November 25, 1985.
13. "The Right to Choose Abortion Makes All My Other Rights Possible," full-page copyrighted advertisement, Planned Parenthood Federation of America, 1985.
14. Ibid.
15. *Facts About the Threats to the Supreme Court Decisions on Abortion*, Planned Parenthood Federation of America, 1973.
16. Marie Bass, "New Birth Control in the Next Century," workshop outline, Planned Parenthood Federation of America, annual meeting, October 19, 1990.
17. "Nine Reasons Why Abortions Are Legal," full-page copyrighted advertisement, Planned Parenthood Federation of America, *New York Times*, October 17, 1988.
18. Ibid.
19. "Five Ways to Prevent Abortion (And One Way That Won't)," full-page copyrighted advertisement, Planned Parenthood Federation of America, *New York Times*, October 18, 1988.
20. Ibid.
21. "Poverty Doesn't Come Cheap," full-page copyrighted advertisement, Planned Parenthood Federation of America, *National Journal*, January 28, 1989.

22. "To Stop the Spread of Sexually Transmitted Diseases, Just Say KNOW," full-page copyrighted advertisement, Planned Parenthood Federation of America, *National Journal*, February 4, 1989.
23. Gloria Feldt, *Planned Parenthood Press*, Planned Parenthood of Central and Northern Arizona, Spring 1987.
24. Ibid.
25. Based on a report from Arizona Right to Life, Spring 1987.
26. "Repro Woman," interview with Faye Wattleton, *Ms.*, October 1989.
27. Ibid.
28. Ibid.
29. Ibid.
30. Philip F. Lawler, "Counterpoint: An Issue This Paper Can't Sidestep," *Wall Street Journal*, August 29, 1991, p. A13.
31. Katherine McDonald, fund-raising letter, Planned Parenthood Federation of Canada, September 1990.
32. Ibid.
33. *PPA-Planned Parenthood Alberta*, Planned Parenthood Alberta, undated (circa 1990).
34. "President Reagan, Why Are You Silent?," advertisement, Planned Parenthood of Metropolitan Washington, D.C., *Washington Post*, December 3, 1984.
35. "Should a Woman's Private Medical Decisions Be Made By a Man With a Bullhorn?," full-page copyrighted advertisement, Planned Parenthood Federation of America, *Time*, January 23, 1989.
36. "'I Don't Think Christians Should Use Birth Control,'" full-page copyrighted advertisement, Planned Parenthood Federation of America, *Time*, February 6, 1989.
37. Leila Hall-Smith, "Opposition Update: T-Shirts Available," *INsider*, Planned Parenthood Federation of America, February 1,1991, p. 2.
38. Alan F. Guttmacher, M.D., editor, *The Case for Legalized Abortion Now* (Berkley: Diablo Press, 1967), p. 9.
39. *Boston Globe*/WBZ Poll, *Boston Globe*, March 31, 1989.
40. Bernard N. Nathanson, M.D., *Aborting America* (Toronto: Life Cycle Books, 1979), p. 189.
41. Stephanie Ebbert, "Planned Parenthood Rapped," *Reading Eagle*, February 1, 1992.
42. James Neel, "Get the Facts on Figures Straight," letter to the editor, *Reading Eagle*, February 8, 1992.
43. Ibid.
44. Teresa K. Brown, "Group Wants to Prevent Abortions," board member, Planned Parenthood of North East Pennsylvania, letter to the editor, *Reading Eagle*, February 10, 1992.
45. Ibid.
46. Marti King-Pringle, Ph.D., president, Planned Parenthood of North East Pennsylvania, "Planned Parenthood Reduces Abortion Need," guest column, *Reading Eagle*, February 11, 1992.
47. "CORRECTIONS," *Reading Eagle*, February 14, 1992, p. A2.
48. Rochelle Hartman, "Writer Can't Get Away With Two Sets of Rules," letter to the editor, *Pantagraph*, February 22, 1992, p. A10.
49. Ibid.
50. Ibid.
51. Jennifer S. Johnson, "Defending Planned Parenthood," *Pantagraph*, date unknown (January or February 1992).
52. Ibid.
53. Ibid.
54. Kris K. Soule, "Anti-Abortion Author is Upset By Honesty," letter to the editor, *Pantagraph*, January 24, 1992, p. A6.
55. Diane Eskin, "Social-Agency Bashing," letter to the editor, *Reading Eagle*, February 17, 1992.
56. Jon Kerr, "A is for Abstinence," *City Pages*, March 4, 1992, p. 8.

57. Ibid.
58. Dave Ransom, "Special Report: Right Wing Attacks on Corporate Giving," National Committee for Responsive Philanthropy, Winter 1990.
59. Randall G. Arnold, "More Trust Can Yield More Debates on Abortion," letter to the editor, *Pantagraph*, January 19, 1992, p. A6.
60. Diane Brown, "Book Flirts With Truth on Planned Parenthood," letter to the editor *Pantagraph*, January 17, 1992, p. A8.
61. "Hate" mail sent to Douglas Scott, postmarked September 17, 1986.
62. Envelope for "Hate" mail sent to Douglas Scott, postmarked September 17, 1986.
63. "Hate" mail sent to Douglas Scott, postmarked September 21, 1986.
64. "Hate" mail sent to Douglas Scott, postmarked September 12, 1986.
65. "Hate" mail sent to Douglas Scott, postmarked September 15, 1986.
66. *Facts About the Threats to the Supreme Court Decision on Abortion*.
67. Jan Brittian, public education director, Planned Parenthood Association/Chicago Area, text accompanying a letter send to editors of publications, April 7, 1978.
68. Ibid.
69. Ibid.
70. Ibid.
71. Ibid.
72. Ibid.
73. Ibid.
74. "Since Your Parents Are Afraid to Talk to You and Your School's Hands Are Probably Tied, Here's Some Hard Facts," advertisement, Planned Parenthood, *Dallas Observer*, January 30, 1986.
75. "Professor Daniel Maguire Keynote Speaker at 56th Annual Meeting," Reports, Planned Parenthood League of Massachusetts, Summer 1986, vol. 67, p. 1.
76. Ibid.
77. Ibid., pp. 1 and 5.
78. Ibid., p. 5.
79. Peter T. Knoepfler, M.D., and Lee S. Minto, "A Psychiatrist Volunteers at a Planned Parenthood Clinic," *Papers 1975*, Planned Parenthood Federation of America, 1975, p. 139.
80. Ibid.
81. Boston Women's Health Book Collective, *The New Our Bodies, Ourselves* (Simon and Shuster: New York, 1984), p. 172.
82. Norman Himes, *Medical History of Contraception* (Baltimore: [publisher not cited], 1936), p. 413, as cited in "Abortion: The Nazi Connection," by Michael Schwartz, *Catholic League Newsletter*, August 1978.
83. Jacqueline Kasun, "Sex Education: A New Philosophy for America?," *The Family in America*, July 1989, p. 6.
84. "The Joan Rivers Show," broadcast in 1991.
85. "Family Planning is Moral Duty, Religious Leaders Say," *Planned Parenthood News*, Planned Parenthood Federation of America, Winter 1955, p. 3.
86. Ibid.
87. Ibid.
88. Ibid.
89. "Religious Leaders Stand Up for Choice . . . Will You?," advertisement, Planned Parenthood Health Services and Upper Hudson Planned Parenthood, *Times Union*, March 14, 1990.
90. "Clergy Go Public to Support Abortion Rights," *Times Union*, March 15, 1990, p. B-4.
91. "Pickets Crowd Sidewalk," *Planned Parenthood Press*, Planned Parenthood of Central and Northern Arizona, Summer 1987.
92. "God Had Only One Son . . . ," poster, Planned Parenthood, date unknown.

93. "If God Could Control How Many Children You Should Have . . ." poster, Planned Parenthood, date unknown.
94. Virginia Coigney, *Margaret Sanger: Rebel With a Cause* (Garden City, NY: Doubleday and Company, 1969), p. 16.
95. Ibid., pp. 177–178.
96. *Sexualpedagogik*, magazine of the German affiliate of the International Planned Parenthood Federation, as translated by the Rev. Paul Marx of Human Life International, HLI Reports, as excerpted in "PP's View of Mother Teresa," *ALL About Issues*, American Life League, July–August 1987, p. 53.
97. Ibid.
98. Ibid.
99. Ibid.
100. Press release, Christian Action Council, July 19, 1991.
101. Ibid.
102. Karen Slater, "Vocal Advocate: Abortion Stand Gives Planned Parenthood New Goals, New Foes," *Wall Street Journal*, June 25, 1986, p. 1.

Chapter 13: A Project of David

1. "Taking the Low Road," *Seattle Times*, editorial opinion, September 18, 1986.
2. Marie Bass, "New Birth Control in the Next Century," workshop outline, Planned Parenthood Federation of America, annual meeting, October 19, 1990.
3. "Planned Parenthood Didn't Plan on This," *Business Week*, July 3, 1989, p. 34.
4. Ibid.
5. Ibid.
6. Ibid.
7. "Caving in to Extremists, AT&T Hangs Up on Planned Parenthood," *New York Times*, full-page copyrighted advertisement, Planned Parenthood Federation of America, April 9, 1990, p. A11.
8. Jon Talton, "Companies Can't Duck Crossfire From Abortion," *Milwaukee Journal*, May 4, 1990.
9. Larry Sterne, "Planned Parenthood Chief Says Many Economic Boycotts Are Backfiring," *NonProfit Times*, date unknown (circa 1991), p. 10.
10. Ibid.
11. Alan J. Miller, *Socially Responsible Investing: How to Invest With Your Conscience* (New York: Simon and Schuster, 1991), pp. 255–256.
12. Paul McGuire, *Who Will Rule the Future?* (Lafayette, LA: Huntington House, 1991), p. 156.
13. Ibid.
14. Eldon Knoche, "Planned Parenthood Says Donors 'Attacked,'" *Milwaukee Sentinel*, October 13, 1990, p. 5 (of first section).
15. "Public Affairs Special Report on the Opposition: Christian Action Council," *INsider*, Planned Parenthood Federation of America, December 1, 1990.
16. Ibid.
17. Ibid.
18. Talton, *Milwaukee Journal*.
19. *INsider*, December 1, 1990.
20. Ibid.
21. Sterne, *NonProfit Times*.
22. Tim W. Ferguson, "Forbes 400 Are Paupers When It Comes to Public Policy," *Wall Street Journal*, October 29, 1991, p. A23.
23. Comment made by Congressman Robert K. Dornan on the floor of the United States House of Representatives, date unknown.

24. Jack Fowler, "Big Business and Abortion," *From the Right*, newsletter of Patrick J. Buchanan, vol. 2, no. 8, Quarterly II, July 1991, p. 6.
25. Charles V. Zehren, "Companies in Abortion Crossfire," *Newsday*, August 13, 1989.
26. "St. Antoninus Pro-Life Principles of Corporate Conduct," St. Antoninus Institute, undated (circa 1989).
27. Joel Makower, *The Green Consumer Supermarket Guide*, p. 7.
28. Ibid.
29. Ibid.
30. *NonProfit Times*, January 1992, vol. 6, no. 1, p. 1.
31. "Christian Action Council (CAC), Announces National Campaign to Boycott Companies Who Contribute to Planned Parenthood Education Fund," *NARAL News*, National Abortion Rights Action League, date unknown (1990), p. 5.
32. Ibid., pp. 5–6.
33. "They Make Up for Pioneer Decision on Abortion," Associated Press wire story, March 25, 1992.
34. *The Chronicle of Philanthropy*, as cited in *Action Line*, Christian Action Council, May 24, 1990, vol. 9, no. 3, pp. 2–3.
35. Ibid., p. 3.
36. Ibid.
37. Anne Lowrey Bailey, "Corporate Giving Under Siege," *Chronicle of Philanthropy*, May 1, 1990.
38. George Grant, letter to the Christian Action Council, December 19, 1991.
39. Olga Fairfax, Ph.D., return note to the Christian Action Council, undated (December 1991).
40. Rev. Donald Wildmon, return note to the Christian Action Council, undated (December 1991).
41. Earl W. Essex, Esq., letter to the Christian Action Council, December 1991.
42. Ralph Reed, Jr., letter to the Christian Action Council, December 6, 1991.
43. Gregg Cunningham, *No More Excuses: A Long-Term Strategy to Stop the Killing*, video series/seminar, 1991.
44. "Pro-Life Groups Join to Support Call for Boycott: Unprecedented Unity Displayed," *Action Line*, Christian Action Council newsletter, September/October 1990, vol. 9, no. 5.
45. Patricia Bainbridge, "From the President," *The Nehemiah Report*, Christian Action Council of Western New York newsletter, August 20, 1991.
46. Ibid.
47. Ibid.
48. Letter written by a woman from Winnipeg, Manitoba, Canada (name withheld), addressed to D. Scott of the Christian Action Council, June 21, 1991, p. 2.
49. Letter written by a woman from Townsend, Tennessee (name withheld), addressed to boycott organizers, March 30, 1992.
50. Tamar Lewin, "Abortion Foes Urge Boycott of Planned Parenthood Donors," *New York Times*, August 8, 1990.
51. "20/20" report on the boycott against Cracker Barrel restaurants, broadcast on November 29, 1991.

Chapter 14: A Project of Goliath

1. "Press Statement by Faye Wattleton, President, Planned Parenthood Federation of America, on Anti-Abortion Counseling Centers," news release, Planned Parenthood Federation of America, January 22, 1987, pp. 1–2.
2. "A Consumer's Alert to Deception, Harassment and Medical Malpractice," Planned Parenthood Federation of America and the National Abortion Federation, undated (circa 1987).
3. Ibid.

4. Ibid.
5. Ibid.
6. "Anti-Abortion Counseling Centers," Planned Parenthood Federation of America, January 1987.
7. "Nightsight," KCTS, aired on January 22, 1987.
8. Ibid.
9. Ibid.
10. Ibid.
11. Ibid.
12. Ibid.
13. Ibid.
14. Ibid.
15. Dr. Marvin N. Olasky, "Abortion Rights: Anatomy of a Negative Campaign," *Public Relations Review*, Fall 1987, p. 13.
16. *Women's Legal Guide to Reproductive Rights*, Reproductive Freedom Project, American Civil Liberties Union, 1981.
17. Olasky, *Public Relations Review*, p. 15.
18. Ibid., p. 17.
19. Ibid.
20. Ibid., pp. 19–20.
21. Marvin N. Olasky, *The Press and Abortion, 1838-1988*, pp. 143–147.
22. Olasky, *Public Relations Review*, pp. 20–21.
23. "Would You Lie to a Pregnant Teenager?," full-page copyrighted advertisement, Planned Parenthood Federation of America, *Time*, March 6, 1989.
24. Denise Cocciolone, former national director, Birthright USA, telephone interview, March 1, 1989.
25. Ibid.
26. Telephone inquiry, information provided by receptionist, March 1, 1989.
27. "Crisis Pregnancy Center Statement of Principle," Christian Action Council Education and Ministries Fund, undated (circa 1988).
28. Harriet R. T. Lewis, vice president for crisis pregnancy ministries, Christian Action Council, personal interview, January 16, 1992.
29. Ibid.
30. Lee Minto, "NightSight," KCTS, aired on January 22, 1987.
31. Report and accompanying memorandum of the Subcommittee on Regulation, Business Opportunities and Energy, United States House of Representatives, September 12, 1991.
32. Memorandum from Ron Fitzsimmons, executive director, National Coalition of Abortion Providers, to "NCAP Members and Interested Parties," June 20, 1991.
33. Memorandum from Ron Fitzsimmons, executive director, National Coalition of Abortion Providers, to "All Abortion Providers," September 4, 1991.
34. Report of the Subcommittee on Regulation, Business Opportunities and Energy.
35. Ibid.
36. *The Random House College Dictionary*, revised edition (Random House: New York, 1982), p. 252.
37. Report of the Subcommittee on Regulation, Business Opportunities and Energy.
38. Ibid.
39. Ibid.
40. Ibid.
41. Ibid.
42. "Crisis Pregnancy Center Statement of Principle," Christian Action Council Education and Ministries Fund, undated (circa 1988).
43. *Crisis Pregnancy Center Volunteer Training Manual*, Christian Action Council Education and Ministries Fund, date unknown (circa 1991).
44. Report of the Subcommittee on Regulation, Business Opportunities and Energy.

45. Ibid.
46. Ibid.
47. Ibid.
48. Ibid.
49. Ibid.
50. Ibid.
51. Ibid.
52. Ibid.
53. Ibid.
54. Fitzsimmons memorandum, September 4, 1991.
55. Yellow pages advertisement of a local pregnancy counseling center, 1991.
56. Yellow pages advertisement of a local pregnancy counseling center, 1991.
57. "Phil Hendrie Show," KVEN radio, September 20, 1991.
58. Ibid.
59. Ibid.
60. Yellow pages, Chesapeake and Potomac Telephone Company of Virginia, a Bell Atlantic Company, January 1992–December 1992, p. 25.
61. Kathy Doherty, "Battle Erupts Over Planned Parenthood Critics' Use of Book," *Charlotte News*, June 5, 1985, p. 1B.

Chapter 15: The Threat to *Roe*

1. Marianne Szegedy-Maszak, "Calm, Cool and Beleaguered," *New York Times Magazine*, August 6, 1989, p. 17.
2. Ibid.
3. Ibid., p. 18.
4. "Five U.S. Supreme Court Justices Just Had Their Say On Abortion. Now It's Your Turn," full-page copyrighted advertisement, Planned Parenthood Federation of America, *New York Times*, July 10, 1989, p. A5.
5. Ibid.
6. Ibid.
7. Ibid.
8. Ibid.
9. "What Extremists Couldn't Do With 100 Firebombs, the Supreme Court Might Do With One Decision," full-page copyrighted advertisement, Planned Parenthood Federation of America, *USA Today*, November 30, 1989, p. 9A.
10. Ibid.
11. Ibid.
12. Ibid.
13. Ibid.
14. Ibid.
15. "Abortion, Inc.," *New Dimensions: The Psychology Behind the News*, September/October 1991, p. 19.
16. Ibid.
17. Ibid.
18. Campaign literature for Warren Barry for state senate campaign, undated (Fall 1991).
19. "Survey Results From Delegate Leslie Byrne," undated (February or March 1990).
20. "Governor Richards Appoints 2 Judges," Associated Press wire story, March 26, 1992.
21. "Can Pro-Choicers Prevail?," *Time*, August 14, 1989, p. 28.
22. "Pro-Choice Group Outpaces Anti-Abortion Rival in Fund Raising," Associated Press wire story, May 3, 1990.
23. Faye Wattleton, fund-raising letter, Campaign to Keep Abortion Safe and Legal, Planned Parenthood, undated.
24. Szegedy-Maszak, *New York Times Magazine*, p. 18.

25. Ibid.
26. "Faye Unfazed," *Vogue*, January 1992, p. 197.
27. *Abortion: For Survival*, Fund for the Feminist Majority, aired on WTBS, July 20, 1989.
28. Ibid.
29. "Ted Turner Lambasts Pro-lifers As 'Bozos,'" *Chattanooga News-Free Press*, July 13, 1989.
30. "World Vision Protests Abortion Telecast," World Vision News Release, July 21, 1989.
31. Ibid.
32. Ibid.
33. Ibid.
34. "Abortion: An Issue Forum," discussion following the showing of *Abortion: For Survival*, aired on WTBS, July 20, 1989.
35. Ibid.
36. Ibid.
37. Ibid.
38. Ibid.
39. Ibid.
40. Ibid.
41. Ibid.
42. Richard Morin, "Rally Draws Movement Veterans: Poll Suggests Abortion-Rights March Failed to Attract Diverse Crowd," *Washington Post*, April 6, 1992.
43. Ibid.

Chapter 16: Putting Up a Local Fight

1. William G. Sidebottom, "How to Beat Planned Parenthood," *Citizen*, August 1988.
2. Polly Paddock, "An Ounce of Prevention," *Charlotte Observer*, June 11, 1988.
3. "The Planned Parenthood Vote: Underneath All the Moral Posturing, It's Mostly Politics," editorial, *Charlotte Observer*, June 13, 1988.
4. Lisa Pullen, "70 Sign Up to Take Shots at '89 Budget," *Charlotte Observer*, May 26, 1988, p. 1D.
5. Lisa Pullen, "Emotion Fills Commissioners' Public Hearing: Planned Parenthood Request for Money Draws Opposition," *Charlotte Observer*, May 27, 1988, p. 6D.
6. Sidebottom, *Citizen*.
7. Molly Jubitz-Geraldi, "Planned Parenthood Will Have to Move," *Pueblo Chieftain*, March 24, 1989.
8. Susan Touchstone, "Lease Renewal Denied to Planned Parenthood," *Chronicle-News*, March 24, 1989.
9. Tubitz-Geraldi, *Pueblo Chieftain*
10. Touchstone, *Chronicle-News*
11. Ibid.
12. Ibid.
13. Fran Hansen, "Critics of Planned Parenthood Wrong," letter to the editor, *Telegraph Herald*, October 23, 1990.
14. Confidential list of press conference speakers, Coalition of Parental Rights, November 21, 1990.
15. Kristina Campbell, "Dubuque Group Rallies Foes of Proposed Clinic," *Des Moines Register*, November 22, 1990, p. 3T.
16. Denise Lamphier-Hoffert, "Planned Parenthood Considers Sites," *Dubuque Telegraph Herald*, May 23, 1991.
17. Lyn Hanson, "Group Fights Planned Parenthood," *Dubuque Telegraph Herald*, November 22, 1991.
18. Ibid.
19. Ibid.
20. Ibid.

21. Frances R. Hansen, "Powerful Partnership: Planned Parenthood and the Community," My-View: Point-Counterpoint, *Dubuque Telegraph Herald*, July 12, 1991, p. 4A.
22. Jim Giese, "Planned Parenthood Living a Lie," letter to the editor, *Dubuque Telegraph Herald*, September 25, 1991.
23. John Carlson, "Abortion-Rights Clinics Feel Heat as Competitor Sets Up on Iowa City Turf," *Des Moines Register*, May 13, 1990, p. 1B.
24. Ibid.
25. Ibid., p. 7B.
26. Ibid.
27. Linda Gordon, *Woman's Body, Woman's Right: A Social History of Birth Control in America* (New York: Grossman, 1976), p. 213.
28. Anonymous letter sent to Jim Giese, October 18, 1990.
29. Ibid.
30. Cheryl Eaton, "6 Companies Build Hard-Won Sidewalk," *Belleville News-Democrat*, May 10, 1991, p. 1B.
31. Ibid.
32. Ibid.
33. Ibid.
34. Lynn Baird, "Sex Education in the Schools: A Parent's Guide to Making it Happen (And How to Beat the Opposition)," *Planned Parenthood Press*, Planned Parenthood of Central and Northern Arizona, Fall 1988.
35. Ibid.
36. Ibid.

RECOMMENDED READING

The Holy Bible (any version, any publication date, any publisher).

Thomas J. DiLorenzo, et. al., *Patterns of Corporate Philanthropy: The "Suicidal Impulse"* (Washington: Capital Research Center, 1990).

Paul B. Fowler, *Abortion:. Toward an Evangelical Consensus* (Portland, OR: Multnomah Press, 1987).

Jean Staker Garton, *Who Broke the Baby?* (Minneapolis: Bethany House Publishers, 1979).

George Grant, *Grand Illusions: The Legacy of Planned Parenthood* (Brentwood, TN: Wolgemuth and Hyatt, 1988).

George Grant, *The Quick and the Dead: RU-486 and the New Chemical Warfare Against Your Family* (Wheaton, IL: Crossway, 1991).

Robert Marshall and Charles Donovan, *Blessed Are the Barren: The Social Policy of Planned Parenthood* (San Francisco: Ignatius, 1991).

Josh McDowell, *The Myths of Sex Education* (San Bernadino, CA: Here's Life Publishers, 1990).

Barrett L. Mosbacker, editor, *School Based Clinics: And Other Critical Issues in Public Education* (Westchester, IL: Crossway Books, 1987).

Bernard N. Nathanson, M.D., *Aborting America* (New York: Pinnacle Books, 1979).

Bernard N. Nathanson, M.D., *The Abortion Papers* (New York: Frederick Fell Publishers, 1983).

Marvin N. Olasky, *The Press and Abortion, 1838-1988* (Hillsdale, NJ: Lawrence Erlbaum Associates, 1988).

Marvin Olasky, *Prodigal Press: The Anti-Christian Bias of the American News Media* (Westchester, IL: Crossway Books, 1988.)

Denyse O'Leary, editor, *The Issue is Life: A Christian Response to Abortion in Canada* (Burlington, Ontario, Canada: Welch Publishing, 1988).

Dr. Judith A. Reisman and Edward W. Eichel, *Kinsey, Sex and Fraud: The Indoctrination of a People* (Lafayette, LA: Lochinvar-Huntington House, 1990).

James W. Sedlak, "How to Dismantle Government Funding of Planned Parenthood" (LaGrangeville, NY: Stop Planned Parenthood, 1991).

James W. Sedlak, "Parent Power: How Parents Can Gain Control of the School Systems That Educate Their Children" (Poughkeepsie, NY: self-published, no copyright date [1992]).

Curt Young, *The Least of These: What Everyone Should Know About Abortion* (Chicago: Moody Press, 1984).

OTHER RESOURCES

"A Close Look at Planned Parenthood," audio tape, Focus on the Family, aired October 26–27, 1989 (tape CS494).

INDEX

C

H

I

J

K

L

M

ABOUT THE AUTHOR

Douglas R. Scott is president of Life Decisions International. He is the former vice president for public policy of the Christian Action Council. Mr. Scott has also served as executive director of HUMAN LIFE in Seattle, Washington, and Arizona Right to Life in Phoenix, Arizona.

Mr. Scott has taught middle school and high school students. He holds degrees in political science and education from Western Washington University.

Mr. Scott also has written *School-Based Clinics: A Trojan Horse in Our Schools* and *Inside Planned Parenthood.* He has been on many radio and television programs including "The 700 Club," "The John Ankerberg Show," Cable News Network, "CBS This Morning," "Focus on the Family," "Nightline," "Family News in Focus," "This Morning's Business," and the "MacNeil/Lehrer NewsHour." Mr. Scott is a frequent speaker at pro-life and other public gatherings.

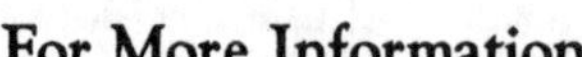

For More Information

LEGACY COMMUNICATIONS is an explicitly Christian ministry committed to help the Church apply the truths from God's Word to every area of life and demonstrate to the Church and Christian community what the practical implications of this effort are: to develop a Christian and Biblical view towards our culture, specifically, and the world, in general.

Through research, publishing, seminars, audio, and video productions, **LEGACY COMMUNICATIONS** strives to bring strategic and substantive focus on the grave dilemmas of our day from the perspective of a distinctively forthright Christian worldview. Creating tools that equip the saints for the work of the ministry, filling the gap where commercial enterprises leave off, and forging ahead into previously uncharted realms, is not just what we do—it is what we are.

To receive a free sample of the **LEGACY** newsletter and information about other books and resources send $1.00 to: Legacy Communications, Post Office Box 680365, Franklin, Tennessee 37068.

LIFE DECISIONS INTERNATIONAL is an educational organization dedicated to providing individuals with up-to-date, accurate information neccessary to empower them to make important decisions regarding sexuality education, abortion, infanticide, euthanasia, and related issues.

LIFE DECISIONS INTERNATIONAL serves as a resource and provides assistance to grassroots organizations and individuals who are using reputable and honorable tactics to defund, limit, expose, and otherwise challenge the impact of Planned Parenthood and other pro-legal abortion groups in North America and worldwide. A boycott of corporate supporters of Planned Parenthood is administered by **LIFE DECISIONS INTERNATIONAL.** For a list of corporate supporters of Planned Parenthood, send a $2.00 donation and a self-addressed, stamped, business-sized envelope to "Boycott List," Life Decisions International, Post Office Box 419, Amherst, New York 14226-0419.